Praise for *The Anxiety Prescription*

"Full of truth and humor, *The Anxiety Prescription* takes the reader on a healing journey, with a deep dive into Dr. Kennedy's own personal recovery from decades of chronic anxiety. This deeply insightful and ultimately practical book gives the reader a new and natural prescription to healing, using an approach Dr. Kennedy has used for himself and countless patients. Russ specifically addresses what many therapies miss: the fundamental role of old unresolved trauma stored in the body as the cause of the anxieties of the mind. Creating that awareness, using strategies effective for both allows the mind and body to reconnect and resolve the mind-body disconnect that fuels and sustains anxiety. The insights and simple practices in this book will put you on the path to self-healing and keep you there. *The Anxiety Prescription* is unlike any book on anxiety and a must-read for anyone who suffers from chronic worry."

—Dr. Nicole LePera, author of the *New York Times* bestseller *How to Do the Work* and social media phenomenon The Holistic Psychologist

"If you are a chronic worrier, *The Anxiety Prescription* is a game changer! Dr. Russ Kennedy's profound insights about anxiety and his practical strategies for healing it have seriously changed my life for the better."

—Mel Robbins, *New York Times* bestselling author and host of *The Mel Robbins Podcast*

"Russell's unique approach to anxiety treatment is truly inspiring. His message has the potential to transform the way we think about mental health and the role of the body in calming the mind."

—Dr. Rangan Chatterjee, host of the *Feel Better, Live More* podcast and five-time *Sunday Times* bestselling author

"*The Anxiety Prescription* by Dr. Russell Kennedy offers a revolutionary and deeply compassionate approach to understanding and healing anxiety. Drawing from his personal battle with anxiety and extensive professional experience, Dr. Kennedy transcends traditional therapy

boundaries, presenting a holistic method that acknowledges both the mind and body's roles in anxiety. His innovative use of the ABCDE process and insights into the energetic nature of emotions provide readers with practical, transformative tools. By addressing the often-overlooked aspect of stored emotional energy in the body, Dr. Kennedy empowers individuals to release the 'background alarm' and step into a life of greater peace and resilience. This book is a must-read for anyone seeking to understand the true depth of anxiety and yearning for a genuine path to healing."

—Dr. Bradley Nelson, bestselling author of
The Body Code and *The Emotion Code*

"Necessary reading for anyone who struggles with anxiety. This is an incredible debut by Dr. Russ Kennedy, certain to help every person who reads it."

—Dr. Chloe Carmichael, PhD, licensed clinical psychologist
and *USA Today* bestselling author

The
Anxiety
Prescription

The
Anxiety
Prescription

The revolutionary mind-body solution to
healing your chronic anxiety

REVISED SECOND EDITION
WITH NEW MATERIAL

DR RUSSELL KENNEDY

Vermilion
LONDON

Vermilion, an imprint of Ebury Publishing
One Embassy Gardens, 8 Viaduct Gdns,
Nine Elms, London SW11 7BW

Vermilion is part of the Penguin Random House group of companies
whose addresses can be found at global.penguinrandomhouse.com

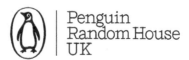

Penguin
Random House
UK

First published by Vermilion in 2024

The information in this book has been compiled by way of general guidance
in relation to the specific subjects addressed. It is not a substitute and not to be
relied on for medical, healthcare, pharmaceutical or other professional advice on
specific circumstances and in specific locations. Please consult your GP before
changing, stopping or starting any medical treatment. So far as the author is
aware the information given is correct and up to date as at June 2024. Practice,
laws and regulations all change, and the reader should obtain up to date
professional advice on any such issues. The author and publishers disclaim,
as far as the law allows, any liability arising directly or indirectly from the use,
or misuse, of the information contained in this book.

Illustrations by Andrea Vásquez Aguilarte

www.penguin.co.uk

A CIP catalogue record for this book is available from the British Library

ISBN 9781785045097

Printed and bound in Great Britain by Clays Ltd, Elcograf S.p.A.

The authorised representative in the EEA is Penguin Random House Ireland,
Morrison Chambers, 32 Nassau Street, Dublin D02 YH68

Penguin Random House is committed to a sustainable
future for our business, our readers and our planet. This book
is made from Forest Stewardship Council® certified paper.

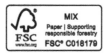

For my Dad,
It wasn't your fault; it's no one's fault.
Your life had meaning; it's here in these pages.
You can rest now.

For my Mum,
You always did what you had to do.
The cost was immeasurable.
Thank you.

For Rusty, my younger self,
I have you now.
I love you now.
You can rest.

Contents

Preface

On a muggy, late summer day in 1973, twelve-year-old me didn't know very much about what anxiety was, but I did know for certain I did not feel safe. My father had attempted suicide, and I was watching the ambulance drive off to take him away to the hospital. Even with the drama and trauma of my father's schizophrenia and bipolar illness, I knew my parents loved my younger brother and me, but the pressures were just too great to provide a stable home life. Looking back, I have often jokingly said my father was psychotic and my mother was neurotic, so my own psyche didn't stand much of a chance.

If you are looking at this book because you have anxiety, chances are you have some old wounding stored in you from your past and you haven't found a way to heal it yet. Anxiety can be the biggest challenge in a person's life. If you had managed to heal from chronic worry and anxiety, you would likely be looking at books on overcoming much easier challenges like becoming a blindfolded bomb diffuser or an amateur astronaut.

If you suffered in your past and you are still suffering now, I feel you. I really, really do. For decades I suffered from crippling anxiety and looked to every type of therapy—and was disappointed at every turn. I know the deep frustration of being promised relief and walking away empty-handed.

I wrote this book as a way to turn my dad's pain and suffering (and the suffering of my mother, brother, and me) into something for good, to create a healing message for others arising out of our pain. When I was a boy, my dad told me of his plans for the future. Mental illness stole those plans and burned them right in front of him. He could only stomp out the flames so many times until he went up in them. Watching the ambulance take my dad away that late summer day in 1973, I swore to myself that his pain, and the chaos, confusion, and heartbreak we suffered as his family, were going to stand for something. Although his potential was taken from him, I have taken that vow of my twelve-year-old self and ridden the energy of his spirit and what he taught me to become a doctor. I told myself that if I was a physician, I could help others in a way I was never able to help my father.

My qualifications for guiding you on this healing journey:

University degrees in medicine and neuroscience.

Master's-level training in developmental psychology at the Neufeld Institute in Vancouver. Over a hundred thousand patient encounters.

Personal insights into anxiety from ayahuasca, LSD, psilocybin, and MDMA. Read hundreds of books on anxiety from highly spiritual to hard-core neuroscience. Lived at a temple in India studying the science of spirit.

Certified yoga and meditation teacher.

Countless conferences on anxiety and mental health.

Many academic and spiritual retreats to explore mind-body mental and physical health. Lived with anxiety every day for many years.

Overcame my own anxiety to become a professional stand-up comedian.

By the way, do you know what they call the person who graduates dead last in their medical class?

"Doctor."

Despite my extensive academic experience above, probably my biggest credential in helping others with anxiety is that I personally suffered from the dreaded condition for decades. The unusual position of being both anxiety doctor and anxiety patient has given me a unique ability to see what works and what doesn't from multiple perspectives. I don't have to go back to the doctor to report my progress; I am the doctor!

What we are currently doing in psychology and psychiatry is taking two very separate things, the anxious thoughts of the mind and the alarmed feeling in the body, and reducing them to one diagnosis: anxiety. Most anxiety treatments have limited success because most treat the anxiety of the mind but neglect the bigger issue—the alarm signals of old trauma stored in the body.

There is a story about the organic chemist Friedrich August Kekulé. He was struggling with finding a chemical formula for benzene, now known to be a six-carbon ring. Try as he might, he couldn't figure out how the six carbons would fit together. Chemical structures were thought to be linear, with the atoms fitting together like the boxcars on a train. Benzene was known to have six of these boxcars, but it was also known that the structure could not be linear. One night while dreaming, Kekulé had a vision of a snake biting its own tail, leading him to the idea that benzene's structure was not a linear but circular one.

In a similar manner, I had a vision while on LSD that went against conventional theory: much of my anxiety was not in my mind but rather in my body. Traditional therapies were looking in the wrong place! That psychedelic-induced vision has allowed me to develop the theory upon which this book is based.

While this book can't change the pain from your past, it can help you perceive it differently, both in your mind and in your body. When you change your perception of your past and especially of your "self," you change your future. This book is as unique as it is practical and not just a rehash of conventional therapies that do not work.

In my own healing from chronic worry, I have had to become my own doctor, therapist, and shaman. This book is exceptional in its amalgamation of the neuroscientific principles of the mind and the spirit of the body. I've spent thousands of hours in scientific training to explain what I found unexplainable in my "out of mind" experiences in India and on psychedelics. What most approaches to treat anxiety miss, and this book addresses specifically, is the critical role of accessing the healing power and wisdom stored in the body. While more "medical," mind-based approaches are important and helpful (and I'll address those as well), you will only fully heal when you commit to a pointed focus on connecting to your body. Finding and soothing the alarm stored in your body is critical to you healing from chronic worry.

We need to know what we are treating to have the best treatments. Anxiety is an endless feedback loop of painful feeling in the body and anxious thinking in the mind. Each energizes the other. I'll show you how to break that destructive cycle so you can get back to living your life.

Leaving your anxiety behind requires a simple shift in your perception from mind to body, so you get out of the frightening predictions of your mind and into the grounded security of your body.

Once you become practiced in this renewal of perception, you may well be able to talk to your doctor about the renewal of your prescription.

My father never got off medication, and in fact, it was medication that ultimately killed him, fourteen years after that summer day I watched the ambulance take him in 1973. It was me who found him, the first of many dead bodies I would see in my medical career. He left a note behind, beside his lifeless body that I found on January 12, 1987.

The note said, "It's not your fault, it's no one's fault."

But I do feel at fault in a way. I could never help him; no one could. He was just too sick. I wasn't even a doctor while he was alive. He died five months before I could tell him that I had gained admission to medical school.

I couldn't help my dad with his emotional pain, but I am fully committed to helping you with yours.

Introduction to the New Edition

With the massive success of *Anxiety Rx,* I am beyond thrilled to be able to create a second edition for this book. While the principles and theories have not changed, I have used and explained the concepts so many times since *Anxiety Rx* was first published in 2020 that my own treatment of anxiety has evolved and I am excited to share that deeper understanding with you. I am certain that this new edition will expand upon the healing generated in the first edition with the addition of new techniques and illustrations. This edition will also provide strategies and practices for reducing anxiety at the beginning of the book, so that when sensitive topics are discussed, you will have tools that will help you right when you need them.

I'll start with the story that began the original version of this book. Many years ago, I had a patient send me an email that said: "Dear Dr. Kennedy, I am almost out of my anxiety medication, and I need you to renew my perception." She had meant to say "renew my *prescription*," but I thought if she could truly renew her perception, she probably wouldn't need the prescription.

I love this story so much and it captures the heart of what I would love to see for you, my fellow worrier, to be empowered to renew your perception of yourself and your anxiety so much that you no longer need to renew your prescription. That said, let me say at the outset that I am not anti-medication; in many cases psych meds are an invaluable part of treatment, and I am not recommending in any way that you stop taking any medications without consulting your doctor. Further, this book is not intended to be medical advice because, frankly, very little of what I am going to share with you has anything to do with what I learned in traditional allopathic medicine. In fact, I believe the traditional medical model of espousing that anxiety is primarily an issue of the mind is inaccurate at best and sinful at worst. The original definition of sin was "to miss the mark," and I believe traditional models of psychiatry and psychology sin because they focus almost completely on the belief that anxiety is primarily an issue of the consciously corrected mind, while completely neglecting the more critical role of the unconsciously directed body. If this doesn't make sense to you now, I assure it will as you go through this revolutionary book.

Another sin of modern medicine may lie in its ineffectual treatments for a condition that affects many millions of people, and then blaming the patient for lack of improvement. I cannot count the number of anxiety sufferers I have seen who blame themselves for their anxiety and assume they are broken and unfixable because traditional therapies haven't helped them. Well, this book is to show you that traditional therapies haven't worked because they are based on the inaccurate theory that anxiety is purely a disorder of the mind. In this book, I propose a new theory that helps you understand and treat anxiety infinitely better, empowering you to heal yourself from a mind-body-spirit perspective, rather than rely on doctors that do not understand anxiety and even blame the patient for lack of progress. I remember getting consultation letters back from traditional medical specialists saying things like, "Your patient failed antidepressant therapy."

What? The patient failed? It is my own medical opinion that it is much more accurate to say that the doctor failed to find an effective treatment, but we can't admit to that as doctors and psychiatrists.

At this point I'll point out that I am a medical doctor but I'm not a psychiatrist. Psychiatrists do at least five years of additional training in psychiatry after graduating from medical school, and in my medical opinion, they are guided down a specific pharmacological tunnel and usually stay within it for their entire careers. As a generalist, I had the freedom to pursue many different ideas that were well outside conventional medicine, and as you'll soon see, I do not think like a medical doctor when it comes to anxiety. I think like a medical doctor when it comes to physical ailments, but when it comes to emotional ones, the medical model misses the mark by ignoring the body in the healing of the mind. I respect the work of psychiatrists because they often get the patients with the most severe illnesses, and often medications are invaluable in those cases, but in general doctors overprescribe medications because they are all they have. It's been said that when you're a hammer, everything looks like a nail, and medical doctors are trained to be pharmaceutical sledgehammers. To be fair, psychiatry is expanding doctors' horizons with the increasing use of psychedelics, and some psychiatrists are starting to accept the role of somatic therapies, but it is the rare psychiatrist that embraces the mind-body connection as I do.

In 2015, I myself came completely off SSRI/SSNI-type medications using the methods I will show you in this book, and I had taken those medications for over twenty-five years. My hope is that when you embrace the hard-won concepts I'll show you, you may well be able to reduce or come off your prescriptions as well. But again, and I cannot state this clearly enough, only reduce or come off your prescription medications under the guidance of your own doctor.

In this book, I want to help you renew your perception and look at yourself and your anxiety in a completely new way. It is what saved my life and just might save yours.

One of the biggest problems I've had as a doctor helping people heal from anxiety is that the term "anxiety" has no consistent definition. Google "What is anxiety?" and you'll see a mishmash of physical and emotional symptoms in a very long list. How are you supposed to treat something when you don't know what that something is? When most people, including doctors and therapists, use the term "anxiety," they refer to a list of worrisome thoughts and painful feelings that you can pick and choose from like some kind of neurotic smorgasbord.

That is not a definition; that's a Costco list—and one that results in a bag of chips, some golf balls, a couple of pairs of green sweatpants, a kid's backpack, and a microwave oven. How do you effectively treat a list of disparate symptoms that you may or may not have? In my medical opinion, you can't. As a doctor, I know the more precisely I define and describe an illness or condition, the better I can treat it.

The opposite is even more true: the less defined something is, the harder it is to treat. And anxiety has been notoriously hard to treat by psychiatrists and psychologists because they have no consistent and predictable way of pinning it down, and the *Diagnostic and Statistical Manual of Mental Disorders* (DSM) is no real help.

What has become even clearer to me since I first published *Anxiety Rx* in 2020 is that what we refer to as anxiety in the conscious mind is much more effectively labeled as a state of survival-based alarm held deeply in the unconscious body. I'd go further to say the reason why so many anxiety patients "fail" therapy is because most traditional therapists are guilty of the sin of focusing on changing the mind while almost completely ignoring the body.

Anxiety, as I define it, is merely anxious thoughts of the mind. Thoughts in and of themselves are not painful, and as such anxiety is not painful.

This may surprise you and may even cause you to doubt my credibility. If you feel resistance to this concept of anxiety being a painless thought process, let me assure you that making this distinction has allowed me (and many others) to heal from chronic, relentless, persistent, worrisome—or fear-inducing—thoughts.

Quite simply, anxiety itself doesn't hurt. The painful part comes from anxiety's evil twin: alarm. And I would tell you that you are confusing anxiety (the process that produces potentially fearful thoughts in your mind) with what I refer to as alarm: a painful feeling in your body.

As this book unfolds, you will clearly see the pain you feel is not coming from the anxious thoughts of your mind but from a sense of alarm stored in your body. This alarm is a combination of misaligned energy of your fight-or-flight sympathetic nervous system, with an activating energy originating from unresolved emotional pain that has been repressed within your body, probably since your childhood. If you struggle with anxiety, your worry aggravates the alarm in your body, and as such the worries of the mind appear to be the source of your pain, but I will show you it is the sense of alarm stored in your body, often for decades, that is the true source of your discomfort.

The worries of the mind play a role, no question, but just because those worries activate the alarm does not mean the worries are the cause.

I'll show you what I call the alarm-anxiety cycle, a self-reinforcing feedback loop, showing that anxiety is not one entity but two. What we refer to as anxiety is a combination of a sense of alarm in the body and the worries of the mind. The alarm activates the anxiety and the anxiety activates the alarm. We must separate each from the other, and when we break this cycle we can start to heal.

ALARM-ANXIETY CYCLE

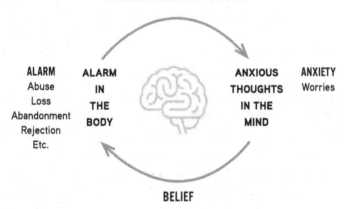

ALARM	ALARM		ANXIOUS	ANXIETY
Abuse	IN		THOUGHTS	Worries
Loss	THE		IN THE	
Abandonment	BODY		MIND	
Rejection				
Etc.				

BELIEF

For one more clarifying example, imagine your toaster short-circuits and starts a fire in your house, and then for some insane reason you throw lit matches on the flames. The matches make the fire worse, but they did not cause the fire in the first place. If you stop throwing matches on the fire, the problem is still there in the form of a fire in progress—started by the toaster, not the matches.

The alarm stored in our bodies is the toaster with the exposed wire. The matches are our worries. To heal, we must address the root problem (the toaster) and stop blaming the matches for a fire they surely aggravated but did not start. Even once we extinguish the fire, the problem may reoccur if we don't replace the toaster. But with the illusion that the matches (the anxious thoughts) are the problem, we may direct our efforts at removing all the matches from the house while leaving the broken toaster in place.

In 2015, I was at an anxiety conference in Vancouver, British Columbia. I know that sounds like a bunch of nervous people in the same room, but it was a group of doctors, social workers, teachers, and psychologists listening to various presentations on how to heal anxiety. Much of it was predictable and not new to me, but when developmental psychologist Gordon Neufeld, PhD, spoke, what he said rocked my world.

"All anxiety is separation anxiety."

That, along with many other things Neufeld said, has stuck with me to this day. Anxiety and alarm almost always result from a break in attachment during childhood—in other words, an experience of separation.

When we are separated from our attachment figures, either physically or emotionally, our bodies go into a state of alarm. This is an activated state, a fight-or-flight-type reaction the body mounts automatically when we sense real or perceived separation. However, instead of fighting or fleeing, that activated response is initially not about fighting or fleeing at all. It is an activated reaction to mobilize us to pursue a lost connection. That's right, the reason for our fight-or-flight reactions is usually not about a threat to our physical safety. In our modern world, it is much more often about a threat to our emotional safety. According to Neufeld—and I agree completely—this state of alarm is not about flight (moving away) but about pursuit (moving toward). In reaction to real or perceived separation, we engage in this alarm-based pursuit as a reflexive attempt to reconnect to our attachment figures. If the pursuit fails and, despite our best efforts, we still feel separate from our attachment figures, the alarm intensifies, and the body stays in a state of alarm for an extended period. (As a quick aside, females may have more of this pursuit energy because they secrete much more oxytocin in the "fight or flight" stress response than males do, in what researcher Shelley E. Taylor, PhD, has put forward as the "tend and befriend" response in females. I wonder if this helps explain why women stay in stressful relationships when they are alarming.)

This state of alarm, which started as a reaction to a real or perceived separation in childhood, becomes intensified and potentiated by the anxious thoughts of the mind. Over time, if we are subject to an alarming state of affairs (e.g., abuse, loss, abandonment, or rejection) we are unable to resolve, or if we don't have access to a caregiver that can love and calm us, that alarm state becomes stored in, and stuck in, our bodies.

If you struggle with chronic anxious thoughts, it is highly probable you have a version of this state of alarm in your system, likely from a time in your life where you felt separated from your attachment figures and you were unable to close the gap. For me, my emotional separation from my schizophrenic father caused my body to go into an alarmed, activated state of pursuit to reconnect with him. As I was unable to decrease the separation because his mind was too fractured for him to connect with me, my level of alarm increased and intensified.

This alarm energy became a chronic state in my body, where it would energize more false, worrisome thoughts in my mind. Complicating matters, the alarm energy would create a sense of my survival being threatened, which would impair the rational part of my brain to be able to see those thoughts as false. As a result, I would believe, or give power to, the false worries I had created, thus increasing the sense of alarm, which then created more worrisome thoughts that could not be debunked by my impaired rational brain. I was trapped in a self-reinforcing feedback loop of the alarm-anxiety cycle, where the alarm in my body generated anxious thoughts in my mind and those thoughts generated more alarm in my body.

Countless people have told me this concept of the alarm-anxiety cycle is the first time someone has explained anxiety in a way that feels right to them.

At its essence, what we call anxiety is a combination of an alarm state in the body and anxious thoughts in the mind. I have found immeasurable relief in myself, as have my patients, by addressing the alarm of the body separately from the anxious thoughts of the mind. A considerable part of my healing was due to using the term "anxiety" simply to refer to the anxious thinking in my mind and "alarm" to refer to the painful feeling in my body. To be clear, in distilling alarm and anxiety down to their essence and divorcing them from each other, I was able to break the cycle by clearly showing the component parts were separate and therefore separable.

The reason why most treatments for anxiety have failed or been of limited benefit is they have focused on treating the anxious thoughts of the mind (which is only the effect of the alarm in the system) and virtually ignored the true underlying cause—the alarm stuck in the body. In other words, we have been trying to get rid of all the matches in the house while ignoring the short-circuiting toaster! Said another way, traditional therapies fail because they believe we can reach into the mirror to change the reflection, and they fail because to truly fix an issue you can't just change the way it appears on the surface, you must go deeper.

When I was living at a temple in rural India and later teaching yoga classes in downtown Vancouver, I saw a lot of people with a string of prayer beads around their necks. These strings of beads, called japa malas, are often used by Hindus and Buddhists to help maintain focus during meditation and prayer. (They are also used by hipsters to appear spiritual.) The traditional japa mala has 108 beads. The number 108 is held as a sacred number said to be found in the ratios of our solar system, with the diameter of the sun being 108 times the diameter of the earth and the distance from the earth to the moon being equivalent to 108 diameters of the moon. (I did the math, and it's very close but by no means exact.)

What I can say for sure is 108 is a three-digit multiple of three (three times thirty-six) and its components add up to nine (three times three). Three is also purported to be the number of balance, as you can see with the tripod base on any drum stool. The drummer may be all over the place, but he sits in a place of balance to do that.

This book is about me going all over the world in search of emotional balance as a salve for my unending anxiety. The farther I traveled out into the world, the farther it took me inside to myself. To quote Elizabeth Gilbert in her book *Eat, Pray, Love*: "Stringing these stories along the structure of a japa mala . . . is so . . . structured." Although it may not be popular for a guy to say this, I really loved that book. I thought if I ever wrote a book, I was going to use that structure as well, and here we are.

In the first thirty-six chapters, we travel to the land of Awareness of Mind. I'll show you that you must be able to see your anxious thoughts with a new outlook because you can't change what you can't see. I'll show you how to use awareness to examine your anxious thoughts in nonjudgmental curiosity to make the conscious choice to let those worries flow by, rather than contracting around them and holding them tighter. I'll show you how anxious thoughts cannot survive in the light of awareness and flow, which disarms the anxiety half of the anxiety-alarm cycle.

In the middle thirty-six chapters, we visit the faraway land of Awareness of Body, which is devoted to recognizing and relieving the alarm part of the cycle. I will show you techniques and strategies that I have used in myself and my patients to calm the nervous system to maintain the mind-body connection. I'll teach you simple ways to stay in the present moment sensation of your body so as to keep you out of the (always future-based) worrisome thoughts of your mind. This sensation-based process helps disarm the alarm half of the anxiety-alarm cycle.

On the last leg of the journey, Awareness of Self, we go back in time to the place our connection to ourselves was interrupted. We will focus on reconnecting and cultivating a compassionate connection with ourselves. Anxiety at a fundamental level is a separation of mind from body and a separation of our adult self from our child self. To heal anxiety at its core we must join the mind to the body and our adult self to our child self. The reason you became anxious is that once upon a time you separated from yourself, and that split created a deep sense of alarm inside of you that is still there to this day. To heal the alarm you need to reestablish this secure attachment to yourself so your mind and body get back in sync and you become more whole within yourself.

The last thirty-six chapters are devoted to strategies to resolve the split that created the alarm in the first place. Once you heal the split, you can then connect the mind and body in a constructive, adaptive, and fulfilling way.

In short, we go from surviving to thriving.

As we take this journey together, you'll learn how to remove those blocks your mind creates. We will isolate and expose the inner critic that judges, abandons, blames, and shames you (what I call

JABS), and perhaps for the first time, you'll learn how to be truly connected to yourself. As your relationship with others can be no better than the relationship you have with yourself, your own mind-body connection allows you to become connected to others, which in turn provides you with the long-term attachment you need to soothe the alarm permanently. Since anxiety depends on the alarm created by the mind-body separation and cannot survive without that separation, once you are truly connected within yourself, what you call your anxiety has no choice but to retreat because the old alarm energy is no longer there to feed your worries.

Healing in the body leads to healing in the mind and vice versa—and each opens a new door for the healing of the other. If you try to heal just one (as in doing yoga ten hours a day for the body or psychotherapy ten hours a day for the mind), you won't heal nearly as effectively or efficiently as when you do an hour a day of each.

Seeing the difference between anxiety and alarm will help you immeasurably in understanding how they form a reciprocating loop, each one feeding off the other like two siblings fighting in the back seat of a car. And once the anxiety of the mind is separated from the alarm in the body, each loses its respective energy source. At that point, the anxiety of the mind and the alarm in the body can be treated separately and the fight stops, just like the two siblings who are now separated by a caring parent. As you'll learn, that compassionate parent is you.

If you claim to "suffer from anxiety," it is imperative for you to know there is nothing wrong with you or your nervous system. In fact, your mind and body are working exactly as they should based on how you grew up, which might sound weird to you, especially if you have been suffering for a long time. You have simply learned to automatically believe your thoughts because a part of you thinks that indiscriminate belief in your worries is keeping you safe. You are being tricked by your own perception—an internal conditioning that says you must be hypervigilant and keep on worrying to keep yourself safe. That may have had an element of truth in your childhood, but you are not a child anymore, and that vigilance that once appeared to help you survive is now incredibly harmful.

You do not have a DSM-categorized disease. You have simply learned a pattern of fearful perception that is creating what you call anxiety. As I'll show you, what you call anxiety of the mind, I call alarm in the body, and you must treat the right entity if you are to truly heal. Anxiety likely started when you were a child, when everything became dysregulated after you experienced a separation of some kind that was too much for your conscious mind to process. Then that pain was pushed down out of your conscious mind and buried in your unconscious body, where it remains stored as a state of alarm to this day.

> This book is about showing you ways your body and mind can unlearn that trauma pattern and renew that faulty perception with a healthier one based in greater truth and awareness. In doing so, you can learn to accept that you do not have to believe everything you think, and come to see and know a peaceful place in your body where you need not think at all.

Returning to *Eat, Pray, Love* for a moment: "Every japa mala has a special, extra bead—the 109th bead—which dangles outside that balanced circle of 108 like a pendant. When your fingers reach this marker during prayer, you are meant to pause from your absorption in meditation and thank your teachers."

As I reach the 109th bead and publish this book, I acknowledge Elizabeth Gilbert for inspiring me to create the framework for this book and all my teachers who have gone before me on the path. Looking for truth in my search to heal from chronic anxiety has been a bit of a disjointed free-for-all, for I, too, realize I am a seeker and a writer. Perhaps most important, as I reach the 109th bead, I must acknowledge anxiety as my greatest teacher. I am grateful for the trust the universe has placed in me to experience it in the presence of so many other teachers. I am grateful for the learnings, both scientifically and spiritually based, in the hope I may be the teacher for others to help heal the root cause of anxiety in both individuals and across the world.

One of the criticisms of the first edition of this book was that it was repetitive. You may well find repetition here in the second edition as well. I wrote it to be repetitive, and this is why: I can change how you *think* about anxiety very quickly as the cognitive mind can readily understand a new perspective, but the greater issue is to change the way you *feel* about anxiety. Ironically, worry and hypervigilance formed in an attempt to keep you safe when you were a child and that program has had years to ingrain itself within you. As this hypervigilant pattern is tenacious, I cannot show you the way out of anxiety by merely showing you how to think differently in your conscious mind. To create long-term healing, I need to make you *feel* differently in your more unconscious body, and that requires repetition. In other words, if the concepts feel repetitive, and you are even getting a little frustrated with the repetition, that's a sign I am changing your deeper unconscious and therefore accomplishing my goal!

Before we get into the new edition, note that you may not fully understand what I am talking about in the early part of the book. In neuroscience, there is a concept called priming, a type of foreshadowing that primes you to understand and absorb more of the concepts I will show you as the book goes on. Because this book operates on a very different premise from traditional models of treating anxiety, I work to change the way you feel about your anxiety, rather than just change the way you think about it, and that requires some priming for the new concepts. Note that you don't have to fully comprehend the concepts presented right away, but rest assured the material will make more and more sense to you as you go through the book. When you finish this book, you will not only think differently with respect to your anxiety but most important, you will *feel* differently. Most therapies attempt to change anxiety by simply changing thinking and those therapies tend to "wear off" over time. Anxiety is a feeling issue and can only be resolved in the long term with a feeling solution.

I get messages every single day about how this book has changed someone's life for the better, so let's get into the *better* edition of *Anxiety Rx*.

The Anxiety Toolkit

Use these tools and strategies as you move through this book.

THE PHYSIOLOGICAL SIGH

This is a quick and effective way of calming the alarm system in your body.

Take two quick, deep breaths in through your nose, followed by a long, slow exhale through your mouth.

Do three to five rounds of this and it will immediately lower your alarm.

With my anxiety patients I show them how to supercharge the effect. Take three quick, deep inhales through your nose, hold for two to three seconds, and then exhale through pursed lips with your teeth together so that the exhalation makes a hissing sound.

While you hear the hissing of your exhalation imagine in your mind's eye an overinflated tire or balloon deflating.

Repeat for three to five rounds.

The more you do this, the more you teach your system to calm, so don't just wait until you are stressed to practice it!

AM I SAFE IN THIS MOMENT? *OR* I AM SAFE IN THIS MOMENT

When you find yourself in a state of alarm, put your hand on your heart or over the place you feel alarm, and ask yourself, "Am I safe in this moment?" or tell yourself, "I am safe in this moment."

Anxiety is *always* about the future, and future-based thoughts and worries, so when you lovingly bring yourself into the present moment you bring yourself out of your imagined catastrophic future.

To supercharge this effect, think of someone you love or a pet you have love for and put that same love into *yourself* while you affirm that you are indeed safe in the moment (and you *are* always safe in the moment you are in).

Like right now. Are you safe right now? Even though your body may feel alarmed, *you* are still safe.

PS, this is my favorite strategy for the middle of the night.

OBJECTING WITHOUT CONTRACTING

I adapted this from the work of Kathy Kain, PhD.

Allow yourself to feel your alarm and feel the pain of whatever worry you are dealing with.

Then notice the automatic urge to contract around it. I notice this contraction in my lower chest and upper abdomen. Sometimes it takes a moment or two to see and feel this contraction, but I assure you, it's there.

This contraction is the first automatic and unconscious step in the alarm-anxiety cycle and it happens so insidiously that we don't even notice it.

But the cycle needs your contraction (resistance) to the worry to rev up the alarm, so if you consciously decide not to contract and just breathe, with the intention to stay present and open, you teach yourself to be aware of this critical first step in the cycle.

When you are aware of this triggering urge to constrict, you can make a conscious decision to just stay open and not contract, because when you contract around your anxiety and alarm it begins to activate the alarm-anxiety cycle.

To supercharge this effect you can add touch to the area you feel the contraction, and see how long you can stay with the uncomfortable sensation of contraction by just staying present with it, even if it hurts (actually, *especially* if it hurts).

WHAT IS WORKING?

When we are overcome with alarm, our brain's confirmation bias looks preferentially for what is painful or scary in our lives.

This is the mind's confirmation bias, the tendency to give credibility to what you already believe. I also believe that the mind will also confirm what the body feels, so if the body is alarmed, the mind preferentially looks for, and gives credibility to, our worries.

So when our body is in a state of alarm, our mind pays more attention to scary things, to the point that good things fade so deeply into our emotional background we cease to become aware of them.

In a process I call stacking, worrisome things pile on top of one another and begin to take us over. Even if there are good things and good people to connect with, our brains don't let us "see" them.

So, this tool is about consciously looking at what in your life *is* working well, and it doesn't have to be a big thing, we are just trying to help you see that there *are* positives, but your brain just won't let you see them.

This always reminds me of a story of a man who would hit himself with a hammer over and over, and when asked why, he simply said, "Because it feels so good when I stop." Sometimes we move toward a positive direction when we simply stop moving in a negative direction.

To supercharge this effect, put on a favorite song and *really* feel it. This will create a different state in your body that will start to shift the confirmation bias in a more positive direction so you can see other things that *are* working.

DON'T BE A VICTIM

This is parallel to what *is* working. Victims stack worries on themselves and it happens so insidiously, and usually begins as a pattern in childhood, that they don't see how automatically they assume the worst and expect the worst and then create the worst in their worries.

This victim mentality shows up in the mind and body and becomes a neurologically self-fulfilling prophecy. The victim, via their worries, creates cortisol and adrenaline which prepares the system for stress and pain, so the victim preferentially learns to look for, and see, stress and pain.

As a result, people get trapped in a helpless victim mentality for their entire lives, and victims never escape anxiety and alarm because they become addicted to the chemicals of stress. Victims literally cannot get enough of what hurts them, and that includes worries.

One way I get myself out of victim mentality is to incite some mobilizing anger in me. Victim mentality is a paralyzing state, but anger is an activating state. Human beings feel anger as a form of protection when they are being victimized or taken advantage of. However, often as children we learned our anger did not help (or we were punished for it), so we dropped that tool, and a child without protective anger has no option but to become a victim.

I am not saying to rage—that is very different—but I would often use anger as a way to get out of bed or prime my system to activate instead of wither and show myself I was an adult and not a powerless child. This anger is meant to be directed *for self* more than to be *against other*.

One of the best statements I have used is: "I now use my anger to stop being victimized by myself or anyone else."

(There is a whole chapter on victim mentality later in the book.)

RECLAIMING FAITH

This doesn't necessarily mean religious faith, although people with religious faith often have lower levels of anxiety.

So how does reclaiming faith help as a tool to alleviate anxiety? When we experience trauma as children and that trauma is not resolved by a parent or caregiver, we lose faith that the world is a safe place. As a byproduct of that loss of faith in the inherent safety of the world we become hypervigilant and adopt the (false) belief that if our parents can't protect us, then we must do everything ourselves.

In addition, as a result of this childlike egocentric view of our world, we become very controlling of our environment and this hypervigilant, excessively worried attitude often provides a false sense of being able to influence what "might" happen.

In a vicious cycle, when we lose faith in the safety of the world, hypervigilant worry swoops in to try to protect us, and the more we believe our worries, the more those worries reaffirm that the world is not safe.

Worries remove faith, but the reverse is also true, faith removes worry.

In a leap of faith, we can remove the controlling need for worry. Even if it's just faith that we don't need to do anything. When we combine faith with objecting without contracting, we find a place where our worries are suspended by a power and a peace that are greater than us.

Cultivating faith in the world as a safe place is hard because it is the exact opposite of the coping strategy of worrying we adopted as a child.

Faith is one of the most powerful antidotes to worry. But more on that later on!

SELF TOUCH

Many of us didn't get enough loving touch as children.

Loving touch deeply wires the brain to cue toward safety and thriving. Lack of touch wires the brain to cue toward danger and surviving.

As you will see in this book, what we call anxiety of the mind is much more a state of alarm in the body, and I will show you that it is much more effective to use the body to calm the mind than to use the mind to calm the body.

When you feel anxious, get out of your head and instead see if you can find an uncomfortable place of alarm stored in your body. For many it shows up as a pain or pressure sensation in the throat, heart, solar plexus, or abdomen, often in the midline of the body.

I'll let you in on a little secret. That pain in your body is a remnant of your younger, wounded self. This is the true source of what you call your anxiety.

Put your hand over this sensation, breathe into this feeling of alarm if you can, tap over it, rub it, and make the intention to lovingly connect to it. In many ways, this sensation is the wounded child in you that wanted to be seen, heard, protected, and loved, so give that to them now with your touch and attention. Don't be too concerned if you can't find this sensation right away, but rest assured you'll be able to very soon.

SENSATION WITHOUT EXPLANATION

I saved the best tool for last. This is the hardest of all the tools to implement and also the most effective for your healing. Don't worry (haha) if this concept doesn't make a lot of sense right now, but I am priming your mind (and body) with this critical concept early, because it is essential in your relief from chronic anxiety.

To break the alarm-anxiety cycle, you must learn to separate the worrisome thinking in your mind from the painful alarm feeling stored in your body. This unconscious cycle is at the root of what we refer to as "anxiety." The alarm in the body activates the worries of the mind, and the worries of the mind aggravate the alarm in the body; so to heal, we must learn how to separate each from the energy source of the other.

Again, the alarm is a sensation in your body. I will go through this in detail as the book progresses, but when you are caught up in worry, see if you can pause your thinking and switch your focus into the feeling in your body. Look for a physical sensation that is intense and uncomfortable. In me I found my alarm in my solar plexus, but common places to find it are your heart, throat, or belly—but it can be anywhere. It may feel like a pressure or a pain or an ache. Some describe it like the heartache we feel when someone has died or a romantic relationship has ended.

If you can't find this right away, that's fine. As I said, I'll show you how to find this alarm as the book progresses. As another option, my online program MBRX goes into great detail on how to find and resolve your alarm. Once again, I am priming you to be familiar with this invaluable tool right away, so it gets more ingrained as you go through the book.

If you can find this uncomfortable energy in your body when you are caught up in worry, and then focus on the feeling of the alarm in your body, you begin to teach yourself the skill of specifically and directly moving your attention away from your thinking mind and into your feeling body. I imagine a "pause" button for my thoughts in my forehead and actually press it with my fingers and then let my hand fall down to connect with the place I feel the alarm in my solar plexus, as this acts as a signal that I am consciously and intentionally changing the source of my attention from thinking to feeling.

This is also a great time to engage the tool Objecting Without Contracting, where you feel the sensation but don't resist and contract around it. I cannot emphasize enough how crucial these tools are to your healing. I call this last tool "Sensation Without Explanation" as the conscious act of being present with the uncomfortable feeling of alarm in your body instead of allowing your mind to go nuts with Warnings, What ifs, and Worst Case Scenarios (aka the three Ws of worry).

In short, when you find yourself in compulsive worry, press the pause on your thoughts and refocus your energy to the sensation in your body, even if that sensation is uncomfortable. When you consciously move from thinking to feeling, you are starting to functionally metabolize the root cause of your pain (the alarm stored in your body), rather than being trapped in the endless assumption the three Ws of worry will magically find a solution. They won't.

Again, you likely won't be able to separate feeling from thinking very well to start, but the more you develop the skill of moving away from your worrying mind and toward your feeling body, the more you will break the alarm-anxiety cycle for good.

These tools will help you as you go through life, and as you go through this book. So, if you're ready, let's show you exactly what anxiety is and how you can heal from it.

Acronyms

ALARMS (abuse, loss, abandonment, rejection, mature too early, shame)

JABS (judgment, abandonment, blame, shame)

MADD (medication, addiction, distraction, dissociation)

SHOULD (see, hear, open to, understand, love, defend the child in you)

PART I

Awareness of Mind

1

My Trauma

In the summer of 1973, I was a super skinny, distraught twelve-year-old with yellow-blond hair, buck teeth, and bell-bottom jeans, watching through my bedroom window as an ambulance was preparing to take my father to the mental hospital. I had had a suspicion something was not right about my dad for a few years by then, but like most children, I took what I was given for parents as I didn't know anything different. Many have said I made the best of my dad's illness. I would say right up until his suicide fourteen years later that I made the worst of it. Almost fifty years after that summer day, this book is my attempt to finally make the best of it by using my father's pain to help myself and others who suffer from anxiety.

My father was loving and caring, with a great sense of playfulness and humor. He was a relatively small man, about five feet seven, but he had a big voice. So big, in fact, that he had his own radio show around the time I was born in 1960—no mean feat for a man of twenty-six years. The famous newscaster Peter Jennings, I'm told by my mother, said my father had the smoothest voice he had ever heard.

Now, it is 1973 and he is on his way to yet another admission to the mental hospital because, along with his own smooth-as-silk radio voice, he heard other voices too.

My dad was never abusive or violent, but he would lose touch with reality and believe things like he was the smartest person in the world or that he was able to talk directly to world leaders or that he was a cat. Okay, I might have made up the part about the cat, but only to make the point that he was certifiable. In fact, he was "certified" (the term we doctors use to commit someone to a mental health facility against their wishes) on more than one occasion.

I had always been a sensitive child, but I believe seeing my father descend into psychotic depression as a preadolescent and feeling so separate from him is when my anxiety really began to take root.

It wasn't his fault. I loved him, and I knew he loved me, but over time his behavior became too erratic for me to develop any sense of security. Often he was quite lucid and nurturing for months at a time, showing me how to hit a ball, ride a bike, and play chess—you know, dad stuff. However, it's like accidentally being bitten by the family dog; it takes a hundred positive encounters with the dog to counteract that one negative one, and if the pooch bites you one more time, you'll likely never trust that dog again—especially if that dog truly believes he's a chess-playing cat.

I was "bitten" many times by my father. He would regain my trust only to lose it again. If you had a parent or caregiver who was sick, addicted, an alcoholic, or just plain not there—or worse, mentally, physically, or sexually abusive—you know what I mean by being "bitten." The more bites you sustain, the more you are at risk of developing anxiety or a host of other emotional illnesses. For me, my anxiety developed because I lost my sense of self and my boundaries—the lines became blurry and I lost sight of where my parent ended and I began. When a parent sucks the energy out of a family, the children often divert attention from learning who they are and, instead, devote that attention to reading and caring for the needy parent (or caregiver) because children know this intuitively: "If my parent isn't safe, neither am I."

Many of us have anxiety because we gave up our secure, thriving, authentic self in exchange for a surviving, reactive self. We are called things like highly sensitive people, empaths, and people pleasers. We are often praised for taking on adult roles while we are still children. We lost touch with what we needed because we perceived our survival was predicated on someone else being okay. Many of us are good at giving other people care and attention, but the sense of what we ourselves need has atrophied from disuse. We adopted those caregiving roles with our parent or parents and honed them because it gave us a sense of power in situations where we otherwise felt powerless or immobilized. Over time, we lost touch with what we truly needed, and slowly but surely lost touch with ourselves. Then a split occurs inside of us where we consistently choose surviving (attachment to a troubled parent and giving to them) over thriving (attachment to ourselves and giving to ourselves).

When you are attached to a parent in a healthy way, you develop a sense of knowing and caring for yourself because your parent expresses an interest in knowing and caring for *you*. In secure attachment with an attuned parent, parts of your brain develop so you can self-soothe and see the big picture. When conditions get stormy, you can go into the deep, still part of yourself that is unaffected by the rough waves on the surface of your life. Without that foundational, soothing care as a child, the best you learn is how to surf the waves, and you get tossed around. A lot.

Point to consider: What adult roles did you take on before you were ready?

2
Challenges

The year 1987 was the toughest of my life. In the span of nine months, I lost my father, had to finish the final term of my neuroscience degree (and get exceptional grades in order to make the cut to enter medical school), got married, moved four thousand kilometers away, found a new home with a new wife and an eighteen-month-old daughter, and began medical school. And I was a complete nervous wreck throughout.

I still look back on this time of my life with a combination of pride and incredulity that I actually made it.

To start the year, my father's bipolar disorder and schizophrenia had devastated his mind and body to the point that he took his own life by intentional prescription drug overdose on January 12, 1987. I had an ominous sense that morning that something was wrong and called my brother.

Scott and I went over to his place, and it was no surprise to either of us when we found his body. I was not yet a doctor or even a medical student at the time, and my father's was the first dead body I had ever encountered. I remember saying to my brother, "Well, that's it for Dad."

When a boy loses his father, there is a sense of losing a protector, even though it was probably more accurate to say that I had been my dad's protector for many years prior to his death. Even though I was a twenty-six-year-old man at the time of his passing, the little boy in me never stopped hoping my dad would come back and be the man who had taken me fishing and taught me to ride a bike and hit a baseball. His death sparked a deep conflict in me. I remember simultaneously feeling incredible pain and tremendous relief that he was gone. Pain that I'd lost my father, and relief that his suffering had come to an end.

The first few months of 1987 I distracted from the pain by focusing my energy into finishing my premed science degree and applying to medical schools across the country. It felt strange that I wasn't grieving my father, and looking back I now know that I had completely dissociated into a profound numbness. But as you might have experienced yourself, emotion, like energy, cannot be created nor destroyed, only changed in form. I could only suppress the grief for so long until I felt a growing sense of impending doom mixed with my first experiences of terrifying panic attacks.

In May, the first round of acceptances went out, and a few of my friends had been granted early admission to various medical schools. I had not. I felt vulnerable and weak and inferior. I was barely eating or sleeping, and with the stress of exams over, I had started having flashbacks about seeing my father's dead body. In my anxious and fractured state, I wondered if the same fate of psychosis and suicide awaited me.

Looking back now, I remember obsessing that if I could get into medical school and become a doctor, that would prove once and for all I wasn't mentally ill like my dad. I became progressively more fixated on the story that becoming a doctor would be a profound testament to my mental wellness, when in reality becoming a physician would create profound anxiety and mental illness in me.

That spring in 1987, I clung to the idea that being Russell Kennedy,

MD, would save me, but it was looking less and less likely that a medical school, any medical school, would be my rescue. By June I was desperately checking the mailbox many times each day to no avail. (There was no email back then!) As my dream was dying, amongst daily panic attacks, I would have periods of what is called depersonalization, which is essentially the feeling that you aren't inside of yourself. It is like you are hearing your own voice as someone else would or watching yourself drink a glass of water—as if you are outside of yourself, watching yourself do things. This sent me into a complete panic because I had convinced myself I was becoming schizophrenic or bipolar.

The days dragged on, and as each day passed, my psyche was becoming more and more fractured. As the next medical school class would be starting in less than three months, time was running out. Then I got a break. On the morning of June 5, 1987, I got a phone call from the admissions office at the University of Western Ontario asking me if I was still interested in a position in their incoming class. They said I was on the waitlist and they were checking to see if everyone on the list still wanted to be considered.

Here is another reason why 1987 was so hard. One of the hallmarks of anxiety is being caught between two opposing paths. If I didn't get a spot, I would be in limbo, left in doubt of whether I would ever get into med school. If I did get in, there was a good chance I would be doing it without my daughter present with me, as my daughter's mother and I were not married and she was strongly opposed to the idea of moving far away from her family. To say I was pulled in different directions would be an understatement.

To make a long story short, I got accepted, and my partner and I decided to marry and form an official family unit that would uproot and make the journey from warm Victoria, British Columbia, to freezing-cold London, Ontario.

In your life, I'm sure you've faced huge obstacles—times when you felt completely overwhelmed. Hell, having a seemingly insurmountable challenge that completely overwhelmed you is probably why you developed an issue with anxiety in the first place, especially if that challenge occurred while you were a child or a young teen.

If you were to ask me ten years ago what had been the biggest challenge in my life, I would have pointed to my childhood wounding, or medical school, or my two divorces. But I know now none of those are it. The biggest challenge I have faced in my life is dealing with uncertainty.

Those of us with excruciating uncertainty in our childhoods will do just about anything to maximize our sense of certainty in adulthood. As you'll soon see, worrying is seductive and habitual because (1) worry makes us feel we are not frozen in fear and are at least doing something, and (2) a worry appears to make the uncertain more certain.

Many people who experience anxiety had a lot of uncertainty in their lives in childhood or at a time they were least able to handle it. Uncertainty is a huge unconscious trigger and is unbearable for many of us worriers because it reminds us of a time when we experienced tremendous, excruciating, destabilizing confusion and pain. When uncertainty revs up my worry, I know now this is the reactivation of the uncertainty of the child in me who did not know what was coming next or what his father was doing and feeling. Because we will do anything to avoid it, worrying is often seen as preferable to staying with uncertainty.

Uncertainty often created an unbearable feeling for us as children and still does for us as adults—and that discomfort in our body makes us feel we must avoid uncertainty at all costs. The other name for minimizing uncertainty is control. As children, we tried to control the pain of uncertainty by trading the immediate uncomfortable feeling in our bodies for the temporary escape of worrisome thinking in our minds.

In our attempt to control and limit uncertainty, we don't go out. We avoid places, people, and things that may create an undesirable reaction in us. Not only do we avoid things that are uncertain but we then confirm our avoidance by ruminating and worrying about why we shouldn't do those things!

Consciously, we are aware that control and certainty are an illusion, but unconsciously, where much of our motivation originates, we revert back to a time when we struggled to achieve a sense of control. Our childhood coping strategy of worrying becomes the preferential pathway as adults, because we still prefer the certainty of worry over the uncertainty of, well, uncertainty.

Point to consider: Notice your relationship with uncertainty and how much of your mental energy is devoted to minimizing it.

3

Becoming a Doctor

As a child, I never felt like I mattered. My father's tentative wellness and obvious sickness usurped most of the family's energy and attention. In an attempt to matter to my family, I adopted the role of caregiver for my parents and got some positive affirmation and identity that way. I have seen that many of my patients with anxiety carried responsibilities as children that were too much for them and made them grow up too fast. On one hand, you are inflated by the feeling of having a sense of usefulness and importance. But on the other hand, when you carry too much responsibility too soon and part of you knows you're in way over your head, your nervous system goes into a state of chronic alarm.

I didn't know this back then, but by becoming a doctor, I was looking to recapture the inflated sense of importance I received from the caretaking responsibilities I had taken on prematurely as an adolescent. I was going back to a well that had initially given me relief from my thirst for attention, but I couldn't see that the well was not full of pure water—but rather a mixture of water and toxins. All that responsibility I thought was feeding me as a teenager was in reality slowly poisoning me. As I continued to place caring for others above caring for myself, the mix became more poison and less water, and not only couldn't I stop drinking the poison, I had chosen a profession that would assure an endless supply of the responsibility I found so toxic.

As I'll say many times, you can't change what you can't see, and further, what you can't see you are destined to be. So many of my anxious patients learned to look after others' needs before their own. (Most still do, and I want you to see how you abandon yourself to look after others.) For me, I just couldn't see that my compulsive pattern of caring for others before myself played a huge role in my increasing anxiety and alarm.

Just like my addiction to worry was hurting me, but I couldn't stop, I couldn't stop caring for others over myself, and each of those childhood patterns supercharged the other. As I will also say many times, when you start to *see* it, you don't have to *be* it. I want to show you where you are making your anxiety worse in your adulthood by going back to a dysfunctional (but seductive and often invisible) pattern from your childhood.

It's like the old joke where a man goes to see the doctor and says, "Doctor, I broke my leg in three places," and the doctor says, "Well, stay out of those places!" It is important to see how to stay out of the familiar behaviors (and places) that are causing you pain, because, like automatically putting others' needs ahead of your own, there are many anxiety-producing patterns (and places) you compulsively fall into without even seeing how you got there.

Along these lines and patterns, Freud had a concept he called the repetition compulsion. I'll talk more about this later, but in short, the repetition compulsion is the powerful urge to reproduce the circumstances and patterns of your childhood in your adulthood, even if those patterns caused significant pain and anxiety.

Becoming a doctor was the "perfect" profession for me, because compulsively looking after others over myself was par for the course (and we all know how much doctors love golf). The repetition compulsion was my childhood addiction to caretake my parents (now patients), but it just about killed me because I couldn't let go of what was hurting me, mostly because caretaking was such a habit that I couldn't even see I was doing it.

Point to consider: What patterns from your childhood are you replicating in your adulthood? People pleasing, putting others' needs over your own, chronic worrying. (Don't worry! I'll show you how you can see these things so you no longer have to be these things.)

4

Let Go of the Banana

There is a parable about how to catch a monkey. There is a see-through wire fence with a series of holes in it. The holes are just big enough to fit a monkey's hand and forearm. On the other side of the fence is a banana. The monkey can reach in and grab the banana, but the hole isn't big enough for the monkey to pull his hand through while still holding on to the banana.

The monkey sees the banana and grabs it—and then someone walks up and grabs him. The monkey could easily escape if he would let go of the banana, pull his hand through the fence, and run. But because he can't bring himself to release the banana, he is trapped by his own hand and unable to see the simple solution to his predicament.

When people tell you, "Well, just stop worrying," in essence, they are saying, "Just let go of the banana." One of the reasons we worriers can't just stop worrying is because it has grown to be part of our identity. Indeed, it is so familiar that we start to worry when we are not worried! Most of the things we worried about as children (and indeed as adults) did not come to pass, so we drew the erroneous conclusion that the bad thing did not happen *because* we worried. For many of us, hypervigilance and worry were parts of our childhood that we (falsely) grew to believe were keeping us safe. We worriers feel that if we let go of the banana and stop worrying, we are giving up something we have conditioned ourselves to believe is beneficial to our very survival. Consciously we know that worrying about a biopsy result has no influence on the outcome, but deep in the childhood unconscious, we magically believe that it might. As a result, we become afraid not to worry, and we couldn't let go of the banana even if we wanted to.

By 2010, after almost twenty years of being a doctor, I knew that I was burned out and I needed to leave the medical profession—but I couldn't bring myself to do it. For me, being a doctor was like holding on to the banana. Some part of me thought it was serving me when in reality it was entrapping me.

Being a doctor is one of those jobs where they brand the title into your identity by making it part of your name. Instantly upon graduating med school, I became Doctor Russell Kennedy. I was in*doc*trinated, you might say. For some reason, they don't do this with other jobs. You don't become Plumber Jones or Jackhammer Johnson. (Actually, I think Jackhammer Johnson is the name of an adult film actor, but I digress.)

My point is that once you're holding that banana in the form of your anxious and worrisome thoughts, it's very hard to let go of—even though you can clearly see it is hurting you.

I knew that being a doctor was hurting me, but I just couldn't let go of that poisoned banana and leave medicine on my own. The compulsion to care for others was a very old habit, and one I had associated with being seen and heard in my family of origin, so the child in me believed if I gave up being a doctor, I would go back to my childhood perception of being unseen and unheard and unloved.

On February 8, 2013, I fully ruptured my left Achilles tendon because, like the arrogant doctor I was, I injected it myself with cortisone and lidocaine. But, as any doctor will tell you, although the relief from Achilles tendinitis is virtually immediate from the anesthetic (and it was), the tendon is weakened by the cortisone part of the shot and there is a serious risk of rupture (which mine did).

That was the shot that broke the doctor's back. I was out, and I knew it. I haven't practiced medicine as a traditional allopathic doctor since that day, not because of my Achilles rupture (although it never fully healed), but because that rupture forced me to let go of the banana and admit that my mental health couldn't take practicing medicine anymore.

Have you ever heard the saying "You can't see the label from inside the bottle"? I was so overwhelmed that I was unable to see I was trapped in my own (repetition) compulsion to help others at the expense of looking after myself. If you'd asked me back then, I would have told you I was a good doctor and helping others was my life's work. But my body was in a constant state of fight-or-flight alarm, and my mind had become overwrought with anxious thoughts.

The irony was I believed that becoming a doctor would show me that I wasn't mentally ill, but being a doctor drove me so deep into anxiety and mental illness that I considered suicide.

I was a mess. As I faced the idea of giving up being a doctor, I had flashbacks to those dismal days where it was a very real possibility I would never get in to medical school. I remember thinking back then I wasn't a doctor and really wanted to be, and now I was a doctor but really didn't want to be. However, being Dr. Russell Kennedy was so much a part of my identity that I felt I'd be lost without the title that came very close to killing me. Talk about a blind spot!

If addiction is not being able to get enough of what you don't want, I was addicted to the title of "doctor" along with the compulsion to worry—and both were killing me.

The first stage of my escape from this vicious cycle of worry creating more worries (and I'll show you how to do this too) involved developing a sense of awareness—a sense that I could witness and truly feel what was really happening inside my emotional body rather than escaping up into the thoughts and worries of my mind. It is getting outside of the bottle and truly seeing the label "Looks after others before himself."

One of the most critical and consequential parts of this book is to show you that the feeling in your body can be separated from the thinking of your mind. When you can't see the worries of your mind as separate and separable from the feeling of who you are, those worries become a self-fulfilling prophecy, locking you in the false perception that you *are* your worries. In other words, when you can't *see* your worries, you are destined to *be* your worries.

Point to consider: Entertain the idea that the feeling in your body and the thoughts of your mind can be two separate entities.

5

What Is Awareness?

In my own healing journey from anxiety, one of my greatest tools wasn't a technique or a doctor or a therapy or a pharmaceutical medication. It was a sense of awareness. One of the hallmarks of the repetition compulsion is it's notoriously hard for us to see. We just keep repeating the same childhood patterns (worrying, people pleasing, avoiding conflict, etc.) as if we don't even see them anymore. Some of the most valuable substances that helped me create a much deeper awareness of my own anxiety (and how to heal from it) were the psychedelics and I'll tell you those stories soon.

Entire books have been written on awareness, but in this book, I'd like to cover the aspects of awareness that have helped me the most in my search for relief from anxiety.

So, what is awareness?

We all have an awareness of the taste of our food, the touch of the steering wheel on our hands, and the sound of someone calling our name. This is the basic level of awareness that we use to experience the world. What I mean by awareness is a deeper level of being, typically called conscious awareness.

There is a major difference between unconscious awareness, which is rapid and automatic and directs attention in a reactive way, and conscious awareness. Unconscious awareness is feeling something, like the sensation of water as you are swallowing it. Conscious awareness is specifically directing your attention to that feeling, really honing in on it and savoring the specific sensations like the temperature of the water and feeling the liquid run down your esophagus. In unconscious awareness, or just plain awareness, time just flows by. In conscious awareness, there is a sense that time stops at that moment to allow a slower, more deliberate process of focusing specifically on an experience or object. Conscious awareness is being aware that you are aware.

As another example, you are breathing right now and likely aren't conscious of it. In conscious awareness, you would deliberately say, "I'll take a conscious, focused breath." You may even close your eyes and focus on how the breath feels going in and out of your nostrils. Try it right now: take a slow, conscious breath in and out, savoring the gamut of sensations a single breath provides. Now repeat the process and elongate the little space as the breath changes direction between inhalation and exhalation, and now you are really creating a sense of awareness of your breath.

In going from unconscious to conscious awareness, you go from daydreaming to awake, from past or future to present. In fact, the hallmark of conscious awareness is that it brings you firmly into the present moment.

Awareness can be seen as a skill, a practiced way of observing with nonjudgmental curiosity. With practice, meditators develop the skill of seeing their thoughts as mere expressions of the mind, without believing the thoughts or automatically giving them the weight of truth. In a state of conscious awareness, thoughts can appear and be observed simply as by-products of the mind.

Without the objective curiosity about our thoughts that conscious awareness brings, the mind unconsciously and automatically equates our thoughts (anxious or otherwise) with who we are. Until conscious awareness showed me these thoughts were only a part of me, I was not able to separate from them. Again, if you are not aware of the ability to see your thoughts, you are destined to be your thoughts. Without knowing you have an option to see things another way, you assume your singular perception of the world is how the world actually is. You never think to question your perceptions because you have never seen any reason to question your own experience and your interpretations of those experiences. Fish don't see the water they swim in.

The child who grows up with an abusive or neglectful parent can often see this childhood experience as the totality of who they are. After all, this is the whole world as they know it. It is not until that child gets older and sees other models of parenting that are not abusive or neglectful that they understand there is another way. With new awareness that not everyone sees the world the way they do, they understand for the first time that there are different ways to view their subjective experience, and this is the beginning of seeing they have a choice.

From this point forward, when I discuss awareness in this book, I mean conscious awareness. Conscious awareness is specifically and intentionally turning the intensity of your observation and curiosity to a singular source, as you might focus on your breath in meditation. To become aware that you are aware—that is conscious awareness, and it is the foundation of breaking free from the automatic negative thinking that has probably ruled your life for a long time. Awareness allows you the space to see a reality separate from your habitual worries. Awareness creates options that were always there but were previously invisible to you.

Before I developed this empowering sense of awareness of my childhood patterns, I felt like a passive victim to projections of my painful past. Just because a situation turned out a certain way in our childhood does not mean it will repeat itself, but unless we commit to seeing it we are likely to wind up being it. I was blind to how I was automatically reaching back to the blueprint of my past to build my future. I was tripping over my projections of doom and gloom, and I felt life was living me, not the other way around.

Point to consider: What is a pattern from your childhood that you are recreating in your adulthood?

6

Awareness of Victim Mentality

It is rare that I see anyone with chronic anxiety that is not recreating a victim state from their youth.

One of the tenets of the human mind and brain is that whatever you focus on (consciously or unconsciously), you will get more of. Using your mind and thoughts to amplify the ways you're a victim not only prevents you from moving away from the chronic worry you desire to heal but actually traps you deeper in that worry. Instead of holding on to a banana, you are now holding a hot potato that you won't let go of because you assume it is protecting you. But it's burning you—and it's the worst kind of injury because you are doing it to yourself.

As a family doctor, I saw patterns in families. I often observed that people treat and talk to themselves the way their parents treated and talked to them. The external messages become the internal messages. As an example, children of perfectionists often adopt that same voice and attitude and apply impossible standards to themselves. Victim mentality is also handed down from parent to child, perpetuating that chronic sense that the world is a dangerous place. Interactions in these families displayed a self-fulfilling prophecy by oppressing themselves by preferentially focusing on how the world was unsafe.

I have a friend whom I'll call Mitchell. He and I met at a personal development retreat and had an instant connection. He was in his late forties, with salt-and-pepper hair and a friendly face with an easy laugh. He laughed harder than anyone at a joke I had made to the group, so at that point, I had to be friends with him.

We talked at length about our childhood, mostly about our dads. Mitch had been physically beaten by his father from the time he was about seven years old. His father never once beat Mitchell's slightly older sister. Mitch had a poor view of himself. He had addictions to medications, marijuana, and sex. He told me he felt like a victim and that he could never win. That must have been exactly how that little seven-year-old boy felt.

Mitch had every right to feel victimized by life. Being beaten as a child is victimization. But as an adult, you have a choice to continue seeing yourself (and your life and the world) as a hapless victim or to develop awareness of how you continue to victimize yourself and turn it around. There is no more damaging program in anxiety than adopting a victim mentality; and unless you see how you are a victim you will always be a victim, and you will always be anxious.

Cultivating awareness that you are in a victim state gives you the option to see it clearly—and then gives you the choice to act another way. True awareness not only allowed me to see how I exacerbated my anxiety by adopting a victim mentality, but it also gave me the ability to truly see that if I did not allow myself to be a victim, my anxiety had nothing to feed it.

Seeing how I made myself a victim made it so much easier for me to understand how anxiety took me over. I'll talk much more about how victim mentality can be understood and resolved later on, but suffice to say at this point that without giving in to victim mentality, anxiety has no way of worsening.

Point to consider: How do you see yourself as a victim?

7

What Is Anxiety Not?

I was deeply confused by my anxiety for a long time. It felt like this amorphous blob of pain that I could never isolate.

When I was in med school, I quickly learned that the more I knew about a particular syndrome or condition I was treating, the better my treatment would be. In other words, the more defined something was, the easier it was to treat. That is just as true of the condition we refer to as anxiety. In my opinion, anxiety is very poorly defined.

If I talk to ten different people and ask them, "What is anxiety?" I'm going to get ten different answers—and of those ten, four of them won't know what anxiety is at all. Maybe the only thing I do like about the word "anxiety" is that if you rearrange the letters, you get "any exit." When I was in the depths of my anxiety, I would take any exit to get out of it. So maybe we should change the name to "generalized any exit disorder" or "social any exit disorder" because I know when I get a bit of social anxiety, I'm looking for any exit out of there.

In an effort to narrow down and make an effective definition of what anxiety is, I'm going to talk about what anxiety is not. The first thing anxiety isn't: it's not a disease. (And this is coming from a medical doctor; and doctors love to make diseases out of everything!) Anxiety is a normal coping mechanism that has gotten out of control. It's like putting a smoke detector in a cigar lounge.

Anxiety is a natural part of the human experience. It is there to warn us of potential dangers. It is meant to rise up to activate our nervous system for threat, and then immediately go back down as the threat resolves. However, if threats are chronic and ill-defined, or those threats don't get resolved fully (as in childhood trauma), the normal anxiety reaction gets stuck in the "on" position. Chronic worry is a maladaptive and hyperactive coping strategy of the nervous system in reaction to a perceived danger that may or may not happen in the future, not a disease.

The next thing anxiety is not: it's not a character flaw or a weakness. Many of my patients express this feeling that they are somehow inferior or defective because they worry too much. They worry (haha) that there is something wrong with them and that their worrying will stop them from doing the things they need and want to do, but most do those things despite the alarm they feel. Counter to their opinion of themselves as weak, people with anxiety are among the strongest people I know. Not only do they do the things they are afraid of, but they do them with one hundred pounds of fear on their backs. I can tell you that becoming a stand-up comedian was something I never thought I'd be able to do because of my anxiety, and I've had countless anxiety patients get on a flight, speak at their child's school, and otherwise do things they never thought they could do.

I had to point out to them (and myself) that if you have anxiety, you're actually pretty strong. You do everything everyone else does—go to work, go to school, raise your kids, go to the grocery store—but you do it while you are sandbagged by worry! If you change your perception of this perceived weakness, you can see having anxiety is not a flaw but a testament to your resilience under adversity.

Medical school is a challenge for people with the fittest of mental health, and I made it through (and even did well) even though at times I was afraid to leave my home. So if anything, having anxiety and living your life is a sign of strength of character. Once I realized this, I started to describe my character as sensitive and powerful versus anxious and weak.

By the way, if you're wanting to build more of this skill of perseverance through anxiety, I highly recommend the book *The 5 Second Rule* by Mel Robbins. It's all about conditioning yourself to do things that are difficult or instill fear but that you know you need and want to do. As soon as you have the sense to do something helpful for yourself, try counting down 5, 4, 3, 2, 1, and immediately taking action before your overprotective ego steps in to immobilize you. This skill, which many anxiety sufferers have already developed to some degree as a coping mechanism, will come in handy as you're working on new habits to help you "drop the banana," so keep it in the back of your mind!

The next thing anxiety is not—and this one's really important: it's not real.

Why? Because anxiety and worry are always about the future. Since the future hasn't yet happened and is strictly in the realm of the imagined, anxiety is by definition about something that is not real.

At this point, you may be experiencing some resistance to these ideas. I'm trying to establish anxiety as clearly as I possibly can so you can see you don't have to (and in fact shouldn't) fight with it, try to overcome it, beat it, or do anything else to it. In fact, the more you fight with it or try to overcome it, the more real it appears, because the more you fight with something, the deeper your system moves into a fight-or-flight state and the less rational your mind becomes. The less rational and more impaired by worries your mind becomes, the more likely you will lose the grounding and awareness of the present moment and be transported into the future because all worry is future-based. When your mind loses its rational faculties and you are removed from the grounding of the present moment, even outlandish worries can seem very real. Anxiety is not reality, although it seduces us into believing it is. Remember that you always have the choice to drop the banana and escape instead of continuing to fight to hold on and be trapped by your own actions.

The last thing I'll tell you anxiety is not—and this might blow your mind: anxiety is not a feeling. I'm going to say that again: anxiety is not a feeling. Look, I get it. You picked up this book because it seemed like I knew what the hell I was talking about, and now I go off and make a ridiculous statement like this. I know how you feel if you have anxiety. Or perhaps more correctly, I know how you think. To truly heal my anxiety, I had to realize that it is purely mind-based thinking of projections, expectations, stories, and thoughts of the future. Anxiety is a thinking process, not a feeling one.

As you embrace this new perspective of anxiety as purely a thinking issue, and not a feeling one, you have taken a giant step forward in the understanding of your dis-ease.

8

Anxiety Is Not a Feeling

Before I move on and talk more about what anxiety is, let me say a bit more about what you might be thinking after that last bomb I just dropped. "You keep telling me anxiety is not a feeling. But my anxiety hurts so much." I am showing you a critical concept in my own healing from anxiety—specifically, seeing that anxiety is only a thinking process, only a series of thoughts.

I am about to introduce you to the most important part of healing from anxiety. The pain we feel from our anxiety is not in the mind at all, but in a sense of alarm we feel in our body.

Think of a headache right now. Does that thought hurt? Anxious thoughts are the same: the thought in the thinking of your mind doesn't hurt. The pain you are feeling is a sense of alarm in your feeling body, and that is painful. By the end of this book, you'll fully realize where the pain you attribute to your anxiety truly comes from and what you can do about it. I'm not saying this condition we commonly refer to as anxiety isn't a painful process. I am defining anxiety and breaking it down into its component parts—anxious thoughts in the mind and alarmed feeling in the body—so we can understand exactly what this thing we call anxiety truly is, because once we understand the true essence of anxiety we can address and resolve each of its component parts, the thinking worries of the mind and the feeling of alarm in the body.

Before I address the pain behind what you call anxiety, I need to show you how to break your dis-ease up into manageable pieces because trying to tackle it all at once can feel impossible. So long as we see anxious thoughts of the mind upstairs and the painful alarm feelings in the body downstairs as one and the same, it is virtually impossible to penetrate their defenses.

Think of having two pairs of earphones with their cables twisted together. You are not able to discern which earbuds go with which jack. The whole tangled mess is indistinguishable and therefore unusable. You must patiently pull the two pairs apart so that both become recognizable and useful. Traditional therapies attempt to fix a feeling (the alarm in the body) with a thinking of the mind, and I've learned through decades of unsuccessful (and expensive!) therapy that you can't fix a feeling problem with a purely thinking solution.

In short, anxious thinking and alarmed feeling have become coupled together in a feedback loop. Traditional therapy doesn't see each component part and fixates on the thinking component, which is why CBT won't heal you long term. Until I teased apart and distilled out how the worries of the mind activated the alarm in the body and vice versa, I had no way to break the cycle and heal myself. When we can fully understand, appreciate, and distinguish each component, we can see how to break the cycle by separating and neutralizing each part. Until then, we are at the mercy of the alarm-anxiety cycle—where the anxious thinking in the mind feeds the alarm feeling in the body, and the alarm feeling feeds back into more anxious thoughts.

Incidentally, I didn't become aware of this cycle until I was in my fifties. For decades before that, I was trapped in the fear that my anguish was inescapable, and if it wasn't for LSD I might never have seen the way out.

9

LSD Showed Me What I Could Not See

Despite becoming a doctor and accomplishing assorted other feats, I experienced life as a powerless victim for many years. After more than three decades of trying multiple medications, techniques, and therapies without any significant relief, I felt hopelessly frustrated and resigned myself to the assumption that my anxiety was a life sentence. I have heard this same "life sentence" story from many of my patients who were also frustrated from the failure of many anxiety treatments.

Teasing out the anxiety in my mind from the alarm in my body and treating them separately has been the single biggest discovery that has allowed me to release the compulsive need to worry. It is critical for you to understand my "anxiety in the mind, alarm in the body" theory as you go through this book—even if it is difficult to grasp or believe right away—as the rest of this book (and the rest of your life) depends on it.

Remember that there are two distinct components to what we call anxiety: 1) a sense of alarm in the body, and 2) anxious thoughts of the mind.

There is a sense of alarm that occurs outside of the brain. This fight-or-flight sensation is the remnant of old, unresolved trauma we suffered, typically in childhood. Much of part 2 of this book is devoted to this sense of alarm in the body.

There are anxious thoughts created by the mind. The mind is a meaning-making, make-sense machine that is constantly scanning the body and then automatically and unconsciously making thoughts that match that bodily sensation. Through a process called interoception, the brain constantly reads the body and creates thinking in the mind that is perfectly consistent with the feeling in the body. When the body is in a state of alarm, the mind makes worries or projections that reflect that perceived danger. In this way, the feeling of alarm stored in the body from old, unresolved wounds creates the worries of the mind.

These two entities form a feedback loop where the alarm in the body triggers the worries of the mind, and the worries of the mind exacerbate the alarm in the body in what I call the alarm-anxiety cycle. You will continue to hear much more about this cycle as you go through this book.

I didn't come by the anxiety/alarm distinction easily. In fact, it was a revelation I had while coming off a bad trip I had on LSD in October 2013 (not that I have had any good trips—it was my one and only experience with LSD). But that one experience was all I needed to gain a different perspective, a new awareness that the pain I attributed to my chronic worry had more to do with my body than my mind.

You may wonder, if I am so prone to fear and worry, wasn't I frightened of LSD? You bet I was. I knew that taking a psychedelic is a risk in those with a family history of psychosis, but after thirty-plus years of conventional medical and psychological therapy with no lasting benefit, with thoughts of my own suicide increasing by the day, it was literally do or die. The parallels with my father were not lost on me. He was exceptionally intelligent and exceptionally crazy. I am both less intelligent and less crazy than he was. As I've said, many times I wondered if I was living my father's destiny, and back in 2013, I often thought taking my own life would be my only escape from interminable emotional pain.

Luckily for me, LSD did what I had hoped and gave me a new awareness—an opportunity to see things in a different way when I was "out of my mind." I was so accustomed to seeing things through the lens of my training as an allopathic physician, that anxiety was purely an issue of the mind, that I had lost the ability to see things any other way. I suppose you could say I was able to heal because I lost my mind and gained a new one.

This is what I want for you: to show you how you can see your anxiety in a new way, with a new mind and a new body.

During the psychedelic experience, I didn't see the full distinction of alarm in the body and anxiety in the mind right away. Under LSD my mind was fractured, and thoughts went wherever they wanted, and I did not feel like I had any influence on them at all. A still photo I had of my father in his Air Force uniform I had brought to the LSD experience seemed to have him moving left and right like he was dancing. As soon as I tried to focus on something, it changed. Nothing was static. Most disturbing was that my thoughts "moved" too. The more I tried to hold a thought, the more it would morph into something completely unpredictable. Also, it seemed like there was no distinct "me." While this won't do it justice, the best way I can describe what I experienced is that I had no distinct boundaries. I flowed into everything and everything flowed into me. There was no me; I was everything.

As the drug wore off and the flowing and moving slowed down, some coherent thoughts began to emerge. By no means was I holding on to stable thoughts, but I was shown that my anxiety was centered in my body. I had the distinct image of an irregular, oval-shaped, purple crystalline density that felt like an aching pressure located just to the right of my solar plexus and lower sternum. I don't know how exactly this came to me, but I was told this aching pressure was a type of energy locked in my body. Over time and through meditation, I have come to believe this purple density was the overflow of trauma that my mind was unable to contain and process as a child. I came to know this energy was the source of my alarm.

To this day, I don't know where this knowledge came from, and it certainly didn't come all at once. There were some very rough days immediately after my LSD experience. I fear how odd it might seem, a fifty-year-old traditional medical doctor taking his first trips on various psychedelics to examine his own anxious mind. Usually, it is younger people who experiment with mind-altering chemicals. However, I was truly desperate, and had it not been for LSD, I'm not sure if I ever would have figured out the true source of my pain. To be brutally honest, without the powerful and useful knowledge given to me on LSD and other psychedelics, I doubt I'd still be alive.

In the two years after my psychedelic trips, I still felt alarmed much of the time, but around 2015, something had shifted. I started to see the alarm in my solar plexus as separate and separable from the anxious thoughts of my mind. As I became better at directing my conscious awareness, I alternated between focusing on the thinking of my mind and then the feeling in my body. More and more, I began to see that what I called anxiety was not one entity but could be split into two, the thinking in my mind and the feeling in my body.

Since that experience, the concept of isolating anxiety in the mind from alarm in the body has had such power in my healing from chronic worry. This framework allowed me, with the help of awareness, to break the cycle and begin my recovery from decades of pain.

10

LSD and Me

If it wasn't for LSD, this book may never have been written. I know it may be disconcerting to think of a healthcare professional who has held others' lives in his hands fracturing his mind with psychedelics, and I can assure you it's not typical medical doctor behavior—but I am not a typical medical doctor. I was desperate, and desperate times call for desperate measures. Let me be clear: I do not advocate psychedelics as widespread treatment of anxiety, and please do not assume that because it eventually helped me that it will help everyone.

In short, psychedelic substances take away the ability to use the thinking mind. We anxious people are constantly using our thinking (and worrying) to distract from feeling the pain of our childhood wounds. In other words, *we use our thinking mind to avoid our feeling body*. On LSD, I faced the full force of the pain of my childhood trauma and it was terrifying. But despite the unmitigated terror, I do believe it was my destiny to see that the alarm I had stored in my body was the true source of the worries of my mind.

To date, the most valuable lesson I learned under any of the psychedelics was not some revelation that I was a beautiful and inextricable part of creation or that I was one with everything, although there was a vague sense of that amongst the horror. The biggest and most practical lesson I learned was that my anxiety had much more to do with a storage of old trauma in my body than any thought my mind ever had. At the time, LSD showed me the alarm in my body, but it did not give me a name for it or show me what I was supposed to do with it.

Psychedelics also expanded my consciousness to see that I am much more than my (anxious) mind, but I had to be forcibly evicted from that mind in order to see there was another world of feeling that was separate from my thinking. Before trying psychedelics, my unresolved trauma had me holed up in my head, firmly convinced that I shouldn't venture out of my mind and especially not go into Feeling Town down in my body— because it's pretty rough down there.

The psychedelics also allowed me to see that the feeling in my body was where all the color in life originated. From that revelation, I saw that the key to emotional peace lay in getting out of my thinking mind and into my feeling body. But aye, there's the rub—the feeling holds the pain along with the peace.

Moving into the body can be, and must be, done in order to heal your anxiety, and I'll show you exactly how here in this book.

I only took psychedelics a handful of times, and I don't plan to do it again. It was kind of like a science fair project in Hell. I am grateful for the insights, but I still have semiregular nightmares flashing back to when I lost my mind on LSD, and then there's the unmitigated terror of my ayahuasca experience. (Stay tuned.)

People ask me all the time if they should take psychedelics to see if they will help them understand their anxiety as it did for me. I tell them it's probably best if they study my experience and treat it as though I "took one for the team"—I did it so you don't have to. My own opinion is psychedelics may have some benefit with depression or addiction, but at the time of writing this book, I feel their use with anxiety should be viewed with caution.

11

The Conscious and Unconscious

We may think that what distinguishes humans from other animals is our capacity for conscious awareness and the fact that we are not driven entirely by instinct—but the truth is that humans possess both conscious and unconscious states within each of us, and we are still largely driven, and especially influenced by, the old wounds that are stored in the shadowy parts of our unconscious.

The greatest challenge of the unconscious is that it cannot be commanded directly. The conscious, almost by definition, is under volitional control. If I want to rub my cheek with my fingers, I direct that action voluntarily. But if a mosquito lands on my cheek, I will automatically (unconsciously) reach up to slap it. On some level, we can use the conscious to influence the unconscious (I can consciously decide not to slap the mosquito), but depending on the strength of prior unconscious learning, the conscious may have limited power to change the deeper unconscious patterns of feeling and behavior. This is why (conscious) talk therapy has such a challenge changing unconsciously mediated perception and behavior, especially if that perception and behavior are seen as helping us to survive when we were young. Although you can stop yourself from slapping the mosquito, you cannot simply will yourself into changing a deep unconscious pattern, for example, consciously willing yourself not to love someone anymore.

For the vast majority of human beings, the unconscious is actually in control. The more unstable the environment in which you grew up, the more your unconscious will take over and do whatever it has to do to ensure your survival. Instead of driving you forward into growth toward your hopes and dreams, your unconscious ego (more on this later) will keep you frozen exactly where you are. Fixated on protection, your unconscious keeps you away from perceived danger that, for the most part, your unconscious is actually creating!

Many of us with anxiety and alarm make our lives smaller and smaller, avoiding anything that could potentially cause us pain (and growth!). This avoidance often occurs unconsciously, as we slowly and insidiously shy away from doing things that challenge us.

One of the primary ways the unconscious takes us over is by creating a sense of alarm in our body. A part of our brains called the amygdala, often referred to as the brain's fear center, sounds the alarm when we get close to anything even slightly reminiscent of our old wounding. Another part of our brain called the insula, working in concert with the amygdala, creates what I call an emotional signature of alarm in our body, creating the same sensation now as when the original trauma occurred. As an example, I have a friend who was laughed at by her schoolmates while giving a presentation to her class when she was twelve years old, and to this day—more than thirty years later—she feels a "hot, fizzing, squeezing pressure" in her throat at even the thought of speaking in front of others. Along with the amygdala and the insula, other areas of the brain involved in emotional pain include the periaqueductal gray and the anterior cingulate cortex. When all four of these areas are activated, this alarmed state impairs the rational mind's ability to stay in control. This is exactly where "crimes of passion" come from.

The more the mind is impaired by alarm, the more we will act from an old, unconscious, protective place and our thoughts will reflect the need for protection. In other words, we start to create what I call the three Ws of worry—warnings, what-ifs, and worst-case scenarios—in a misguided effort to keep ourselves safe. As we become seduced by our worries we fall deeper into survival physiology and lose our more rational prefrontal cortex, ceasing to be able to see the three Ws of worry simply as *thoughts.* We imagine a scary story and then frighten ourselves by forgetting that we were the ones who made up that story in the first place.

I often get asked if the thoughts of the mind create the alarm in the body or if, rather, the alarm creates the thoughts.

From my perspective, the answer is both, in other words the alarm-anxiety cycle. But I can tell you straight that I didn't even begin to heal until I embraced that the worries were created by the alarm much more than the alarm was energizing the worries. Of course, the anxious thoughts aggravate the alarm, and the alarm-anxiety cycle takes us over, but as you'll see, for those of us prone to chronic worry, the alarm stored in the body is a much bigger player in the cycle than the anxious thoughts of the mind. The reason most anxiety therapies fail (or fade) is they assume a primary role of the thinking mind over the feeling body.

There are times that the thoughts do come first, like when someone brings up my father or I'm reading a medical paper on bipolar disorder or schizophrenia. When I see the specific anxious thoughts, I can consciously pinpoint where the alarm-anxiety cycle becomes triggered in me as that triggering thought, but for the most part, the unconscious alarm in my body will just hit me, and I won't know where it came from.

Chances are, your old trauma sneaks up on you in a similar way. Most of the (over)reactions of our bodies are beyond our awareness. But once we start using conscious awareness, we start seeing a connection that was previously invisible—and with that new insight, we can start to break the cycle and heal our old wounds.

Here is an example of trauma stored in the body unconsciously triggering an emotional response. After I finished medical school, to become eligible to practice, I first needed to work for a year in an accredited hospital as a medical intern. For my internship, I returned home to work at the same hospital where my father had frequently been admitted to psychiatric intensive care. The first time I was called to see a patient on that psych ward, I was hit with a significant bout of alarm.

I had been so busy going from surgery to cardiology to gastroenterology and then to psych that I didn't have time to think about the implications of where I was. But my body knew. As I arrived on the floor, my body unconsciously went into alarm without engaging thought at all. The ward had a smell to it that I can describe as "body odor and cigarette potpourri." As a neuroscience fun fact, smell is the only one of the five senses that is not preprocessed or filtered by the thalamus and as such penetrates directly into the emotional brain. This is why smell can evoke such strong memories, and that familiar acrid smell evoked old sensations, memories, and images of visiting my incapacitated, drugged, and incoherent father.

As it had only been four years since I was there as a visitor instead of a doctor, the place looked the exact same, and that had its own nostalgic pain, because the last time I was on that floor my dad was alive. My point is that it wasn't the conscious thought "I am on Dad's psych ward" that triggered me, it was the sensations, the unconscious feeling that affected me the most.

Carl Jung said, "Until you make the unconscious conscious, it will rule your life and you will call it fate." I believe he meant our drives and fears that hide in the shadows of our minds will rule our feelings and behaviors until we see them and bring them out of the shadows and into the light of conscious awareness. Until I did LSD, the alarm energy in my body—the real source of my emotional pain—remained unconscious. In making that alarm conscious and localizing it to my solar plexus area, I was able to direct my efforts at the true source of my anxiety, and I will soon show you how to find and isolate the alarm in your body as well.

When you create a sense of awareness, you arm yourself in such a way that you can observe your internal and external environment from a position of power. Without this intentional directive to truly see, you can be blinded by the intensity of your old unconscious programming. Inevitably, there will still be some old patterning and subconscious drives you cannot see no matter how much conscious awareness you employ, but you are infinitely better off having a mindset of openness and active awareness than just living your life as a passive victim to your old unconscious wounds.

When we truly focus on how and what we are feeling, and localize that feeling in our body, we bring in conscious awareness to what was previously hiding in the shadows. We begin to see that *our worries are only a distraction from the pain and are not the pain itself,* and this is why simply changing the conscious thoughts and worries does not heal the anxiety— because the worries are a smoke screen hiding the true root cause, the deeper, unconscious, shadowlike conflicts that Jung talked of.

The unconscious part of us, which I believe has roots in both the mind and the body, holds much of who we believe ourselves to be. But if that was forged by pain, it may not be your authentic self at all—it represents the reactive self you had to be to survive. The more trauma you endure, especially as a child, the more your unconscious gets redirected toward your protective, reactive self and away from your real, authentic self. The more we act from the protective self, the more alarm we feel, and the more we perceive the need to protect ourselves with hypervigilance and worry. We can be in protection or in growth, but we cannot be in both—they are mutually exclusive. The more we find and connect to our real self and commit to our growth by living there, the less alarm we feel, and the fewer worries in the mind we need to create to distract ourselves from the alarm in our bodies.

12

Immobility

HELD IMMOBILIZED

My mother was, and still is, a very sensitive being. Being born sensitive (as I also was), coupled with the experience of heading to the bomb shelters each night as a nine-year-old in Glasgow, made it so she does not tolerate noise or activity well. I do not blame her for her exquisite sensitivity, as I know her nervous system was forged at a very tumultuous time in human history.

Unfortunately, as a child, I was both noisy and active. Had I been born in 2000 instead of 1960, I likely would have been diagnosed with ADHD. I still get frustrated easily, not by people (for whom I seem to have almost infinite patience) but by things. If I have to put together an IKEA desk or a gas barbecue and it's not going well, I will start throwing my toys. My mother showed me in no uncertain terms that being angry and active wasn't okay, so I became immobilized because it wasn't safe to be my real (active and curious) self.

To this day, I hate being told what to do. I was fired from every job I had prior to med school, and my mother said that it was good that I became a doctor because I could work for myself.

Unfortunately, being quickly shut down from the time I was a toddler sent a message to me that my emotionality and intensity weren't welcome. Many of us with anxiety and alarm were made to feel that our attempts at exploring and expressing who we are were not okay. When you take a child's ability to be angry away from them, they feel helpless, move into victim mode, and progressively lose the ability to defend themselves.

Much of the reason I allowed myself to be bullied or mistreated was because my defensive anger had been stripped from me as a child.

How do you feel about your anger? Are you afraid of it? Do you have a temper? Many of us anxiety/alarm sufferers have a conflicted relationship with anger. One of the ways victim mentality weakens you is by paralyzing your sense of anger—as if you feel you don't have the right to get angry, perhaps because you felt denied the ability to protect yourself at an early age and needed to just give up and accept what was given to you. If you were already living in a chaotic environment, you may have suppressed your anger because of the fear of adding more intense emotion to the household.

Anger is a defensive emotion. It mobilizes you to protect yourself. Anger is a response to a real or perceived violation of your personal boundaries. For example, if you hear someone has said something negative or untrue about you, anger is a normal and natural reaction. The anger creates an emotional energy that mobilizes you to protect yourself.

But often, those of us who experienced emotional overwhelm as children do not express that anger energy out of a fear of repercussions. Alternatively, because our healthy boundaries were encroached upon so many times, we gave up mobilizing our anger because it didn't do any good! Instead of mobilizing, we often do the opposite: freeze in immobility and, instead of protecting and sticking up for ourselves, we abandon ourselves. Of course, this inability to protect ourselves and express energy outward reaffirms our victim mentality. Again. When you take a child's anger away from them you leave them defenseless for the rest of their lives.

This thwarted anger energy has to go somewhere in the child and often turns inward, fueling our inner critic and driving us further into victim mentality.

How do you feel about your big emotions today? How were your anger and intense emotions handled by your parents? Were you allowed to express them? Or were you shut down, as I was? Reflect on how this inability to express your emotions may have left you defenseless to bullying, abuse, or neglect throughout your childhood because you weren't able to speak up for yourself.

I once had a patient (whom I'll call Mary) who always appeared cheery and optimistic, even when she was experiencing significant health issues. I once documented forty-three different medical complaints in a single office visit. To this day, it's still a record. Yet during that visit, she was cheery and joking. Mary had adopted a mentality of helplessness. She felt like a victim to her body and mind. I can't say I blamed her. She had so many medical issues I can completely see why she would feel exasperated. Mary had chronic anxiety and alarm, and I really felt for her.

But here's the curious thing. In ten years of being her physician, I never saw Mary get angry. Not once over an entire decade. Even when a long-anticipated medical test was postponed or canceled or her condition worsened, she always remained resigned to her fate. On another occasion, one of the specialists who saw her was quite rude to her in an offhand and insensitive comment about her weight, and she still didn't speak up or show any signs of anger.

Perhaps the worst part of scenarios like this, and countless others I've encountered, is that when we (consciously or unconsciously) adopt a victim mentality in childhood, we accept powerlessness as a way of life as adults. There is no longer a person, external force, or circumstance disempowering us, but we have taken over the role of disempowering ourselves. I saw many of my patients who were overwhelmed in childhood just abandon the fight and give up. In a way, I can't say I blamed them. When you have a history of overwhelm with no history of success or pursuit with no chance of true emotional connection, it's an understandable response to retreat and just accept defeat instead of putting more energy into trying to change your situation. But when we learn to immobilize and suppress ourselves, it sets a very dangerous and damaging precedent, as it fosters a victim mentality that both creates and perpetuates alarm in the body (and the chronic worries in the mind).

One of the most troubling features of victim mentality is that it makes you believe you are protecting yourself, when in reality, seeing yourself as a victim gives you the permission to retreat from your challenges, which endlessly reinforces a sense of helplessness. In this way, victim mentality traps us in a self-reinforcing loop of helplessness and retreat. While you maintain a victim mentality, you can never overcome your anxiety and alarm because paradoxically, you are paralyzed by the victimhood you rely on to keep you "safe" by not challenging yourself. Victim mentality usually begins in childhood when the circumstances of your life seem insurmountable, like when a parent abuses, neglects, or abandons you, despite your attempts to mobilize yourself or even get angry. I would helplessly watch my father collapse into psychosis time and time and time again, literally see the world as a place of persecution. This erodes your faith in the world as a place of opportunity and growth (more on the healing benefit of faith in yourself later), your own abilities, and holds you back from breaking free of the very victim mentality you yourself are perpetuating, all in the name of "protecting" yourself.

Productive anger and mobilization are an antidote to victim mentality and allow you to see aspects of your authentic self that you may have lost as a child. Healthy anger shows you are not helpless—far from it—and that you can gain confidence in and depend on yourself to maintain your boundaries to enable self-soothing and self-care. Worriers perceive themselves as victims and don't have the ability to soothe themselves, and that only intensifies their self-perception as hapless victims.

The starting point, as always, is awareness. It may take a while to notice how you disempower your healthy anger and hold yourself immobile because you have become so complacent in your self-perception as an immobilized victim that you don't even see the option to move toward your challenges anymore.

If you struggle with chronic worry, it's likely you were a victim to a form of abuse, abandonment, or neglect as a child, at a time when you had little power. There is also a good chance you adapted to the futility by repressing your anger and adopting a victim mentality. For many of us, it was just too demoralizing to become angry or try to fight back when we were children and had no power to change the situation, so to minimize stress, we just gave up the fight, like an animal that is cornered by a predator and has no other option but to play dead.

This is the problem with many of our childhood defense mechanisms like adopting hypervigilance, worry, and a victim mentality: we make the assumption that because those defensive adaptations had some protective value to the child in us, that we can "ride them until the wheels fall off" into adulthood. Often nothing could be further from the truth because, while those childlike strategies had some benefit to the child, they keep us locked in protection to the point that we don't even see the possibility of growth as adults. I'll return to victim mentality as a childhood defense mechanism and what you can do about it in its own chapter in part 3, but in the meantime, know that you are not in the powerless situation you were in as a child. It's okay now to mobilize with anger (notice I did not say rage), and it is more than okay to reclaim your life energy, stand up for yourself, and stand up against your worries.

Point to consider: Mobilizing a little anger in your system can break the immobility of victim mentality and help you face down your worry.

13

Issues in Our Tissues

Whether we are aware of it or not, we are guided every single day by our memories. The more intense the memory (good or bad), the more it influences our behavior, perceptions, and beliefs, in both conscious and unconscious ways.

Burning your hand on the stove as a child and never needing to be told not to do it again is an example of implicit memory, or body memory. The memory is in us and unconsciously guides our behavior. The most powerful implicit memories are attached to emotion and pain. The more powerful the emotion, the more powerful the lingering effect. In yoga, we call it having "issues in our tissues." While teaching a yoga class, I would often see a student start to cry, and I don't think it was because I was a bad teacher, but maybe. I've come to know that a certain movement or posture can trigger the release of a strong memory the person hadn't thought about in years, often resulting in an intense emotional reaction. At the end of the class, I would often reassure my tearful student by telling them that some postures are likely to bring out old pain and it's completely normal that tears come, as tears are one of the ways our system heals old pain.

Some of the most powerful body memories are created in childhood when we encode intense experiences that are too much for us to bear. These emotionally charged memories are often shoved down out of our (conscious) mind because they were just too painful or overwhelming, and are exactly the kinds of energies that get stuck in our (unconscious) body as a state of alarm. If we are not aware of them, these old traumas can hold an insidious background energy of alarm in our bodies that can feed our anxiety and worry for decades. I have termed this energy "background alarm." (I'll explore this concept in much more detail in part 2.)

As an example, you may have been bitten by a dog when you were very young and have no conscious memory of it, yet now have an inexplicable aversion to dogs as an adult. For some reason, you just don't trust them. Even though you don't consciously remember the dog bite, it's stored as background alarm and you are still reacting to it.

To use a more emotionally charged and personal example, I developed an unconscious implicit program that it was not safe to love. It took my focused, conscious awareness to see why I had such an inexplicable aversion to relationships. (I've been divorced . . . twice.) The answer? My father's schizophrenia. I loved him dearly, and when he was sane, he was a very attentive protector and teacher, but with each catastrophic emotional collapse and hospitalization, I could see he was progressively leaving me, mentally if not physically.

Losing him to mental illness was devastating. Throughout my early teens, he would bounce back to a level of functionality where I could still count on him, and once I felt his counsel and presence, I would give him my heart, only to have it crushed again in six to eighteen months with the inevitable next episode of psychosis. As I got into my late teens, I went from having a father in him to being a father to him. That's not how it's supposed to work, and my unconscious, protective response was to numb myself and slowly withdraw. I stopped trusting in being his son but, at the same time, resented the loss of him. My protective instinct caused me to start numbing my feelings toward him, as loving him was just too dangerous. But two divorces have taught me that you can't numb to one person without numbing to all people, and this withdrawal from love caused all my relationships to suffer for many years.

Looking back, I know my amygdalae had coupled love with fear, so that when I felt love I also felt fear. For a long time I wondered why I felt so numbed out and disconnected in my relationships, but now I know my system went back and forth between love and fear so often I became mentally exhausted and unable to consistently connect even when I truly wanted to.

I've learned the hard way you can't harden your heart to one person without compromising your ability to love all people. Perhaps even more important, when you stop trusting love for someone else, you limit that same love to yourself. I've also found when you push love out, fear moves in to take its place.

Wow, I got really philosophical there for a doctor and neuroscientist! But now that I'm out on an emotional limb with my own experience of love and life, I am going to share something with you.

What causes alarm and anxiety? Separation. Not trusting love. Lack of connection to yourself and others. Extreme resistance to being and feeling vulnerable. But most of all it's a split from within yourself.

What is the antidote to anxiety and alarm? Trusting and expressing the love I have for myself and others. I had to learn that it was safe to trust love and be vulnerable again. I had to learn to have compassion for my dad. I had to reinstate my love for him. When I stopped blocking love for my dad, I found the compassion and healing I needed for myself.

Staying in victim mode—numb, shut down, and "protected" from vulnerability—cut me off from the very thing I needed to heal from chronic worry: love and connection.

The unconscious pattern or program I was compulsively repeating was "to love means to get hurt," based on my body memories from the pain of dealing with my father's mental illness. Loving someone set off my alarm, and love was the exact thing I needed to assuage that alarm. But how are you supposed to heal when your unconscious won't let you access the very thing you need the most?

> Where did you start to mistrust love and connection, or where did you feel that love and connection couldn't be trusted? How does withdrawing from love and connection show up in your life today? Do you trust the love from your pets more than the love from the humans in your life?

14

The Ego

Imagine something that totally fires you up. It makes you upset, scared, and frustrated, and you can't help but react. Chances are your ego is involved, and the situation is rekindling a painful episode from your past.

Entire books are written on the ego, but I am going to stick with the parts most relevant to anxiety and alarm. The ego is a part of our unconscious that protects us from harm or, perhaps more correct, attempts to protect us from harm. It has other jobs too, but the protection aspect is the part that's most relevant here.

Essentially, the ego tries to prevent us from making the same mistakes again or exposing ourselves to experiences that have hurt us in the past. The protective ego is linked to the amygdala, a structure involved in virtually every fear reaction in the human brain. The amygdalae (we actually have two, right and left) record everything that has ever hurt us, either physically, emotionally, or both. It is the amygdalae that recorded exactly where you were on 9/11 or the Boxing Day Tsunami. The amygdalae never forget anything that has ever hurt us. The ego, in concert with information encoded by the amygdalae, sends our system into high alert when anything even remotely close to the original painful stimulus is perceived. (From this point forward, I use the singular form, amygdala, as it is more common, but know that I mean both left and right.)

Let's say you got bitten by the neighbor's Doberman pinscher when you were five years old. (This book seems to have an inordinate number of dog bites, huh?) Your amygdala and ego will likely sound the alarm in your system whenever you encounter a Doberman (or perhaps any dog) for the rest of your life. In fact, since the amygdala generalizes to anything even close to the original trauma, it may very well sound the alarm and make you afraid of any animal around the same size, or any dog at all. Even the thought of a Doberman might send you into alarm.

The ego reaction doesn't have to make sense, and it often doesn't. Maybe you are in a supermarket and you have a panic attack. You then go outside and the panic attack subsides. Your amygdala and ego conclude that the supermarket is the cause of your fear. The next time you need to go to the supermarket, you walk on eggshells expecting the worst and, lo and behold, get another panic attack. This confirms the evil supermarket as the cause, so you avoid supermarkets. Now your amygdala has inspired you to narrow your world so you can only go to small markets to avoid the ego-based supermarket monster.

This is painfully characteristic of ego protection. It protects you from a danger you made up yourself!

The ego acts automatically, often outside of our conscious awareness. Indeed, one of the biggest challenges we face is actually seeing where we are creating our own pain. The ego shoots first and doesn't ask questions at all. The ego is reflexive, not reflective. It's not interested in solutions or ways of seeing more clearly, or getting along with your crazy relatives. It is fixated on protecting you from harm, oblivious to the mounting list of dangers (supermarkets, buses, doorknobs, open spaces, confined spaces, dogs, cats, trees, wombats, bananas) the ego itself is creating. The more emotional and physical trauma you experienced as a child, the more the amygdala becomes reactive and sensitive and the list of things you react to expands, and the amygdala has been noted to be larger in people who struggle with anxiety. In us worriers, the ego is particularly active, ready to act in an instant. When the ego has its way, we are chronically in an alarmed, defensive state. We may not be overtly aware of it as we become accustomed to its overprotective presence in the background, but make no mistake: the anxious person's nervous system is prepared to jump into action much faster and perceive threat when none is present, much more than that of someone who does not struggle with chronic worry.

The ego has no life in the present moment. It depends on destabilizing you by readily remembering traumas of the past and using them to make scary predictions of the future. Even though we may be safe in the moment in reality, the ego needs you to be on the constant lookout for imagined danger it makes up itself!

Allowing you to feel safe is not in the ego's best interest, even though it is in *your* best interest. Because the ego thrives in the shadows of old fears and unresolved traumas buried in the unconscious past (as well as creating new worries of the future), conscious awareness and grounding ourselves in the present moment are our most effective tools to disarm the out-of-control ego.

It is up to our conscious awareness to ask questions. If we never question why we do what we do, think what we think, or act the way we act, chances are we will stay under the ego's relentlessly protective umbrella, and our emotional and physical lives will become narrower and narrower in a futile attempt to avoid danger that is only real in the ego's warped and overly sensitized perception.

The ego is like an overprotective mother in the extreme. Just as this hypervigilant mother will not let her child explore and have fun playing on the jungle gym for fear of the child getting hurt, your ego will not let you explore and have fun with life because of the perceived danger.

The ego is not inherently bad. It's simply misguided and relentless—much like the Japanese World War II soldier Hiroo Onoda, who hid in the jungle and kept fighting for twenty-nine years after the Japanese surrendered in 1945. He had orders to fight to the death and, not allowing himself to believe the war was over, kept himself in constant battle. The ego is just as tenacious (if not more so). It believes the war we fought so many years ago as children is still going strong, and so it keeps up the fight.

The ego is at its most influential and believable when it takes us out of the present. The ego knows it has no power in the now. It only remembers the past and maps it onto an imagined future. When you bring yourself into the present moment of conscious awareness, the ego is a deer in headlights. Feeling powerless, the ego will try to scare you out of your present grounded state by getting you to emotionally time-travel to past traumas or future worries. Later on, I'll show you how to see your ego with compassion as if it is a big dumb dragon you created to protect you when you were very young, and you don't have to believe everything it tells you.

15

The Fear Bias

Our brains have a bias toward survival, which means they also have a bias to overestimate threat, which is another name for worry.

On an evolutionary basis, our ancestors who were more fearful or assumed the worst were more likely to survive. Thousands of years ago, if you saw a bush move and you assumed it was a predator and made your way to a safe place, you would live to mate and pass on your genes. However, if you assumed it was just the wind that moved the bush, you might become something to eat, and unlike Jackhammer Johnson in the movie *Jungle Bonk,* there would be no mating for you. In a very real way, we were rewarded for being fearful, and parents with a bias toward fear created fearful offspring. Fear became a factor in natural selection, and the fear bias was passed on.

Back then, the main threats were physical and were outside of us, but in modern times our threats are much more mental and come from inside of us. You could say that primitive man feared his predators and modern man fears his creditors, but today, the human brain and body react the same way to both.

The fear bias, a natural feature of evolution designed to make us pay attention to real and specific threats, has now morphed into the unnatural and exaggerated *worry bias* adapted to pay attention to numerous imagined threats. While that cautious mindset was likely to help us survive the hostile environment thousands of years ago, chronic worry, with all the stress chemicals associated with it, has now become a threat in and of itself. In trying to keep us safe with worrisome thoughts, the hyper-protective, worrying ego has become a danger to the very survival it so desperately tries to preserve!

It's like a dog biting his own tail, thinking he is fighting an opponent: as the dog feels more pain from the imaginary combatant, he bites harder, trapped in a cycle that keeps escalating. The good news is that once we become aware we are biting our own tail, we can choose to let go. This book will show you how you are unwittingly biting your own tail, and more important, it will also show you how you can stop. But again, you have to start seeing your worries so you can stop being your worries.

16

You Can't Think Your Way Out of a Feeling Problem

Anxiety is essentially thinking that can't control itself.

The mind thinks. It's what the mind does. From the time we are toddlers, we explore and use trial and error to figure out how the world works. From the time we start to speak, feeling begins to take a back seat to thinking, as the language of words replaces the "language" of feelings.

We've been using the mind since we were toddlers, and we worship it. We see our thinking create amazing things like space travel and Candy Crush and assume it has all the answers. It reminds me of a joke by a comedian I once shared the stage with named Emo Phillips. He said: "I used to think that the brain was the most wonderful organ in my body. Then I realized who was telling me this."

In anxious people, the mind moves faster than the body. The body has a regulating influence on the mind and nervous system, but if we are bypassing the slow, grounding, present-moment wisdom of the body by constantly defaulting into speedy, future-based, anxious thinking, we essentially have become human thinkings instead of human beings.

When we struggle with anxiety, we speed up our thoughts as a coping mechanism in the false belief that we can think our way into feeling safer. This is like saying "eat yourself skinny" or "drink yourself sober." Instead of slowing the mind down and allowing the body to catch up so they can sync together to support us, the mind just goes faster and faster. Unless we stop to feel (versus stop to think), the mind will always take the lead by default, and we'll keep biting our tail harder and harder in a misdirected effort to stop the pain.

I once had a patient who had just lost his wife to cancer. He was clearly distraught and was endlessly ruminating on things he should have done differently. He said to me, "Dr. Kennedy, I'm so depressed and anxious. I just have to find a way to dig myself out of this hole." I told him in the most compassionate way possible, "You can't dig yourself out of a hole. When you see you are in a hole, you need to stop digging."

Trying to think your way out of anxiety is like trying to dig your way out of a hole. You just go deeper! You might feel you are accomplishing something if you keep on digging (worrying). But in reality, you are getting further away from a solution as your hole gets deeper and darker. You would be better off if you just stopped digging.

This is exactly what we are doing when we try to use our thoughts to find our way out of anxiety. The thoughts make the alarm worse, and we move deeper into the alarm-anxiety cycle—yet we sense we are doing something productive by using the only tool we see at our disposal, our thoughts. Distracting away from your feeling body by going into your worried mind might have been your only relief as a child because you had no power to change the situation back then, but you're not a child anymore, and you have awareness and choice now that you didn't have access to back then.

I'll let you in on the secret to healing anxiety, and sure, it's easier said than done. You must learn how to stay more with the feeling of alarm and escape less into thinking of anxiety. When you try to think your way out of a feeling problem, over time, the ever-increasing speed of the mind results in the body and mind becoming progressively more out of sync, which creates more alarm. Instead of trying to think our way out of it, we need to slow down our mind and body so they can join together to allow us to feel our way out. (Stay tuned.)

But many of us are afraid to slow our thinking because we have been unconsciously convinced by our childhood egos that thinking will keep us safe and we become unsafe when we stop worrying. Indeed, one of the most powerful ways we teach ourselves to make our anxiety worse is to believe that if we just keep thinking the answer will come. It's biting your own tail harder and harder and being genuinely confused as to why it's hurting more.

It is akin to this riddle: a man says, "Everything I say is a lie." Having established that, he then says, "I am telling the truth." You end up going in circles because you cannot make this make sense by thinking. The same is true for worry: it is an endless loop, and the only way to escape is to stop thinking (and drop the banana). But the ego's unconscious message tells you the only way out of worry is more worry—and we believe it. We trap ourselves in a cycle of thinking and just keep pedaling faster, believing this will slow us down.

Like your ego, your anxiety is not here to punish you or hurt you or persecute you, although it can certainly feel that way. The anxious thoughts and worries are the ego's attempt to keep you safe by keeping you vigilant for warnings, what-ifs, and worst-case scenarios. These three *W*s of worry your mind creates never truly provide any safety. In fact, quite the opposite. However, as long as you stay unaware that you cannot think your way out of anxiety, you are seduced into the addiction of worry and continue to bite your own tail.

The late, great comedian George Carlin wrote a book in which he calls his incessant and compulsive thoughts "brain droppings." That is a brilliant way of looking at thoughts—as little droppings the brain poops out like a deer as it walks along—except that unlike the deer, we humans fail to just move on. As we consciously or unconsciously stay stuck in those worrisome thoughts, our lives get shitty.

Point to consider: Can you bring to mind a worry of yours and then give yourself the option to simply not believe it, or withdraw all of the energy you have put toward it? Just let that worry sit in suspended animation, observing how badly your mind wants to believe it.

17

Ninja Worries

We must be conscious of our thoughts in order to see that the only power they hold is the power we bestow on them. It reminds me of a saying attributed to Robin Sharma: "The mind is a wonderful servant but a terrible master." If we believe everything we think, we are the servant. If we see the thoughts as brain droppings, with only the power we give them, we are the master.

Like a ninja, worries gain their power by not being seen. Worrisome thoughts are often habitual and slip beneath our awareness. As a result, we believe everything we think and fail to see intrusive thoughts like "I have a fatal disease," "I'm going to lose all my money," and "My family will leave me" as mere thoughts that we ourselves have simply made up. The trouble starts when, instead of seeing our worries as mere intrusive thoughts, we unconsciously and automatically accept them as true. We create these imaginings of the future, then magically believe and act as if they are real in the now. Our worries seem to have some sort of diplomatic immunity where they can cause all sorts of damage but not be held accountable. We do not critically appraise our mind's warnings, what-ifs, and worst-case scenarios; we just accept the three Ws of worry as true, and this fires up painful alarm stored in the body. That alarm in the body, through interoception (the process by which the mind perceives the state of the body), creates more scary worries congruent with the rising alarm in the body. That alarm/survival physiology (e.g., cortisol, norepinephrine) impairs the ability of our rational prefrontal cortex to see those worries as imaginary projections of the future (aka brain droppings). In other words, when we are alarmed, we are likely to fearfully *believe* everything we think—and that is disastrous to our mental and physical health.

Bringing the thoughts of the mind into conscious awareness (along with bringing the alarm in the body into conscious awareness, which you'll learn more about in part 2) reinstates the full ability of the mind to see worries as only a function of imagination. An unbelieved thought or worry has no power to create alarm in the body, and we can break the alarm-anxiety cycle and let go of our own tail to see clearly into the real world and stop looking into our own butt all the time!

Of course, if it were as simple as being completely conscious of our worrisome thoughts and divorcing them from belief, we could erase anxiety in a matter of a few seconds. Some relatively superficial worries are easily recognized for what they are in the light of conscious awareness, while other, deeper, more emotionally charged ones (typically from childhood) are so familiar they hide in plain sight, masquerading as part of our neural furniture.

The deeper worries that are linked to self-worth (or lack thereof) or guilt or shame are often the most damaging, creating alarm in our bodies before we even know they are there. These are our ninja worries, dressed in the black of the unconscious mind, sliding past the gate of our awareness to do their dirty work.

The overprotective ego believes these ninja worries will keep you safe by preparing you from a painful future. However, that future is not real by virtue of the fact it has not happened. Therefore, worry by its very nature is imaginary, since all worries are about the future that is yet to unfold—and the only place worries have any power is in our automatic belief of them. Once we bring worries into conscious awareness, often simply by labeling them by saying, "This is an intrusive worry," they lose much of their clandestine power to control us. (More on this coming up.)

To paraphrase the Dalai Lama, "If there is nothing you can do about your worry, you need not worry—and if there is something you can do about your worry, you need not worry either."

18

You Are Here (Not There)

When you are in a state of chronic worry, you may think you are worried about something specific that is about to happen, like an examination, a public speech, or a medical test. Even though your mind may be in the future, your body is existing in an alarm state recreated from your past that is being remembered and reenergized through your anxious thoughts.

You might say, "I thought you said worries are always about the future. Now it seems you are saying that your worries also come from the past?" You might also say, "Which is it, Dr. Kennedy, if that is your *real* name?" Well, you don't have to get so angry about it, but I'm glad to see you sticking up for yourself instead of being a victim!

All worries are about the future, but in a way, worries are a way of preparing and protecting you from something that has happened in the past. Worries are a type of "memory for the future." Let's revisit the dog bite scenario. If you were bitten by a dog when you were a child and you see a dog that resembles the one that bit you, you may have the worrisome thought: "I hope that dog doesn't bite me." But you don't worry about the past dog bite. You can't. It's over. You can't worry about something that has already happened. You can be sad or frustrated or angry, but worry is always anticipatory (just as you are likely anticipating more of my dog bite references).

Worry, the way I define it (and it's my book!), is always about the future, and that gives us a conscious and effective way to separate from it. Although the feeling of alarm may be present in the moment, the worry itself is always about what *might* happen in the future. When I say all worries are about the future, I find it is a useful construct to help us disarm the charge of our imagination by bringing ourselves into the real and present moment where the future-based worry is not, well, present. If you are worried about something, by definition it is not happening now.

When we bring our worries into conscious awareness, we also slow them down and bring them squarely into the present moment, and as those worries need to transport you to the future to have any impact, being in the present suspends their power.

Perhaps a better way of saying this is all worry is dependent on your belief in how well you can transport yourself into the future.

We do this mental time travel all the time with worry. We split ourselves from the inside, with our body automatically jumping into the memory of past events and our mind leapfrogging into the future prognostications based on those memories. In this split, we are trapped in our head and locked out of the grounded, present-moment sensation in our body that could help us feel better. This internal split also activates alarm!

When you catch yourself worrying, it's a great time to ask yourself, "Where am I right now?" Worrying about something is mentally firing yourself into the future and then recreating the pain of the past when you get there, and then making it even worse by firmly believing the story you are telling yourself. Bringing yourself into the present moment neutralizes the worry, pulling you out of the ego's time machine, helping you realize you are safe in your body in the present—even if the safety is just for this very moment.

Consciously bringing yourself to the present moment and affirming that you are safe, and actually feeling safe, is a revelation for many (I know it was for me). We worriers are so accustomed to living with an omnipresent sense of danger we don't even think to break that pattern with even a momentary affirmation of safety. So choose the present moment over your future worry and say to yourself, "I am safe in this moment." *Peace is a consciously available choice to you in every moment.* I'll talk more about exactly how to find this peace in part 3, but note that you can always consciously choose to find the safety of the present moment as a respite from your imagined worries of the future. (A quick reminder to review "I Am Safe in This Moment" in the Anxiety Toolkit.)

If you had asked me ten years ago, "When did you last feel safe?" I would have told you that I had never felt safe. The overprotective ego suspended me in a vigilant state of alarm since I was a child, so how could I ever feel safe? For many others who have never felt safe, just to open up to the possibility that in this present moment, right now, you are completely safe, can be a revelation. For many of my patients (and me too!), asking themselves "Am I safe in this moment?" and realizing the answer is "yes" is the first time in their lives that they've actually acknowledged they were safe.

> How about you? Can you see and feel that you are safe in this moment? Even if you are facing impending doom five minutes from now, you are still completely safe in this moment. Many of us worriers never allowed ourselves to feel safe as children, even for a second. We just assumed the next trauma was coming and didn't stop to see that for much of the time we were actually safe.

Perhaps you never knew when your father would get drunk, or your mother would be abusive, or a family member would become sick or incapacitated, or if your caregivers would even be home to look after your needs. When you have to stay in a constant state of vigilance, the human mind and body adopt a strategy that it is best to stay ready for trouble, never letting your system rest. In my early teens, I would let down my guard with my father and believe he was going to return to normal and then get blindsided when he would inevitably become psychotic again. Over time, I adopted the coping strategy of hypervigilance and self-protection—an attitude that by its very nature suspends ever-present danger as its default position.

As children with little understanding of, or power over, our stressors, it made sense to stay vigilant and assume trouble was just around the corner. But now as an adult, when you make the unconscious conscious and affirm to yourself in conscious awareness that you are safe, even if it is only for the next five seconds, you are interrupting that unconscious vigilance. You are breaking the childhood delusion that danger is omnipresent, and once the hypervigilance to danger is broken, it can be broken again.

For many of my anxious patients, asking themselves "Am I safe in this moment?" and drawing conscious awareness that they were indeed safe were difficult because a deep part of their unconscious still believed their childhood danger could arise at any moment. This is how alarm steals our lives from us.

In other words, many of us choose the familiarity of worry over the unfamiliarity of safety. Worry also carries the illusion of making the uncertain appear more certain. Given the choice of worrying or leaving something uncertain, we anxious types will pick the worry because we hate uncertainty more than we hate worrying!

> **Point to consider:** Can you begin to see and embrace uncertainty in your everyday life? Start with the small things! Sometimes I relish the uncertainty in just looking at the choices on a restaurant menu!

19

Worry Makes the Uncertain Appear More Certain

When I was a teenager, my mother (in addition to taking care of two sons and a severely mentally ill husband) worked a lot of evening shifts as a full-time registered nurse. We lived fairly close to the hospital, and she would almost always be home ten minutes after her shift ended at eleven o'clock.

By five past the hour, I was excited to see her and would wait for her anxiously. On the rare occasions that it would be 11:10 and she wasn't home, I would start to get agitated. This was in the days before a quick call or text via cell phone could have reassured me. I simply had to wait . . . and then I would return to my coping strategy: worry.

I'd start out telling myself that one of her patients was very sick or she had to do overtime. But with each minute that passed, the scenario became direr. Perhaps she had fallen? Maybe she was in a car accident? It's dark outside—what if she was attacked or got hit by a bus? As my body would react to the worrisome, painful projection as though the scenario were indeed real, I would be activating a state of alarm in my body.

Then I'd hear her key in the lock. She was home! My body and mind would get a tremendous rush of relief.

Worry releases dopamine, a neurotransmitter that is part of our brain's reward system and is part of what makes drugs like cocaine pleasurable—and addictive. The worry itself becomes an addiction—and to further reinforce this habit, when I would worry about my mother's safety, other highly pleasurable substances of relief would rush in when my worry turned out to be false. So this habit was doubly addictive.

Especially if your youth had more than its share of pain, can you see how you might have adopted worry as, paradoxically, a source of comfort when surrounded by a sea of uncertainty and pain? When the thing you worry about does not come to pass (as is usually the case), the rush of feel-good chemicals can be a welcome change from a chronically hyper-vigilant, protective state. I know this sounds counterintuitive, but much of understanding anxiety and alarm is counterintuitive. As you'll see as you go through this book, much of healing from anxiety and alarm is also counterintuitive.

Here's an even more counterintuitive consideration. What if, on some unconscious level, you believe the worrisome thing did not happen *because* you worried? Consciously, we know worry has no beneficial effect, but unconsciously there is an unwritten belief that worry not only can make you feel good but that it has the power of magically changing events in your favor! Can you see how anxious thoughts and worries insidiously become a part of your coping strategy as a child who believed in magical thinking?

Again, consciously we know that worrying about the results of a biopsy makes no difference to the pathologist's report. But if the biopsy comes back benign, we expert worriers use that positive result and the ensuing joy of relief as unconscious "evidence" that our worry 1) did something, and 2) magically changed the results in our favor. Again, this is not rational, but your unconscious mind is not rational. Again, many of us started to worry as children, and the magical thinking of a child is not too far away from assuming worry had a protective effect.

For many of us, worry was seen as a childhood friend and one we are resistant to let go of, even decades later.

In addition to being a familiar friend, worry is a childlike attempt to control the uncontrollable. Although we are not consciously aware of it, we worriers trick ourselves into believing in our self-created, worrisome stories because they provide a sense of control, a magical way of predicting the future. When we buy into our own illusions of the future, it creates a sense that we can prepare for what is going to happen.

For example, I would often focus on my father and see if I could predict if he was going to need hospitalization. When he would become what I perceived as overly happy or overly sad, I would begin to prepare myself and worry that he was indeed heading for mania or depression. I would focus on the possibility of him being admitted to the hospital and worry about it so much that it seemed like a certainty.

As painful as that was, it seemed less painful than being in limbo as to whether he was truly heading for hospital admission or not. The odd thing was that most times I worried and convinced myself he was heading for a tour of duty on the psych ward, he would improve. It was only on rare occasions that my worrying turned out to be an accurate prediction of psychosis. Even though I was wrong most of the time, I couldn't seem to stop doing it. Crazy, huh?

All human beings have a drive for certainty, but for worriers, that drive becomes an obsession. If you had trauma in your childhood, your drive for certainty becomes exaggerated, and creating a worrisome story is a way of creating a semblance of order where there is none. OCD is, at its root, a drive to make things certain. Typically, the obsessions become more elaborate over time in a fruitless attempt to create certainty where none exists. For the OCD sufferer, the obsessions provide a little patch of certainty in a frighteningly uncertain world. But the obsessions become the problem as the person becomes overtaken by them, just as we worriers are overtaken by our worries. Just as the OCD sufferer becomes afraid not to count stairs or tap the doorknob six times, we worriers become afraid not to worry.

That worry is a source of both pleasure and pain is one of the paradoxes of anxiety. Given the massive amount of pain uncertainty caused me, I can completely understand why I created a worrisome story to make a scenario appear less vague and uncertain. But, paradoxically, my worry compounded the problem my child mind perceived those worries would solve. In other words, to my inner child, uncertainty needed to be avoided at all costs, so it was a worthy bargain to bear the cost of accepting the painful worry as true. In an effort to avoid the familiar, intolerable alarm of uncertainty and not knowing what was going to happen, I created a story of worry that gave me the illusion of *knowing* what was going to happen. By creating a worrisome story, I was fooling myself into creating a fable of what was going to occur because simply leaving the situation to uncertainty was an excruciating reminder of a childhood time when I truly did not know. Imagining and accepting the worst was actually preferable to not knowing, and that is one of the most devastating aspects of the anxious mind.

When you experience trauma in childhood that is not resolved, you lose faith in the world—yet faith is exactly what you need to endure, and even embrace, uncertainty. I'll show you in part 3 how to use faith (not necessarily religious faith) to embrace uncertainty so it no longer seduces you into worry.

It wasn't until I saw worry for what it really was—a magical attempt to make the uncertain more certain—that I ultimately learned how to manage it. Having faith amid uncertainty, and even embracing uncertainty as the spice of life, is worry's undoing.

Being aware of your power and your access to choice, along with calming the alarm in your body, will help you relish and embrace uncertainty, for it is the uncertainty of life that provides the true fun and joy. Developing a sense of awareness is a critical step to learn, and eventually, the space taken up by the negative habit of worry will be filled with this new positive skill of being present in the moment, no matter how uncertain.

Old habits die hard. I still get caught up in worrying sometimes. But with the keen sense of awareness I possess now, I know that I can engage faith to give me the choice to worry or not (more of faith being a neurological antidote to worry in part 3).

20

Wired to Worry

If I could find the guy that invented worry, I would punch him right in the balls. Pointless worry has cost me so much and limited my enjoyment of life more than I can express. I imagine you might feel the same way.

So then why in the world do we do it?

Remember interoception? The neurological process by which the mind is constantly reading the body? The mind is a meaning-making, make-sense machine and will create stories and worries that are completely consistent with how the body feels.

The more worries the mind creates, the more alarmed the body becomes, and over time, the worries of the mind become chronic in response to the chronic alarm in the body. (This is the alarm-anxiety cycle and it holds a tremendous amount of inertia.)

In physics, the concept of inertia states that an object at rest tends to stay at rest and an object in motion tends to stay in motion. This is equally true with anxiety: the more you worry, the more likely you are to keep worrying.

Remember when I said we worriers do not take well to uncertainty?

When we resist and avoid uncertainty by taking a detour into worry, we create a belief that resistance avoids pain, and then resistance becomes a pattern of behavior that holds tremendous inertia. Worry can be described as a resistance to uncertainty. That resistance keeps us frozen in a form of ego-based protection and blocks us from moving away from the compulsion to worry. In other words, using worry as a form of imaginary protection keeps us locked in worry.

When we have bonded or imprinted to resistance and worry as a form of safety, and practiced worry so much that it's gained inertia, we have tremendous resistance to letting it go. Much like the monkey that refuses to let go of the banana and escape, we worriers are resistant to letting go of our worries and escaping our minds. Instead, we become WIRED: worry, inertia, resistance, ego, defense.

Critical point: What exactly is the ego protecting you against by keeping you in your head with worry? The *feeling* down in your body.

In essence, as the child in us becomes afraid to feel alarm in the body, the worry in our heads becomes a convenient substitute. Worrisome thinking is a distraction from painful feeling.

Remember the concept of background alarm, that excess, chaotic energy that spilled over into our bodies when our young minds were overwhelmed? This state of uneasiness, this uncomfortable energy, sits vigilantly in the background, waiting for any reason to rise up. If you've been sitting in a movie theater or at a family dinner or driving to work and you've felt a sense of impending doom when there's no actual danger in sight, you are likely sensing your background alarm.

For our younger selves, the feeling of background alarm in our bodies was too much to bear. We developed resistance to feeling in our bodies because in connecting to our bodies we would need to face the old trauma and alarm energy stored there. So we move out of the feeling body and up into the worried mind as an escape.

As the lesser of two evils, the ego decides that the body is not safe to inhabit and retreats or detours into the mind to avoid pain. The ego-created worries keep us in our minds as a way of keeping us out of the background alarm stored in our bodies. Just as the person with obsessive-compulsive disorder (OCD) counts stairs or turns three times before going through a doorway as a form of distraction from their inner pain of alarm, we worriers obsess with worrisome thoughts as a form of distraction from the old alarm stored in our body. The trap here is that our worried minds appear to be the only "safe" place, and we globally move away from feeling and become locked into thinking.

The more dramatic the thoughts, the more effective the distraction from feeling. This explains why worries tend to get more and more intense over time. Compounding matters, I have often noticed that worriers seem to be quite intelligent and artistic with hyperactive imaginations, so we can conjure up very elaborate and complex worries! Basic worries like the fear of flying are for amateurs; we elite-class worriers can make up a nine-headed, flying, fire-breathing hydra that has cobra venom for blood and sweats syphilis and still have some imagination left over for something really scary. I'm not saying the fear of flying can't be debilitating; I am saying that the worries we can come up with are often much more elaborate and complex. The reason why our worries are so scary to us is that they have to be. If they weren't so scary, we might venture back down into our bodies and revisit the background alarm of our past. As scary as the worries are, that childhood pain stored in our body looms as infinitely more frightening.

So, our worries do serve a purpose in distracting us from the background alarm in our bodies, but they have a devastating side effect. As the worries become more intense and pressing, they begin to increase the alarm in our bodies. Because the body has difficulty distinguishing a thought from reality, the thought in question ("Am I having a heart attack?") is read by the body as a declarative statement of truth ("I am having a heart attack!"). It's like the game show *Jeopardy!* Even if you phrase the thought in the form of a question, your body reacts with an activation of your fight-or-flight response, or your sympathetic nervous system—just as a normal body would when faced with a threat it accepts as real.

Here's where everything begins to worsen. Our coping strategy of worrying to distract us from the alarm in our bodies intensifies the very alarm we are trying to escape.

Point to consider: Can you stay with the discomfort of the alarm in your body and observe how your mind relentlessly tries to redirect your energy into worrying? (Sensation without explanation, remember?)

21

Stronger than You Think

It's worth repeating here: chronic worry and anxiety are a dangerous combination of overestimating threats and underestimating our courage to deal with them—and this programming usually starts in childhood.

One thing about childhood trauma is that it forces you to be tough before you are ready. Ironically, the trauma makes you tougher than you believe yourself to be, not in spite of the trauma you endured but because of it. You are both strengthened and weakened by your traumas.

Anxiety, in its relentless pursuit to shield and protect you, makes you shy away from challenges and tries to convince you to quit, or worse, not even start. It harkens back to the time in your childhood when you were unprepared and weren't able to handle the pressure, and assumes you are in the same place now. Anxiety tells you, "You shouldn't try. It'll be easier if you just avoid this." But as I have seen with many of my patients, once you start to narrow your experience of life in an attempt to avoid pain, it becomes a slippery slope and your life quickly becomes less about experiencing new fun and more about avoiding old pain.

So often I have given in to it, but just as often I have risen to the challenge—and if you are reading this book, I am sure your courage has risen up as well. You might look at what I've become—doctor, speaker, author, stand-up comic—and think, "How can he have a serious anxiety problem if he's done all that?"

It's because I am much stronger than my anxiety would have me think. And so are you.

Again, look back on the times when things really did go bad. Did you handle it? Are you still here?

I thought so.

One of the most devastating effects of anxiety is the double whammy of making you overestimate external threats and underestimate your internal resources to deal with them. I'll talk more about this in part 3, but anxiety and alarm paralyze your rational brain and activate your emotional brain, and if that sounds like a bad deal, that's because it is!

Here is one of the secrets anxiety doesn't want you to know: on the rare occasion that it does go bad, you will handle it. There is this illusion that you're going to collapse if your worries come true. You won't. In many ways, living and coping with anxiety has made you much more resilient than you give yourself credit for. I can't emphasize this enough. In decades of working with anxiety patients, I have seen them rise to the occasion of adversity and surprise themselves with faith and courage they never believed they had. You are infinitely stronger than you believe you are. Please read this paragraph over and over until you really absorb its message. I guarantee you that it is true.

Not only are you much more capable than anxiety would have you believe, but you'll have help. The child in us may have felt that there was no hope and no help was coming. But that is also a misperception. Think of your biggest past challenges. Now, notice 1) how you clearly made it through, and (2) where the universe helped you. There is no reason to believe that is not going to be the case in the future. Don't abandon your faith in yourself and reject the uncertainty of life for the illusory certainty of worry. It's a bad deal every time. But you can't change it until you turn up your awareness and understand that you have a choice. In part 3, I'll show you specifically how to choose a number of options over fear.

The big lie of anxiety and alarm is "You can't do it." Even after you've done it many times before, it still tells you this is going to be the time you fail. For my first five years of doing stand-up, every set I did I was convinced would be a catastrophe. No matter how many times I did well, my child self was convinced that the next set would be a disaster. Your child self is also likely to believe your catastrophic predictions because they are based on your real experiences. But you're not a powerless child anymore, and once you see yourself as a powerful adult, you can break anxiety's hold on your thoughts. You can retreat into being the servant to your worries, or you can expand into being the master of your mind. In the former, you have constricted and regressed into your fearful child self from your past and see the world that way. In the latter, you expand into your wise and resilient adult self in the present and see the world that way. Awareness gives you the choice to acknowledge the child you were then but live as the adult you are now.

"If you are not living this moment, you are not really living."

—ECKHART TOLLE

Our anxious thoughts make us think we are much smaller than we truly are, and the alarm in our bodies makes our challenges feel much bigger than they truly are because we are perceiving through the eyes of our anxious and alarmed child self from the distant past. As an adult, committed to being grounded in the present, you become a powerful force and are much more capable and resilient than anxiety would have you think. And your challenges are there to expose your beliefs. Your child self, who lives in the past, believes he or she can't handle it, but I can assure you from personal experience, your adult self who chooses to live in the faith of the present moment can handle anything.

It really comes down to committing to awareness of the present moment and seeing that at any moment you have a conscious choice to be your present-moment adult self. Alternatively, if you do not see the choice of engaging your empowered adult self, by default you will regress into the victimhood of your child self, and adopt the child's old coping strategy of worry. If we can stay in the present moment and choose faith and courage, we become the master. If we are swept away by our old alarm, we become the servant and fail to even see the choice of staying present. We default back to the anxiety and alarm that characterized our childhood, and we may even regress into a form of our child self. If you unwittingly and automatically fall into the victim mindset of the child you once were, how are you supposed to manage the life of the adult you are now?

Even when we've been practicing awareness for a while, challenges have a way of knocking us back into our old destructive habit of believing every worry we think. Before we are aware of it, our bodies get alarmed, and we are back in that deep, dark hole of our childhood wounding. The only way out is taking a few breaths using the physiological sigh, and seeing that we have the power to choose to stay present and rooted in our adult selves or fall into the hole of our old childhood wounds. This is a learning process, and I have fallen back into my childhood wounding thousands of times. But when you see the choice is always there and you practice staying present in your adult self, the path of the adult becomes easier to see and easier to take. As we practice grounding into our adult selves, we are progressively more able to pick up our scared inner child and move to courage and faith together.

When you say, "I can't go out today because of *XYZ*," that is a belief that is not necessarily true. It is the belief of your child self, and that belief needs anonymity to survive and exert its influence. Bringing your beliefs into the present-moment light of awareness takes away much of their power. Then your present-moment adult self can take over and reassure that worried and alarmed child in a way they never received back when they needed it most.

There is no worry-based belief you can have that is true. How do I know? Because worry is always about the future, and since the future is unknown, anything that claims to know the unknown cannot be true. But our fears sure look like they are going to come true to the child that still lives in us, because it was their truth back then. Worries are predictions we accept as fact in order to avoid the pain of uncertainty, and then we suffer, believing to be real what are only the brain droppings of an anxious mind. Once you see that worries are mere illusions, you break the cycle of worries aggravating alarm in the body and alarm aggravating the worries of the mind. The cycle needs your unconscious belief to operate. Once you make the unconscious conscious, you learn to objectively *see* your worries so you no longer have to subjectively *be* your worries.

22

The Feeling-Thought Cycle

I clearly remember getting home from India at the end of September 2013 and feeling paralyzed in my bed under the crushing weight of anxiety and alarm. The trip to India was to be my salvation, giving me the spiritual answer to my anxiety, but it just wound up giving me more questions.

I was biting my own tail and then biting it even harder to try to get the pain to stop. I was caught in a vicious cycle to the point I considered suicide because not only did I not see a way out, but the anxiety and alarm were continuing to worsen. I felt like I was losing my mind (and my body) along with my hold on reality—there was no safe place. Suicide is not so much about wanting to die as it is seeing no other option to end the pain.

I used to do a joke about this. In a down-south, evangelical Georgia accent, I would say, "Gawd, I say, Gawd will never give you . . . more . . . than you . . . can handle!" I would pause and then say, "Does God meet suicide victims at the pearly gates and say, 'Ah . . . sorry . . . um, dude, my bad, I really thought you could handle it.'"

When I look back now, part of me was glad it got this bad, as I don't think I would have taken my transformative trip on LSD had I not had my back squarely up against the wall. Even though I was on my knees, I was strong enough to go deeper, and that is my point when I say we worriers are much stronger than we think when *we are actually faced with what we worry about.* As much as I was absolutely terrified of LSD and was already in a desperate state, I knew I had to do it, so I did. As I alluded to earlier, on October 5, 2013 (my father's birthday), under the supervision of my guide, I took my first hit of acid. I did not know what to make of the massive change in perception I experienced under the influence of the psychedelic right away, but what LSD did do for me was allow me to see my anxiety as a feeling state of alarm in my body as opposed to a thinking state in my mind. This revelation was fundamental to my healing, and for the healing of countless other chronic worriers. Over time, observing the alarm in my body as different (and separable) from the anxious thoughts of the mind allowed me to see I was trapped in a feedback loop of thought (worry) and feeling (alarm) that I eventually labeled the alarm-anxiety cycle.

Although I didn't immediately know how to feel and think better, after the LSD trip I was no longer dealing with a ghost. I now had the earliest inklings that anxiety had two distinct elements (thought and feeling) that the doctor in me was trained to believe were one and the same. Not only were these elements different, but they were separable from each other. For the first time, I had the very real sense that I was dealing with a process that could be eased by identifying and then separating the component parts.

> **Point to consider:** The worries of your mind and the alarm in your body can be two distinct entities.

23

Awareness Gives Choice

Simply put, the feeling-thought cycle states that how you feel dictates how you think. It is also true that how you think is how you are going to feel, but an integral part of my healing was realizing that feeling influences thinking much more than thinking influences feeling.

When we are in a state of alarm, negative thoughts and worries that are consistent with the negative feeling of alarm are accentuated, encouraged, and magnified, while positive thoughts that are inconsistent with our feeling state of alarm are discounted, discouraged, and diminished. This selection bias for the negative is how a state of alarm in the body can overwhelm us by only paying attention to negative thoughts, and why it is so hard to think positively in our minds when our bodies are steeped in a state of background alarm.

Personally, I find it extremely difficult to try to think in opposition to how I feel. Another way of saying this is feelings are more powerful than thoughts. Furthermore, with both myself and my patients, I've seen it is much more effective to change your thinking state by changing your feeling state than the opposite. Thoughts and thinking states can be reversed in a matter of seconds by simply consciously focusing on the exact opposite of the thought. Whatever you are thinking right now, I can guarantee you the exact opposite of that thought has some truth to it. In this way, thoughts are more changeable than feelings and have less momentum. You can change your thoughts, but unless your state of feeling changes to support them, those thoughts don't tend to "stick," and they will default back to closely mirroring your feeling state. Feelings are denser and carry more energy to create long-lasting change and, thus, are a more effective focus for our interventions. With respect to healing anxiety, it is much more effective to focus on changing the feeling state of the body than trying to redirect the thoughts of the mind.

This example may sound trivial, but it makes a point. Let's say you believe that Toronto is the capital city of Canada. You call me and it comes up in conversation, and I correct you by saying it is actually Ottawa that is the capital of Canada. From that point on, you have switched the erroneous thought of Toronto for Ottawa.

Simple.

Now say you are feeling down because your pet has passed away. Does telling yourself "Don't be sad" significantly change your emotion? No, because emotions have more power and momentum than thoughts do.

So contrary to what most "positive psychology" advocates will tell you, simply having people change their thoughts is not likely to carry much power to change their feelings. I'm not saying it is not helpful to change thoughts of the mind, but changing feelings in the body is a much more effective way of making long-term change. Typically, it is hard work to stay aware enough to consistently try to think new, happy thoughts in your mind that are in contradiction to the old alarm feeling in your body. Not saying it can't be done, but I have found adopting the approach recommended by positive psychology requires tremendous commitment and perseverance, and I simply can't keep it up. People who are chronic worriers have a significant amount of alarm stored in their bodies, and relentlessly trying to think positively while feeling a panic state in the body is as impossible as it is exhausting. Personally, I have found it much more beneficial to devote the energy I was supposed to use to change the thinking in my mind, to change the feeling state in my body instead—but more on that soon.

To illustrate how feeling is more powerful than thinking, I remember being in Las Vegas with my daughter, Leandra, when she was about ten. (I'm not an irresponsible father. In 1996, Vegas was really focusing on family fun, with waterparks and kids' shows.) Leandra has never been comfortable in hot weather. She likes warm weather, but she hates it when it gets hot. We were on an open-air shuttle bus going down the Las Vegas Strip in August. Did I mention it was noon, in August, in the Nevada desert?

Lea was not happy.

She was sitting on a bench on the little shuttle bus and I was standing above her holding the grabrail. I can still remember the tilt of her head, looking up at me with those big brown eyes, with the *What the he** did you get us into here?* look on her face. If you don't think an otherwise genteel ten-year-old girl can gun you off with a look, you are dead wrong. As we were going to be on this shuttle for another twenty minutes, I told her to imagine she was in an ice-cold swimming pool. That bought me a little time, but in another three minutes she "convinced" me to get off the bus, and we found an air-conditioned cab to take us the rest of the way.

Leandra has always been a happy-go-lucky kid, so to see her mad like that was atypical for sure. As soon as we got into the cool cab, Leandra's sunny disposition returned. That is to say, once she felt better, she thought better.

As you'll see as you move through this book, you'll get the most bang for your emotional buck by directing your energies into improving how you feel rather than improving how you think (although I'll absolutely show you how to do both).

It is an uphill battle on the scale of Mount Everest to think in a way that opposes the way you feel. This is not to say that consciously changing your thought processes is not helpful, but trying to think in constant opposition to how you feel is demoralizing and self-defeating. Unless you are hypervigilant about thinking more positively, simply changing your thinking will give you only short-term relief. And neuroscience tells us that your rational brain shuts down as your emotional/survival brain revs up, so when you feel like you're in survival mode you can't think effectively anyway!

Feeling states like alarm, anger, and frustration have much more inertia in the body and take more time to turn around than thoughts of the mind. I often think of thoughts as a speedboat and feelings as a freighter.

Once a feeling takes hold, especially the feeling of alarm, it's like trying to get a thousand-ton ship to turn on a dime.

Here's another way to look at it: the heart exerts an electrical field five thousand times stronger than that of the brain. Given that biological reality, it feels rather futile to try to use thoughts to strong-arm our feelings into submission, doesn't it?

Now, here is where it gets more complicated: thinking positively does tend to have a positive effect on how you feel, but typically the effect is not that powerful. However, thinking negatively has a much more robust effect on how you feel, probably due to energizing the inherent fear/survival bias of the brain. In other words, a positive thought tends to make you feel only a little better, but a negative or scary thought can make you feel much worse!

I am not saying thinking is unimportant and cognitive strategies for anxiety relief are not helpful. It is very important to see your negative thoughts and worries. But once you see them, it is a much more effective course of action to direct your energy into changing the way you feel than trying to address the way you think. Changing your thoughts may only give you a few seconds of relief, but changing the way you feel lasts considerably longer and addresses the issue at its root cause. When you are trapped in worry, it is a much better use of your time to abandon thinking altogether and focus on changing your feeling state. The best way to change Leandra's discomfort was to change her feeling state by getting her out of the hellfire shuttle and into an air-conditioned taxi. Although having her think and imagine she was in a cool swimming pool helped a little, changing how she felt helped a lot!

Typically, how you feel and how you think are remarkably consistent with each other. If you feel alarmed in your body, it's likely that will be reflected by anxious thoughts in your mind. In fact, without awareness, chronic worriers very quickly default to the state of alarm in the body and anxiety in the mind that you'll now recognize as the alarm-anxiety cycle. This is the unconscious feedback loop I followed automatically for decades before I saw another way of feeling and thinking.

Even in non-worriers, the feeling-thought cycle operates unconsciously and automatically; feelings feeding thoughts and thoughts feeding feelings in a self-reinforcing loop. To break the cycle, we first need to be aware that it is operating. When we know we are feeling alarm, we can anticipate our mind handing us alarming thoughts. Our best defense is awareness of the cycle's existence and the knowledge that we can break it by separating the two components.

I don't mean to give the impression that thoughts don't have power. Both thoughts and feelings are powerful in their own right. Some thoughts are more disturbing and "heavier" than others, but that also depends on how much belief and subsequent feeling they are granted. At the end of the (anxious) day, however, changing the feeling state is what will give us the deepest and longest-lasting form of relief from chronic worry.

When you become aware of the thoughts as simply thoughts (or brain droppings!) and separate them from their energy source of feeling, you have taken a crucial step toward healing. What you are aiming for, by practicing awareness, is to see and isolate the thoughts before you believe them.

Again, my goal is to show you how to see your thoughts so you don't have to be your thoughts. Seeing your thoughts (especially your worrisome thoughts) as groundless, transient, and inconsequential helps you avoid turning a painless thought in the mind into a painful feeling in the body.

Just to emphasize (and to save me putting a diagram in here), imagine the thoughts of your mind traveling down to your heart area and influencing your feeling state. Then imagine your feeling state around your heart traveling up to your mind and influencing your thoughts. There is no beginning and no end to this cycle or feedback loop—thought can create feeling and feeling can create thought. This is the feeling-thought cycle and it operates in all humans. The alarm-anxiety cycle works in the exact same way in us worriers, with anxious thoughts of the mind generating alarm feelings in the body and alarm feelings in the body generating anxious thoughts of the mind.

As both cycles operate unconsciously, conscious awareness is the key to seeing them so we don't have to be them. We don't have to charge either cycle by believing in every thought we have and staying unaware of every feeling that we feel.

Even in our minds, worries have no power to hurt us until we bestow them with the power of belief. Once we see it's up to us whether we believe our worries or not, we can make real progress in breaking the cycle. But as you'll see, your energy is better spent connecting to and changing your feeling state versus simply trying to change your thinking.

Perhaps the most powerful aspect of awareness is that, in slowing down and becoming aware of the anxious thoughts of the mind, you create the space that wasn't there when you automatically believed everything you thought. It is in that space that you create choice—and choice is power.

As Dr. Viktor Frankl said: "Between stimulus and response there is a space. In that space is our power to choose our response. In our response lies our growth and our freedom." This is the space I'm talking about, and it holds the key to your liberation from chronic anxiety.

That space is the gift in the practice of awareness. With conscious awareness, you see options that were not available to you previously, and in those options rests the power of choice—including your power to choose not to be a victim of your old wounding.

Dr. Frankl also said, "Everything can be taken from a man but one thing: the last of human freedoms—to choose one's attitude in any given set of circumstances, to choose one's own way." When I learned I had a choice—that I had the power to see my thoughts without believing them, that I could take the energy I had previously funneled into rumination and worrying and divert it into staying with my feelings—from that point on, I was choosing my own way, and that way was to value feeling, however painful, over thinking. My choice became to see the thoughts with a curious detachment, suspending them while I focused inwardly on sensation (without explanation). Starving anxious thoughts of the energy of credibility allowed me to break their spell by not bestowing them with the power of belief. Not believing my worries took practice, but it was fueled by a sense of agency over this condition called anxiety that had ruled my life for decades. Since I could see my anxious thoughts and chose to focus on something else, starving them of belief, I was free from being my anxious thoughts.

24

Family and Liar

The vast majority of patients I see who suffer from excessive worry felt distinctly unempowered and victimized as children—and in a nasty glitch in our wiring, whatever was familiar to us as children is what we tend to replicate in adulthood. This is Freud's theory of repetition compulsion. It is built into the human brain to equate familiarity with security. This means that whatever was familiar for you as a child, there will be an unconscious push or compulsion to repeat as an adult—even if you are repeating something that caused you considerable pain.

One of my own quotes that I am proud of is: "If you grew up in a dysfunctional family, the word 'familiar' can be broken into two words—'family' and 'liar'—because your family essentially lies to you about what is safe." As a result, we will often reproduce the negative events from our childhood in adulthood in an attempt to recapture a sense of security that was never really there in the first place!

If you felt victimized as a child, a part of you will often unconsciously and automatically gravitate toward that victim state as an adult. In other words, we will unconsciously and compulsively select for experiences and thoughts in our adulthood that replicate that familiar victim mentality of our childhood. Add to that a felt sense of fear in our bodies, and you have the perfect environment for the alarm-anxiety cycle to form and thrive. If we do not apply conscious awareness to the alarm-anxiety cycle, it will take us over—and that is exactly what happened to me.

But it's not just me. Let's look at a patient of mine, Jane, who would tend to pick men who were abusive alcoholics. Whenever she met a man who fit that profile, she was drawn to him like a moth to a flame. Jane was on autopilot, seduced by her unconscious drive to replicate her past, exchanging her abusive alcoholic father in childhood for her abusive alcoholic boyfriend as an adult—endlessly trying to recapture a "security" with her father that was never there in the first place. I always felt Jane was hoping the new boyfriend would take care of her in a way her father never did. (As an aside, I believe the child in us is always waiting for the parent to "come back" and be the parent they were supposed to be. Consciously we know it's never going to happen, but unconsciously the hope remains alive in us.)

Of course, it always ended badly for Jane. Yet for many years she persisted in attracting alcoholic after alcoholic, with no awareness of why she repeatedly put herself in harm's way. Since you can't change what you can't (or refuse to) see, Jane's unconscious and destructive pattern of victimizing herself continued for as long as I knew her, although in the latter stages of our doctor-patient relationship she did start seeing her self-destructive repetition compulsion with more awareness.

Many of us worriers became familiar (aka secure) with worry when we were young. Just like Jane embraced alcoholics and replicated that pattern, we worriers embrace worry (even though it is toxic) in part because it is familiar to us. Perhaps, like me, you had a parent or caregiver who was a chronic worrier and modeled that behavior for you. When we worry, along with making the uncertain seem perversely more certain, we also get a perverse sense of comfort from the sense of familiarity it provides. In my case, I saw my mother worry a great deal, and it became a familiar ally of mine. In times of stress, I will still feel the compulsion to replicate that old pattern of hypervigilance and worry, in search of a familiar sense of security that was never actually there.

It's time to take your power back. There's an old saying that goes: "If you do things the way you've always done them, you'll get what you've always gotten." If you aren't aware of your actions and don't see that you have the power to consciously and objectively observe your impulses and desires in awareness, you'll never be able to change them. Without awareness, we just repeat the same old familiar patterns of our formative years, and if those patterns involve you being a helpless and unwitting victim, your anxiety and alarm can never resolve.

Point to consider: Did you have a parent who modeled worry? Or could you just *feel* their anxiety?

25

Is It a Belief Problem or a Problem of Belief?

Here's one for all you hypochondriacs out there. During medical school, I would create an anxious thought about having a fatal disease and then try to argue with it, attempting to reassure myself that I didn't have the fatal disease. But here's the rub: the more energy and attention I gave to arguing with the thought, the more credibility I inadvertently gave it. In trying to convince myself that I didn't have to believe the thought, I was paying more attention to the possibility that I really could have the disease!

It's like telling yourself not to think of a pink elephant. Pink elephants are not real; everyone knows that. Who thought of the idea of a pink elephant anyway? Ridiculous. There is no such thing. Pink elephants do not exist. I should just stop thinking about it. Unless, I guess, you sprayed an elephant with pink paint, but why would you do that? In that respect, you could paint an elephant pink and create a pink elephant, but in that case, it's artificial, not real. Though I guess it would be real to someone who saw it and didn't know that it was painted. Or a child, a child would definitely believe it was real . . .

I think you get the picture. The more I tried to tell myself my thoughts were not to be believed, the more real and believable they became. This is exactly why I say you can't think your way out of anxiety.

During the stress of medical school, my muscles began to twitch involuntarily. The medical term is "fasciculation." They twitched all over, even the muscles of my tongue. Of course, I looked up fasciculation in a medical text and it told of a horrendous disease called amyotrophic lateral sclerosis, or ALS (also known as Lou Gehrig's disease), where your muscles literally waste away until you die.

And one of the early signs? Fasciculations. So I was off! I completely freaked out.

One of the cardinal signs of ALS is weakness or discoordination in the hands. Guess what—I became fixated on my hands. Anytime I did something clumsy I convinced myself that this was the beginning of the end.

It. Was. Awful. The more I tried to convince myself that I was okay, the more worried I got. It was the pink elephant situation all over again. I cannot tell you how terrified I was and how I pestered my wife every day asking her if she could see changes in my hands.

Luckily, I got to see one of the most caring doctors I have ever had the good fortune to meet. Dr. John Noseworthy was a staff neurologist at the University of Western Ontario Medical School and went on to be CEO of the world-renowned Mayo Clinic. Dr. Noseworthy gave me a thorough exam and reassured me that he had seen many cases of ALS, and although he could not tell me with 100 percent certainty, he was 99.9 percent sure I had a condition called benign fasciculations.

Do you think that ended it?

Although I felt immeasurably reassured, that 0.1 percent still haunted me. It's like the old joke about the man who asks a prospective mate on a date by saying, "What are the chances you'd go out with me?" The response comes: "Ha! One in a million!" And he answers, "So you're telling me there's a chance."

Despite the reassurance of a world-class neurologist and additional tests that showed no sign of degenerative disease, I held on to that fear for another year. After twelve more months of no additional symptoms other than the fasciculations (which I still have thirty-plus years later), I was finally able to acknowledge that I probably wasn't dying.

At the time, I had no awareness of what was going on. I was deep in alarm, and as I'll show you soon, an alarmed brain is one that defaults to survival mode and redirects its energy toward avoiding danger and potential threats and (perhaps most destructive) away from rational thought. As a result of being in survival mode, my threat-focused brain was unable to see and accept the overwhelming evidence that I was fine.

The critical error people with anxiety make is attributing their pain to the thoughts of the mind, since the fight-or-flight alarm reaction occurs immediately after the thought. The thing is, the alarm reaction is not a thought problem—it is a belief problem.

Don't believe me? Let's say you are a female (XX chromosome pattern) who does not want to be pregnant. Let's also say you have the thought "I might be pregnant." Your body will go into a fight-or-flight alarm reaction when you believe that thought. It is not the thought but, rather, the belief of the thought that creates the alarm and the subsequent pain and discomfort.

Still don't believe me? Okay, let's say you are male (XY chromosome pattern) and you have the thought "I might be pregnant." Your male body will not go into alarm because you simply do not believe the thought (because it is impossible). Same exact thought—"I might be pregnant"— but no belief, so no bodily reaction. It is therefore not the thought that causes your pain. Thoughts and worries are collections of words in a particular order. Thoughts themselves are painless brain droppings—until we believe them.

Incidentally, I once had a psychiatrist tell me in reference to my hypochondriac tendencies, "It seems to me you're not afraid of dying—you're afraid of living." He told me that more than thirty years ago and it still sticks with me. With hypochondria and other phobias, fear of death can be a convenient scapegoat that obscures the fact that our fear of death is actually preventing us from feeling and enjoying life. When we *fear* life, we are unable to *feel* life—and as you'll see, that is the whole point of the fear. The phobia is there to block us from feeling—and from living— because feeling life in the present opens us up to the reminder of what feeling life meant in our painful past.

Recovering from anxiety is less about feeling better and more about getting better at feeling. Healing is about being open to the nuances of life instead of railroading all intense emotions into fear and worry.

Point to consider: Your health anxiety or hypochondriasis is a way your mind devised to distract you from the alarm in your body. You don't have a health anxiety problem, you have an alarm problem.

26

The Alarm-Anxiety Cycle

In my book, anxiety, anxious thoughts, and chronic worry are synonymous. They are all activities of the mind, and none have any feeling attached to them—until we believe their content. When we believe the content of the worries, our bodies react with a form of alarm. As I will show you in part 2, much of that alarm comes from your present-moment sympathetic (fight-or-flight) nervous system—which I call foreground alarm—in contrast to an activation of the old, unresolved traumas that you still hold in your body—which I call background alarm. We'll explore these in greater depth later, but for now, just know that alarm has two components—one reactionary and new (foreground alarm), the other anticipatory and old (background alarm)—and each acts to energize the other.

It is the alarm that we experience as painful, but again, since the thoughts immediately preceded the alarm sensation, the mind incorrectly assumes the thoughts are the source of the pain. As you'll see in part 2, the background alarm stored in your body—the energy of your old, unresolved childhood wounds—can flare up at any time, even in the absence of conscious thoughts. You may see, hear, or even smell something you aren't even consciously aware of that can trigger a state of alarm.

I remember being at a big band–style concert many years ago, the type of music popular in the 1940s, and really enjoying it. Then, seemingly out of nowhere, I got really angry and stopped enjoying the concert. Not only did I stop enjoying the concert, but I wanted to leave—pronto.

It was the strangest feeling to be enjoying something and then, in a matter of seconds, almost hating it. I was stunned by this sudden turn of events and just stood there in frustration, thinking the music was too damn loud and there were too many people there and I should go. Then the trumpet player stood up to play another solo, and I had an immediate flashback to my father playing that same solo in that same song, many years ago.

My father was a trumpet player and he would practice in the house, often playing the same short phrase fifty times in a row. The trumpet is not the most soothing (or quiet!) instrument, and it has always been an irritant to me. Okay, my apologies to all you trumpet players out there, but I hate the trumpet. Not for the musical instrument it is but for what hearing the trumpet does to me. It always takes me back to my father imposing himself on the rest of the family.

The trumpet is an instrument you can't just practice unobtrusively in your own room; the sound penetrates the entire house like body odor and cigarette potpourri. Played well, it can be tolerated, but when the same phrase is played (poorly) over and over and over again, it's a form of torture. When I saw a hostage taking on TV, I often thought the FBI should bring my dad in to play outside so the perpetrators would give themselves up quickly.

Let's get back to the sound of the trumpet triggering my old background alarm at the big-band concert. Even though it had been twenty years since I heard that same phrase, it fired me right back to the same frustration I had felt with my father decades before. In other words, it triggered my old background alarm, flaring me into a full-body reaction.

After the fact, I figured out it was the sound of the trumpet that had triggered me. However, it was not the thought "Oh, this is the same phrase my father used to play" that sent me into alarm. Rather, it was the sensation in my body that alarmed me, before I cognitively recognized the particular musical phrase. I had an implicit memory (aka a body memory) of old pain, and even decades later it reignited a significant alarm reaction in me.

I've heard it said that all stress comes from our thoughts. I disagree. There are old wounds that become activated in us that have nothing to do with conscious thinking but still cause considerable alarm and pain—and they often occur well before the brain has time to process what's happening into a coherent thought. Many of my patients who had trauma before they could speak well (before the age of seven) can be triggered by a feeling or a smell or a touch that had nothing to do with thought. Cognitive, or talk, therapy has little benefit for these people as their trauma is in the unconscious "feeling" more than the more conscious "thinking." These patients respond much better to feeling therapies like somatic experiencing or therapeutic touch than they do to cognitive therapies like CBT.

People with a fear of spiders have a full-body reaction of alarm to the sight of a spider, or even anything that resembles a spider, and their body will recoil instantly—much faster than the brain can process the thought "This is a spider." Neurologically, this recoil reaction occurs almost instantly, well before the conscious thought has had a chance to form.

There are at least two parallel pathways for alarm to be activated, one conscious and one unconscious, and the latter has very little to do with thinking and everything to do with feeling. So while stress and alarm can absolutely be made worse by our thoughts and worries, thoughts are not always a prerequisite to the creation of stress. Again, all stress does not come from a thought. I did not create my reaction of getting upset by thinking to myself, "Oh, this is a trumpet solo." I *felt* it. Anyone who has had an intense panic attack seemingly out of nowhere can attest to this.

Often, though—and especially where chronic worry is involved—we do have a thought or worry that perpetuates the alarm-anxiety cycle. How we feel reflects and perpetuates what we think and vice versa. As I said earlier, the feeling-thought cycle is directly analogous to the alarm-anxiety cycle, and you will soon know both like the back of your hand. The two cycles are so similar as to be virtually interchangeable. Just like the feeling-thought cycle, the alarm-anxiety cycle also runs on a type of autopilot, automatically operating outside of our conscious awareness. To break the cycle, we must first be intimately aware of how it operates beneath our awareness, with the cycle insidiously becoming our emotional master. When we adopt an attitude of nonemotional, nonjudgmental awareness, we can return to a place where we are in control of our minds, as opposed to our minds being in control of us. As Dr. Frankl shows us, awareness creates a space between stimulus and response, and that space is an omnipotent place of power and choice.

Seeing the space between anxious thoughts and the alarm in the body, and in turn between the alarm in the body and the anxious thoughts of the mind, was crucial in my own healing from the cycle because it gave me a place to stick in a crowbar and break the cycle apart.

When we unconsciously assume the anxiety of the mind and the alarm of the body are inextricably linked, or one and the same, we see them as one impregnable and invincible enemy. I know that over many years of conventional therapy, I felt extreme frustration with my lack of progress, like I was fighting an indomitable giant. After my LSD experience, where I visualized my anxiety as a state of alarm in my solar plexus, I knew that thinking and feeling could be separated because they were different entities. Once I sat in awareness and saw that space between emotion and thought, I knew I had a way to break the alarm-anxiety cycle. Awareness of that space between the alarm in my body and the anxious thoughts of my mind showed a vulnerability in the reverberating loop that was previously invisible to me. I surmised that if there was a space between the anxiety of the mind and the alarm in the body, they must be separate and therefore separable—and separating the components of the cycle might very well be the Achilles' heel of the previously indomitable giant.

If we do not see alarm and anxiety as distinct, we have no entry point—no place to "break in"—and we are victims to the effect of the cycle's destructive power. You can't change what you can't see, and when we use awareness to see alarm and anxiety as separate and distinct entities, we are able to divide and conquer.

In part 3, I'll show you specific ways to break the cycle by using the space between the thoughts of the mind and the feeling in the body, but I will give you a little foreshadowing now. The best way is to use the space to redirect your attention away from thinking in your head and into the feeling in your body, and when you get out of your head, you starve the anxious thoughts of attention and energy.

Once we have awareness that we can use the space to choose to detour our attention away from the relentless thinking of our mind and into the grounded feeling of our body, we see a chink in the armor of the indomitable monster of anxiety that was previously invisible.

Unconsciously and automatically, we give our thoughts an omnipotent status they do not deserve. I'll show you that in using your awareness you will see there is simply no anxious thought that is worth having. Period. It is time to consciously use awareness to take that power back and break the alarm-anxiety cycle forever.

27

You Are Not Your Thoughts

The common saying "You are not your thoughts" captures the idea that when you can see your thoughts, you don't have to be your thoughts. So many of us go through life identifying with our thoughts, but when you can learn to see them as mere machinations of the mind that you can observe with curiosity—and without reacting—that's when the realization dawns; while you are the entity that thinks the thoughts, those thoughts are separate from your essence. They are just thoughts—just brain droppings.

Seeing yourself as separate from the thoughts you think is crucial—but this is often easier said than done and is virtually impossible if you don't consciously employ the power of awareness. In conscious, intentional awareness, we apply a nonjudgmental air of curiosity to our thoughts. If we are in alarm or intense emotion, we may lose the ability to engage our awareness, as our emotionality drives us into survival brain and away from the rational brain we need to employ awareness in the first place. Adopting a framework of curiosity in our awareness can strip the emotionality from a thought, because curiosity engages a rational, non-emotional part of our brain. In other words, adopting an attitude of the curious observer to our worries keeps us connected to our rational brain.

For me, the hallmark of conscious awareness is this curiosity, a calm and rational place where I see the ability to slow down and stay focused and discerning without being emotional and judgmental. It is a place where I can observe my anxious thoughts from some distance and don't have to be taken over by them. The catch here is the thoughts I need to see with the most curiosity and rational, nonjudgmental awareness are the very same worries that fire my system into a state of alarm, simultaneously shutting down the rational brain I need to access that awareness in the first place! The emotional intensity of some thoughts puts me in a place where I lose my rational mind and pulls me away from my nonjudgmental awareness. It's much easier for me to be a curious observer of the thought "I need to eat less sugar" than of the thought "I'm going to die from diabetes," because in the former I am not as emotionally triggered and I can stay in my rational mind. Coming soon, we'll explore some ways to stay present in awareness so you don't get swept away by worries of your mind.

Conscious awareness is being aware that you are aware. It is a sense that you are a curious, conscious observer of the events of your life, not a hapless, unconscious victim of circumstance. With this nonattachment, as Buddhists call it, you can be the observer of both the anxious thoughts of your mind and the alarm feeling in the body, and in deciding to be the observer, you gain a degree of separation from both those automatic thoughts and feelings. You can then (consciously) see the alarm-anxiety cycle and not have to (unconsciously) *be* it. From that separation and curious observation, you can literally see a space where you can catch your breath and stop short of activating the alarm in your body. (This is the essence of the "Objecting Without Contracting" exercise in the Anxiety Toolkit.) As the alarm is diffused and your system moves away from survival mode, you regain access to your rational brain so that you can see your worries are irrational and unlikely to occur. It's a win-win.

With practice, as your rational brain increasingly sees you as separate (and separable) from your worrisome thoughts, that space creates an atmosphere of choice. Awareness and presence allow you to stay in your rational brain so you no longer automatically believe your worries and exacerbate your alarm. Without conscious awareness, we unconsciously believe everything we think, especially our scary predictions of the future. This unfortunate and automatic belief of our worries is a major player in activating our alarm which, in a vicious cycle, impedes the thinking mind so needed for a rational assessment of those worries!

Without our conscious awareness, we stay unconscious and fail to see our worries as simply scary prognostications of the future that we ourselves have created. When we automatically believe our worries, we energize the alarm-anxiety cycle. When we commit to curious, objective awareness, we see those worries as something that is not an integral part of who we are but just brain droppings that the mind has created. When we become less attached to our worries in this way, those worries lose much of their power to intensify the alarm in our system, and we can begin to heal.

With the core tenet of nonattachment, Buddhists are very skilled at detaching from their discomfort. When I visited a Buddhist monastery in India in 2013, I noticed there was dirt in the corners of their temple. I asked one of the monks, "Why don't you vacuum in the corners?" and he said, "Because we are Buddhists. Even our vacuums don't have attachments."

(Sorry, all this talk of alarm was getting a bit heavy, so I had to lighten the mood.)

28

Power of Belief

Why would we do such a thing as believe alarming thoughts? Why would we make ourselves sick with worry? Why would we accept thoughts we hate as true?

Remember that if we had a lot of trauma and uncertainty growing up, we will avoid uncertainty at all costs, and the certainty of believing our scary worries appears to be the better option than leaving the future uncertain. Given the choice of believing a scary thought or living with complete uncertainty, our automatic, protective reaction as worriers is to believe the thought because we hate the uncertainty of not knowing more than we hate the anxious thoughts. Another way of saying this is in fixating on our worries, we accept the certainty of misery in favor of the misery of uncertainty.

Here's one more example. You are supposed to have a coffee with a new friend and she doesn't show up. Then you see her out with someone else at the same time you were to meet. The pain is unavoidable and a consequence of being human. But in an attempt to make the uncertain certain, your mind makes sense of the situation by telling you that your new friend probably thinks you are unworthy and boring. You go on to tell yourself that you'll never find a good friend and you'll end up cutting your ear off and dying alone like van Gogh.

Too much? Okay, let's back up, Vincent. Looking at that situation with conscious awareness, she missed your coffee meeting. That's it. You can be curious as to a potential reason why without adding all sorts of emotionality that only creates suffering.

This is how anxious thoughts work. We allow thoughts to snowball into massive amounts of emotionality and suffering simply because we fail to see that we can create a curious space where we have a choice whether or not to believe those thoughts. When we unconsciously and automatically accept and believe everything we think (especially our anxious thoughts), we suffer. We take alarm-created suggestions of the mind and elevate them to the level of truth. When those worries are believed, we get fired into survival mode which paralyzes our thinking brain. With our rational mind impaired we are unable to critique the onslaught of those worried and self-critical thoughts as false, which creates more alarm and survival physiology to further impair our rational prefrontal cortex's ability to see reality—which is that she simply forgot. Can you see how this sh** gets so easily out of control?

If you can become aware of the space between stimulus (getting stood up) and response ("I must be a boring person"), in that space you can bring in "Don't believe everything you think."

Here's a non-fun fact about your mind. Your mind is a compulsive meaning-making machine, and in us worriers, the mind strives to make sense (and limit uncertainty) more than it strives to make you feel better. For worriers, the mind's mandate is to limit uncertainty, even at the cost of accepting a painful thought or worry as truth. In other words, the anxious mind places making sense first and foremost, and if it creates collateral damage to you in the process, it accepts that as the cost of doing business. In this case, telling ourselves we were stood up because we are boring and/or unworthy is yet another way we use our mind to victimize ourselves. We do this to ourselves but it is unconscious, so it's kind of not our fault. Now that you know about developing conscious awareness, if you victimize yourself by compulsively and automatically allowing yourself to believe your worries, it *is* your fault.

That may sound harsh, but I genuinely don't mean it to be. On my YouTube channel called *The Anxiety MD*, I used to end all my videos by saying, "Don't believe everything you think." I know how challenging it is to not believe your own mind and its compulsive warnings, what-ifs, and worst-case scenarios. If you are a worrier, at some unconscious level your overprotective ego has tricked you into believing your worries are keeping you safe. I am telling you the complete opposite. To paraphrase Maya Angelou, "When you know better, you do better." Doing better is a gradual process, but the first step is seeing that your mind is not always accurate and it's not always your friend.

Sometimes it craps on you with brain droppings.

Let me remind you that you are not abnormal in your tendency to worry and be alarmed, and in fact, your mind and nervous system are operating exactly as expected if you have unresolved trauma. What you have is a compulsive habit of believing (and being) your thoughts in a misguided (childhood) attempt to keep yourself safe.

Another way of saying this is: your mind tries to avoid one pain by distracting you with a different pain. It sounds ridiculous, right? But until I saw what my mind was doing, I could not change it. Until I saw the choice and space in my commitment to curiosity and awareness, I unconsciously just kept going with my childhood coping strategy of believing every worry I crapped on myself. Until I saw the space between the alarm I felt in my body and the thoughts I created in my mind, I had no way to break the alarm-anxiety cycle because I couldn't even see the cycle. And (all together now!) when you can't see it you are destined to be it. Are you ready to learn the way out of chronic worry? One of the best ways to break the alarm-anxiety cycle is to learn how to detach from your thoughts. Learn how to see your worrisome thoughts as simply thoughts, or better yet, brain droppings. Learn that you do not have to believe everything you think. Learn how to be the master of your mind and not its servant. Learn that your anxious thoughts are not protecting you or making things more certain. Learn that when you are in alarm, your brain is in survival mode and those thoughts are poisoned by fear and should not be consumed. Learn that when you are feeling alarmed, you can create space to move into the sensation of the body and away from the thoughts of the mind. Learn to create a pattern of awareness so you avoid continuing on with the old coping strategy of worry and pain. Stop blindly making sense of the feeling of alarm by automatically and unwittingly turning it into the thoughts of anxiety. Learn that between stimulus (alarm in the body) and response (anxious thoughts) there is a space, and in that space there is a choice to make a new reality, breaking the unconscious and maladaptive habit of the alarm-anxiety cycle.

Jerry Seinfeld has a joke about the use of helmets relating to why humans want to carry on with old habits even though we know they are bad for us. He asks: "Now why did we invent the helmet? Well, because we were participating in many activities that were crackin' our heads. We looked at the situation, we chose not to avoid these activities, but to just make little plastic hats so we could continue our head-crackin' lifestyles."

You do not have to carry on with your head-crackin' alarm-anxiety lifestyle. Your coping strategy of escape from your alarmed body into your feeling mind had some adaptive advantage when you were a power-less child, but you're an adult now and have much more effective options.

I'll talk more about this in part 3, but many therapists suggest to crit-ically and rationally appraise your anxious thoughts on the spot so you can show yourself they aren't true. I do not agree. I've learned the hard way that trying to assess my worries while I am alarmed just gives more credibility to those worries. When I am alarmed, my survival brain takes over and I lose my rational brain, so why would I try to rationally look at my worries if the rational part of my brain was offline?

I've found the best way to deal with anxious thoughts is to immediately redirect the energy that was going into believing or analyzing the worry into a focus of grounding safety in the body. In this grounding, we can focus on faith and a knowing of the inherent safety of life. Once we have grounded ourselves and our rational brain is back online, *then* we can crit-ically appraise our worries, if we feel we still need to do that.

I've lived well over twenty thousand days, and I can honestly say that at least one thousand of those days I was absolutely convinced I was dying. This is not a joke or trying to make a substantive, literary point. I have spent months convinced that I had some neurological, psycholog-ical, or cardiac condition (among many other organ system disorders) and truly believing it might kill me. I have the journal entries to prove it.

And I am still here, still healthy.

We can use belief for us or against us. We get to choose what we believe, but only if we see the space that allows that choice to actively be made. Seeing that space between thought and alarm, between stimulus and response, between alarm and thought has been invaluable in the healing of chronic worry in myself and in countless numbers of my patients.

Point to consider: Don't try to reason with your worries while you are still in alarm, because you can't beat thoughts on their own turf. (More soon.) When you see you are in the hole of worry, stop digging. Get out of your head and into your body.

29

Power of Belief

Many of my patients describe a powerless, helpless state of being tortured by their own minds. Perhaps this resonates with you? I, too, have spent much of my life in this unconscious, unaware autopilot state where my mind automatically and compulsively believed every scary thought created by my emotions.

I kept automatically believing my anxious thoughts in this autopilot state. There was no chance for the pain of alarm in my body to release or pass through me, because I kept metaphorically throwing matches on the fire of alarm in the form of my anxious worries.

When we move out of autopilot and commit to curious awareness of our thoughts, we can separate those thoughts from the power of belief. Notice I said "separate thoughts from belief" and not "analyze thoughts for accuracy."

You need to use your awareness to see your anxious and intrusive thoughts and then make a conscious choice to separate from them by moving your attention out of your head and into the grounding in your body. Again, there is no point in trying to wrestle with a worry while you are in survival brain—it will pin you every time. Remember how our mind jumped quickly from ludicrous to possible with the pink elephant example?

When people tell you to get out of your head, believe them! When you are stuck on autopilot, believing every worry you think traps you in a prison of your own making. The key to getting out of worry jail is committing to conscious awareness over unconscious autopilot. I will show you exactly how to do this in part 3.

Point to consider: Take one of your worries and see it only has power if you believe it.

30

In Survival, We Lose Our Minds

When the body is in alarm and the mind goes into survival mode, we literally lose blood flow to the more cognitively oriented "thriving" parts of the brain. When you are being chased by a lion, you don't need to cognitively know if the lion escaped from the zoo or if the lion is Asiatic or Southwest African or if he just wants to play. You just need to get the heck out of there.

This descent from our "newer" (evolutionarily speaking) brain, called the neocortex or rational brain, into the older, more primitive lower brain areas, called the limbic or emotional brain, is a remnant of a time when our thoughts were more likely to be about predators or mortal threats. In that world, we did not need reason as much as we needed to escape a clear and present danger. The reaction to thoughts of threat became hardwired: channeling energy into focusing on immediate danger and deciding to flee or stay and fight. This fear is real and must be acted upon immediately. But in modern times, most of our thoughts are of delayed and/or imagined danger, like running out of money or getting a divorce (or two). The difference between fear and anxiety is timing. With fear you must act immediately, like if someone is approaching you in a hostile manner, but the hallmark of anxiety is that action can wait. If you ever question whether you are dealing with fear or anxiety, ask yourself if you can wait five seconds. Often what we call fear is really anxiety, and the latter is made up in our minds. This is one reason why telling yourself "I safe in this moment" is so helpful, because when we see that we can wait, we also see we are not in real danger.

However, our brain and body still react to imaginings of threat by acting much as they did fifty thousand years ago. In other words, the brain and body react to nonurgent imaginings in the same way they would to urgent realities. One of those reactions is to prioritize (perceived) survival by moving us away from rationality and into emotionality, making us feel we must act immediately, on limited information—on a mere perception from an alarm-impaired brain that is highly distracted by imagined fears.

Sound like trouble?

By shunting energy from our rational brain into our survival brain, we lose access to our reasoning minds. In this process of losing our minds, the worrisome thoughts appear more real than they truly are, and this overestimation of danger creates an even greater alarm reaction in the body, endlessly triggering the alarm-anxiety cycle. In other words, the more we default into the cycle, the stronger (more potentiated) the wiring that perpetuates alarm and anxiety.

From this survival-focused state of alarm, it can be very difficult to become aware of the possibility of simply observing your worries in awareness and making a conscious choice to move away from the thinking of your mind and into the sensation in your body. Without awareness you don't see the choice to change the direction of your energy, and in the potentiated autopilot of the alarm-anxiety cycle you compulsively redouble your efforts to try to stay in your head believing you can think (worry) your way to safety, even though your mind isn't rational enough to realize that you aren't rational. You increase both your anxiety and your alarm as you become more frustrated at your inability to think your way out of a feeling problem.

This is why cognitive and talk-based therapies are limited in their effectiveness. They try to use the mind prematurely, assuming the mind is in a capable state to immediately grasp cognitive solutions.

When you are in an alarm state, your mind is far from capable—it's downright impaired. More on this soon, but a more effective approach is to immediately move away from thoughts altogether and focus your energy on grounding yourself in your body. Once you have moved your body out of alarm and your rational brain has returned, then and only then is it safe to make the ascent back up into the heady land of thoughts.

31
There's a Hole in Your Boat

Most traditional therapies go after thoughts, believing that all stress comes from our thoughts and that if the thoughts are fixed, the condition will resolve. That has not been my experience personally or professionally. While cognitive or talk therapies may help for a while, research shows the effects of talk therapy often fade significantly over time. If the alarm in the body is not addressed directly, it is only a matter of time until that alarm rises up and begins skewing your perception (and your subsequent thoughts) right back to worry.

If there is a hole in the floor of your boat and you learn better techniques of bailing water, things will appear to get better, but you still have a hole in your boat. Trying to fix the anxious thinking alone is like bailing out the water and ignoring the hole. The underlying cause and main source of emotional pain is the alarm feeling in the body, so fixing the thoughts will not fix the problem. The alarm must be "repaired" before any strategies designed to address the worries will be able to "hold water." Here's a massive point: the worrisome thoughts of our mind are not the cause but the effect of the alarm stored in our body that originates from our unresolved (typically childhood) wounds. Those worries are not the root cause of our pain but they sure trick us into believing they are.

While talk therapy and learning not to believe everything you think are still valuable, focusing on the feeling/alarm component of the alarm-anxiety cycle holds the most promise for long-term relief. I am not saying you just need to do yoga and stand on your left ovary twelve hours a day to heal. You do need to have some ability to "tell your story" in a way that makes sense to you, what interpersonal neurobiologist and child psychiatrist Dr. Dan Siegel calls having a "coherent narrative" of your life. In my own journey to relief from anxiety and alarm, I needed a combination of a visceral/feeling/body strategy and a cognitive/mind/thinking strategy to make sense of what happened with my father, but ultimately, it was addressing the alarm in the body that made the most difference in finding real peace. Once I resolved the alarm in my body, I created a space where CBT and cognitive therapies could "stick," but doing cognitive work without a place for the learning to ground is like trying to build a skyscraper without first creating a concrete foundation.

My approach here in this book goes against the current dogma suggesting that cognitive therapies are the most effective remedies for anxiety disorders. I spent over twenty-five years in therapies that operated under the assumption that changing the thoughts of my mind would help me find peace from chronic worry, but I did not experience lasting relief until I embraced the critical role of my body in the healing of my mind. After decades of limited success with conventional therapy, I had to go well outside of traditional therapy to heal, and it's likely you will too.

Skeptical that alarm in the body is at the root of your pain? Consider this. There is a procedure called a stellate ganglion block (SGB) in which local anesthetic is injected into the stellate ganglion, a mass of nervous tissue in the neck. This ganglion transmits information from the body to the brain, and the SGB is typically used to reduce the sensation of pain. When this procedure is done on combat veterans with post-traumatic stress disorder (PTSD), between 70 and 80 percent of them report immediate improvement of their PTSD symptoms. They state it is like having a weight lifted off them and they can think calmly and clearly again. Their families say it is like witnessing a miracle. The vets are able to experience a state of calm in their minds, and connect with family and friends once the constant alarm signals from the body have been blocked. Further, the cognitive (talk) therapy they do receive is much more effective because their body-based alarm is no longer overwhelming their rational brain and nervous system. It seems that the talk therapy these vets receive "sticks" better post-SGB because the deafening noise from the body has been silenced (or at least turned way down). They are now able to move out of survival brain into thriving brain and actually integrate the good information that talk therapy provides. This highlights the overpowering force the alarm in the body exerts on the mind. Once the body's alarming influence is taken out of the equation (as in the SGB procedure), the mind can think clearly again and better absorb the cognitive strategies that are offered. Once we repair the hole in the hull (calm the alarm in the body), we can more effectively stop the flow of worry in the mind.

32

The Body Trumps the Mind

For us worriers, our conscious minds know it is okay to relax and let our guard down, but our bodies won't let us, just like the monkey who can't get his arm to release the banana. When our bodies have learned to stay in vigilant attention regardless of what our minds are saying, simply talking about our stresses won't change them.

Since the body has learned to reproduce the alarm, the body is the better place to focus our healing energy because it carries much more weight than the mind in the calming process.

To use a computer analogy, imagine the operating system that runs the mind is made by Windows and the system that runs the body is made by Apple. You can get complicated programs that will convert the information from one into the other, but an Apple computer runs best with Apple programs and a PC works best with Windows programs. In other words, it's a lot more complicated to calm down the body by starting with the mind than just starting with the body directly.

Changes to the mind alone cannot heal our alarm, but the power and intention of the mind are used to direct the calming of the body. We use the mind to start the process—for example, by directing ourselves to do a few rounds of the physiological sigh or by focusing our attention on calming and relaxing our muscles. Once the body moves into calm, the mind follows, moving out of survival mode. Once the body is calm we can start using more complex, mind-based approaches. Trying to reason with a mind in alarm-based survival mode is like trying to use objective reasoning with an upset five-year-old who has just been told they cannot have an ice cream cone as it will spoil their appetite for dinner. (Or explaining to an overheated ten-year-old in the middle of the desert that she should think of a cold swimming pool.)

> **Point to consider:** If you have to go into a tough conversation or speak in front of an audience, do three to five rounds of the physiological sigh to regulate your body first. This is infinitely more powerful than using your mind to say "hey, relax!" or "it will be okay" to yourself.

33

On Alarm in the Body

Like the second-nature groove the body falls into when we drive a car, the body has learned to launch a fight-or-flight alarm response without much input from the cognitive mind.

When I heard that trumpet solo, my body went into instant alarm; it was only later my mind figured out why. This preloaded firing pattern is a form of implicit memory, also called body memory—a pattern or framework that is automatic, repetitive, and unconscious, akin to the patterns we ingrained when learning to drive a car or ride a bike. The purple, hot pressure alarm pattern in my solar plexus is also automatic, repetitive, and unconscious and fires up when I am reminded of a time in my life when I felt helpless and hopeless—and alarmed. When I heard that trumpet solo, my amygdala recognized the old pain and fired my body into alarm, regressing me back to a powerless and angry thirteen-year-old boy who was frustrated by a father who seemingly paid more attention to a brass instrument than to his own son. (You, too, have your own alarm pattern with its distinct emotional signature in your body, and we'll find it in part 2.)

Upon examination of my own alarm, in times of stress, my body replicates the same alarm state I felt as a teenager watching my father lose his mind. I believe my insular cortex recreates the same sensation in my solar plexus area *now* that I felt back *then*. I call this an *emotional signature* because the sensation in the insula that was occurring at the time of the original trauma is the same sensation we feel today. The same is likely true for you—when you are alarmed, in part mediated by your amygdala and insular cortex, your body feels today the same way it did when the original trauma occurred. (More on this later too.)

For many years, I woke up with an alarm in my solar plexus. It felt the same way every single day. I believe this early morning alarm is an implicit body memory precisely recreated by the insula and the amygdala among other brain structures. This "memory" was encoded at a time when I was seven years old and being woken up at 5:30 A.M. by a stressed-out mother who needed to get to work by seven. This would send me into a state of alarm because Mom had to drop my brother and I off at our babysitter who, frankly, I was afraid of. My wakeup alarm (forgive the double entendre) is a form of implicit memory and a throwback to my childhood. My body did it every day for many years—it did not need the mind. As a medical intern, if I got a call around 5:30 A.M. it would set off the same alarm reaction in my solar plexus from twenty years earlier. Curiously, if I got called at 1 or 3 or 4 A.M., I would not get this alarm reaction—only if my pager woke me around the time my mother used to.

I started to consciously bring my mind into my morning alarm. I saw that by playing with believing scary thoughts, I could consciously increase the intensity of the alarm sensation in my solar plexus. I also observed that as the alarm would increase, I had a tremendous desire to explain it with more thought. In other words, there was a compulsion to attach thinking to the painful feeling.

In conscious, pointed awareness, I observed that if I separated the alarm in my solar plexus from the thoughts in my mind, by directing my intention and attention into putting my hand on my chest, focusing on my breath, and generally directing all my attention to the feeling in my body, my scary thoughts didn't seem so scary. When I put my hand over my solar plexus and consciously directed my focus of attention into my body and breath, there was markedly less energy left over to pay attention to, or to create more negative thoughts.

I was on to something.

I also observed that the longer I focused on the present sensation in my body, the more it seemed to starve the thoughts of energy, and as a result, those thoughts often wouldn't go down without a fight, and they tried to get louder. It was as if the pain of alarm in my body needed an explanation, dammit! The urge to worry increased, I believe, because those worries were a helpful distraction in childhood. But I intuitively knew I needed to stay the course, and I would redouble my efforts to get out of my head and focus on the pure sensation of the alarm. With practice, the more I focused on the sensation of my body in the moment, like putting my hand on my chest and focusing on the pleasant sensation of my breath going in and out, the more distant (and less powerful) the thoughts would become. But I had to stay focused on my body because the worries tried to rise up, wanting to regain the childhood "security" they once had by firing me up into my head and distracting me from the alarm pain in my solar plexus. It was almost like when the thoughts finally saw they wouldn't be believed, they gave up. But there was a whole lot of "sensation without explanation" going on before the worries retreated. By making this unconscious alarm-anxiety cycle more conscious, I was shown how to break the cycle by holding my ground and staying present with my body, but early on the worries tenaciously fought on, like Hiroo Onoda. Disciplining myself to move my attention away from my mind and into my body took time and practice, and I still get sucked up into my worries to this day, but I cannot express to you in words how valuable this practice of staying in my body and out of my worries has been for my mental health.

I want to show you the same thing—how to break the cycle and stop feeding the alarm by directing your conscious attention into the sensation in your body and away from the thinking of your mind.

Point to consider: Review the tool "Sensation without Explanation" in the Anxiety Toolkit.

34

Intention and the Power of It

So many times, I felt like giving up. The fight with anxiety and alarm seemed never-ending as therapy after therapy failed miserably. Maybe you've felt that exasperation too. I tried so many medications (legal and not), therapies, retreats, and procedures and processes of all kinds. You name it, I probably tried it. When nothing really helped and I was still waking up every single day with unbearable alarm, I lost hope that I would ever recover. After years of intense alarm, not just in the mornings but often throughout the whole day, not only did I not think I would recover, I was sure it was going to kill me the way mental illness killed my dad.

But the tide started to turn when LSD showed me there was a source of pain in my body that was distinct and separate from my mind. I named the pain I felt in my solar plexus "alarm," and I honed the concept of alarm, contrasting it with the condition doctors refer to as anxiety.

Although the alarm was aggravated by my worrisome thoughts, I slowly began to see that the alarm in my body could be separated from those thoughts. Learning to set an intention to allow myself to just sit in awareness with the alarm without having to compulsively add worries to it was life-changing for me. One of the most valuable lessons you can learn in healing your anxiety is to allow yourself to feel the alarm sensation in your body (which we will find just around the corner in part 2) and observe your mind's compulsion to add worry in an effort to distract you from the pain of alarm. Then we break the feedback loop of the alarm-anxiety cycle by learning how to separate its component parts, each starving the other for energy to break the cycle apart.

When you truly see you can separate the alarm in your body from the thoughts of your mind, you gain a decisive advantage—the ability to break out of the prison of your own making.

You cannot change what you cannot see, and the awareness that it is you who is unnecessarily adding thought to a feeling begins to make the unconscious conscious and the invisible visible. For so many years I assumed my thoughts and worries were the cause of my pain, and I couldn't "see" the alarm, although I surely felt it. I spent so much time and money for some therapist to help me change my thoughts when I couldn't see that my thoughts and worries weren't the true underlying source of my pain. I wish I knew forty years ago what I am telling you now. My life would have had so much less frustration and pain. As you go through this book, I will show you how to direct your awareness toward addressing and healing the alarm in your very real body instead of being misdirected by the illusions of your mind.

Where awareness goes, energy flows. We can use that energy as power to start to make real changes to unconscious patterns that were previously both destructive and invisible. When you find yourself in the alarm-anxiety cycle, you'll set the intention to focus your awareness and attention on the feeling of alarm in your body and learn to intentionally and deliberately ignore the incessant worrisome propositions of your mind.

Point to consider: When you find yourself in worry, can you intentionally direct your attention downward and just start the process of beginning to look for a place of discomfort (or alarm) in your body?

35

You Can't Think Your Way Out of a Feeling Problem

If you've ever been super tense and had someone say to you, "Hey, relax," did it help? Probably not, because you cannot effectively calm a fight-or-flight feeling with simple words and thoughts.

Learning coping strategies in our higher brain centers during psychotherapy is valuable, no question. But we must learn techniques not only with our thinking minds but also with our feeling bodies. We cannot fight a feeling armed only with a thinking.

I'm very close with my fourteen-year-old, eighty-five-pound blond labradoodle, Buddha. I estimate that I have given "BooBoo" close to half a million kisses on his snout. In contrast, he's not one for displays of affection, public or private. Buddha's internal ranking of things is: 1) breakfast; 2) dinner; 3) snacks; 4) any ball; 5) my wife, Cynthia, and my daughter, Leandra (it's a tie); 6) swimming; and 7) me. I got Boo on my birthday in 2009, and he has seen me through a lot of transitions and changes. Some days, I felt so alarmed that the only reason I would get out of bed was because I needed to take him outside.

Boo started to have seizures when he was eight years old. Now, as a doctor for humans, I know there's a good chance the onset of seizures in an adult is caused by a tumor. I would tell myself it could just be epilepsy and then I would argue with myself and say "It's not a tumor!" like Schwarzenegger in *Kindergarten Cop*. Then it would be a benign tumor, then a malignant tumor. (As a fellow worrier, you know how it goes, the "don't think of a pink elephant thing" again.) The more I believed my catastrophic predictions, the more alarm I felt in my body, which activated my survival-focused brain and paralyzed my rational brain. I wouldn't allow myself to be reassured because allowing myself to think Buddha pup was going to be okay was not consistent with the feeling of alarm in my body.

So, in the days leading up to his MRI scan, whenever I caught myself thinking those catastrophic (dogastrophic?) thoughts, I would put my hand on my solar plexus area, focus deeply on connecting to myself, and visualize breathing into the area of alarm, only allowing myself to focus on the sensation in my body. No thoughts: only sensation, no explanation. I had to make a concerted effort not to be seduced back into thinking and to focus completely on the feeling, *even if the feeling was uncomfortable*. Focusing on the uncomfortable sensation of alarm in my solar plexus and then putting my hand on my chest, or breathing into the feeling with an attitude of compassion for myself, shifted my perception from a projected painful future thought to a consciously connected present-moment sensation. It also gave me a sense of control, in a milieu of uncertainty, about what was going to happen to my beloved Bubba (Buddha has over one hundred nicknames). Even if my alarm was painful, which it was, I could stick with it and not acquiesce back into worry, and that showed me I could handle the pain as long as I didn't keep throwing matches on it.

One of the tenets of the brain is whatever you focus on, you get more of. When I focused on connection to myself, I got more of that. When I focused on the worries about my dog, I got more worries about my dog. Your attention will fall into a groove, and the groove it falls into can be conscious, willful, and constructive, or it can be unconscious, chaotic, and destructive. In a very real way, the brain doesn't care, so it's up to you to direct where you choose to put your attention and your energy.

If you aren't paying attention, and the feeling in your body is one of alarm, the groove of your attention and perception will fall into looking for things that are completely consistent with that feeling of alarm, which is where your worries will enter with a vengeance. To use a different metaphor, if you don't direct your focus consciously to something productive when you are in a state of alarm, your attention will be hijacked to what they refer to in *Star Wars* as the "dark side." When your system has been hijacked by alarm and taken over by the dark side, your perception will follow. You will actually start to perceive more negativity (and ignore positivity), because the alarm in your body will trigger your mind to see what you already feel. Then, per your old childhood habit, you will look for certainty in your worries, and you will believe those worries and get trapped in the alarm-anxiety cycle forever.

I'm going to emphasize this critical point: *your mind will see what your body feels.*

When I consciously chose to break the hold that worry had on me and instead focus on connecting—putting my hand on my chest, concentrating on my breathing, and moving from a focus on worries to a focus on the pleasant sensation of self-connection and self-care in the moment—my worries fell into the background. Not right away—this self connection took practice and conscious attention, and it is not that those worries disappeared completely, but as I gave my worries less attention they had less energy, and I was able to develop a conscious awareness of the signs I was falling into my childhood pattern of being sucked into worry. In other words, I taught myself to be in charge of my worries and triggers, instead of the other way around. By disconnecting the scary thoughts from the alarm sensation, I broke the unconscious thought-feeling cycle and derailed the runaway worry train. I was learning to be the master of my body and not the servant of my mind.

As I said earlier, "You cannot beat thoughts on their own turf." If your mind has been seduced into worrying and the subsequent yea-or-nay back-and-forth that ensues, you've already lost. You can't find your way out of worrying and rumination with more *thinking*; you must learn how to feel your way out by going into your body, even if it hurts.

I am a little hard on talk therapy (mostly out of frustration with my own lack of progress with it) but it's not so much that talk therapy for the mind isn't effective; it's that it's not effective when the patient and the doctor ignore (or simply do not see) the significant alarm in the body. This is why we need to calm the body first, and then—when the brain is receptive, open, and fully available to absorb information—work with the cognitive mind. There is little point trying to learn rational concepts when your alarm is drowning your rational brain in stress chemicals of cortisol and adrenaline. I'll soon show you how to understand and calm the alarm in your body so you can go back to thinking with your rational mind, but for now, let's understand why the dark side of the mind takes us over when we are alarmed.

36

When It's Not Safe in the Body, We Retreat into the Mind

The scientific law of conservation of energy states that energy cannot be created nor destroyed, only changed in form. When the acute energy of our childhood wounds becomes too much for our conscious mind to bear, as a protective measure, that painful energy gets exiled down into our body. Our nervous system transmutes the acute pain from the thinking in our mind and "hides" it in the chronic feeling in our body. And my nervous system hid it so well in me that it took a trip out of my mind on

LSD to finally see it. That chronic energy, hidden in our bodies, is what I've been referring to as background alarm. If you've read the book *The Body Keeps the Score* by Dr. Bessel van der Kolk or are familiar with Eckhart Tolle's concept of the "pain body," I'm referring to the same thing.

When there is trauma in your home and you don't feel safe in your emotional, feeling body, the only option left to the helpless child is to distract with worry up in their thinking mind. When trauma makes us move away from being grounded in the present moment in our body into the fractured and compromised future-based mind, this is called dissociation. We will explore this concept in greater depth later, but for now, know that dissociation is akin to a daydreaming state where you are not connected to yourself. The bigger the trauma experienced, the more likely a person is to dissociate or fragment. Classically, dissociation is described when someone separates from (or rises above) their body during a trauma, but there are more subtle forms of dissociation where the mind and body separate from each other.

So why am I telling you about dissociation? Because I see compulsive worrying as a form of dissociation, and before we leave this section on awareness of mind, I want you to be aware of this trick your mind plays on you. When you cannot stay in your alarmed body, you fragment and escape into the only other place available, the worries of your mind. Your rational mind is impaired by the alarm in your body so you are unable to see the worries as false, which perpetuates the worries as a perennial distraction from the pain of alarm in your body. In dissociating up into your mind you escape the alarm in your body, and that is exactly how your ego "protects" you, but this is the proverbial robbing Peter to pay Paul situation where you are held in a state of pain in an attempt to avoid pain! When you see your signs of dissociation—zoning out, daydreaming in worry, being unavailable to others, forgetfulness, and absent-mindedness—you can use that as a signal to use your awareness and choose to get back into the present-moment sensation of your body. Of course the paradox is that when you go into dissociation, by definition you don't see you are in dissociation, and you can't see how to get out of something you don't even see you are in! But you can train yourself to see early signs of dissociation before you get too deeply taken over by it. More on this later.

Can you can relate to zoning out into worry? I love the T-shirt that says, "I'm in my own little world, but it's okay . . . they know me here."

(As an aside, I believe this seduction to dissociate into the daydreaming state is why trauma, anxiety, and attention deficit disorder [ADD] occur so frequently together.)

Growing up, I felt safe physically, but I didn't feel safe emotionally. I didn't know when my father was going to lapse into a deep depressive state or stay awake for days in a manic state with that damn trumpet. This had the effect of keeping my body in a chronic state of alarm, waiting for the other shoe to drop. As a coping strategy, and to escape from the alarm sensation in my body, I began to overthink and worry up in my mind. Some part of me felt that if I stayed vigilant with warnings, what-ifs, and worst-case scenarios, I would be prepared for my father's next flight over the cuckoo's nest.

Worrisome thoughts acted as a temporary distraction. Worry diffused some of the uncertainty energy by giving me something to do. Also, ruminating on what could go wrong kept my focus on the machinations of my mind and away from the alarm that I couldn't bear to feel in my body. I would think things like, "He seems a bit down today, he must be diving into depression," or "He seems in a good mood, I wonder if he is winding up into a manic phase?" But again, I was essentially robbing Peter to pay Paul. Those worrisome thoughts initially distracted me from the feeling of alarm, but over time they created more alarm as I invariably and unconsciously believed those worries.

Worries are like a drug we develop a tolerance to. Over time, my anxious, ruminative thoughts had to become more frequent and more intense to maintain their ability to keep me up in my head. This is why worries tend to get more and more catastrophic over time, as they need to ramp up the intensity to keep you in your head and out of the alarm scored (ahem, stored) in your body. Of course, as the worries gain strength, this intensifies the alarm-anxiety cycle.

Because of my trauma, I had retreated into my head and lost the grounding potential of my body. When you perceive your mind is your only safe place, or, at the very least, the safest place available, you try your best to stay there. I had lost faith that my body was a safe place because of the pain stored there, and that left me with my mind as the only port in my (childhood) storm.

This overidentification with the mind (believing your thoughts and believing that you are your thoughts) is one reason I believe people ascribe anxiety solely to their anxious thoughts.

Perhaps, on some level, we don't even feel like we have a body. As an aside, for a long time, I didn't feel hunger or the need to go to the bathroom until it was urgent. I postulate that is because I had denied my body for so long that I was numb to the messages it sent me. Now that I have done a lot of work to reestablish a connection with my body, I can feel its nuances. I can feel a little hungry, or get the message I'll have to pee in the next hour or so. I've also learned that many of my anxious patients were bedwetters as children, or had disordered eating, which may be a sign of this same dissociation from the body and its signals.

I find anxious people, as a rule, quite smart. A possible reason for this is when mind-based thinking is your only option (because body-based feeling is too painful), you get very good at it. When thinking (and worrying) becomes a coping strategy, you get better at it. But you fall under the illusion that rumination and excessive thinking are productive. Nothing could be further from the truth. Rumination and overthinking do distract us from the pain and alarm in our bodies; with repetition this dissociation becomes a familiar groove, and we tend to distract into worry when we are stressed. Worrying gives us a sense of making the uncertain more certain and temporarily distracts us from the pain in our body. But the cost comes when we do not realize we are biting our own tail, and like an addiction we keep giving ourselves more of what we don't want. This is how we worriers get trapped in our minds with chronic worry.

The more you can see *why* you worry, the less you'll be tricked and trapped by it. Before we move on, let's take one more look at worry and what purpose it serves.

Anxiety/worry is an attempt to keep you safe. The worry is there as an attempt to warn you and prepare you for potential danger. But, in constantly warning you, it feeds the alarm in your body. Once you feel ease in your body and feel you no longer need to worry to stay safe, you can begin to release it.

Anxiety/worry is always about the future. This is where you can unmask worry. When you know it depends on you being mentally transported into the future, you can neutralize it by focusing on the present moment.

Anxiety/worry is a way of avoiding uncertainty and creating a sense of control. When we worry, we are creating a story of the future that makes the uncertain appear more certain. There is nothing worse for a worrier than uncertainty because of what uncertainty meant in our childhood. When we can start to accept and, I dare say, even embrace uncertainty as the spice of life, we can release the need to worry.

Anxiety/worry is a way of explaining the alarm felt in the body. When we feel alarm in the body and there is no obvious cause for it, this creates dissonance—a state of conflict between thinking and feeling. If you are standing at the edge of a cliff and your body goes into fight-or-flight mode, that makes sense to you and there is no dissonance. However, when your body is reacting like you are standing at the edge of a cliff while you are lying safely in your bed, that dissonance only adds to your uncertainty and consequently to your alarm. When we feel alarm in the body, worrying is a way of creating congruence between mind and body. But that worry, although it appears to make things more congruent in the short term, only adds to the alarm in the long term.

Anxiety/worry distracts us from the painful alarm in the body. There is a misdirection to worry. On one hand, it redirects the painful alarm energy by distracting us into thinking, with a very temporary reduction in the perception of alarm. But ultimately, when we believe our worries (consciously or unconsciously), the worry creates more alarm and we get trapped in the never-ending treadmill of the alarm-anxiety cycle.

Anxiety becomes an addiction. Your brain doesn't have a need to make you feel better, it has a need to resolve uncertainty—especially if you had trauma as a child. All worries are an answer to uncertainty in some way, and our brains get a shot of motivating dopamine when the uncertain appears more certain. This may be the neurological explanation why worriers prefer the certainty of misery (the worry) to the misery of uncertainty. This addictive quality of worry is one of the reasons it is so hard to stop it.

To recap, the worries of the mind aggravate anxiety, but the painful part comes from a sense of alarm stored in the body, often from decades ago. By all means, we should draw awareness around why we worry and neutralize those worries to the best of our ability, but our ultimate relief lies in healing the alarm that is "keeping the score" in the body. I will show you the means of doing both.

As I said earlier, this book may feel repetitive, and it's specifically written that way. I can change your explicit cognitive understanding by giving you facts about your anxiety, but my goal is to help you heal it on a deeper, feeling level. Explicit, cognitive understanding helps you cope with anxiety in the short term, but changing your implicit feeling state allows you to heal the anxiety in the long term. By the end of the book you will have a deeper, more implicit understanding of your anxiety so you can resolve it at the level it was created and encoded in your nervous system. My goal is for you to have a different felt sense of your anxiety, because *feeling* is the only place where real, long-lasting *healing* can take place.

To sum up part 1, akin to the saying "don't believe everything you think," I would encourage you to open to the idea (and here's me priming your brain again) that *you don't have to think everything you feel*. Indeed, learning how to separate feeling from thinking is exactly how you'll heal from chronic anxiety! Now let's learn how to truly heal by turning to the true cause of our pain: the feeling of alarm that flowed into our bodies when our minds were overwhelmed.

PART II

Awareness of Body

37

The Source of Your Pain: Waking the Tiger

I was trapped in my worried mind for many years. I also believed, because my worries were so easy to see ("I sure hope _____ doesn't happen!"), that my worries were the source of my pain. Healing anxiety by focusing on changing the worries of the mind was, and still is, the predominant narrative in psychiatry and psychology, so in a professional sense as well as my lived experience, I was just going with the flow. As a doctor, I had been trained in this worry-centric view that anxiety was best treated by talking about and modifying our way of thinking.

But decades of therapy (at hundreds of dollars an hour) focusing on changing my thinking did very little to help me feel better. How about you? Perhaps assuming my mind was the main source of my pain was a very expensive mistake. What if the pain I felt was a sleeping tiger rooted in my body and no therapist had thought to wake that tiger up to examine its behavior and see what it kept inside? What if, in being hyperfocused on changing my mind, my therapists completely missed the aspect of feeling caged in my body?

Remember the male who thinks "I might be pregnant." Thoughts are just collections of words that are painless until they are believed to be true. Worry, in and of itself, is painless. The pain we attribute to it is in reality coming from a state of activation or alarm in the body when we *believe* our worries. This is why the body is where we should be directing more of our energies in treatment, as the body keeps the score and is the ultimate source of the pain we feel.

A body-centered treatment focus tackles the root of the issue, essentially cutting off worries' power supply. With body-centered approaches, I finally got to the "guts" of true healing because I went back into my body and faced the alarm that had been stored there for decades. It was messy, but I had to feel it to heal it.

To understand where our pain truly comes from and start to heal from the source, let's learn more about this entity I call alarm.

Point to consider: The next time you feel anxious, make the intention to leave your mind's worries and redirect your awareness to where you feel the discomfort in your body.

38

The Two Types of Alarm

Recall that there are two types of alarm: foreground alarm and background alarm.

Foreground alarm is a function of the sympathetic wing of the autonomic nervous system (see diagram below).

The autonomic nervous system is the "automatic" nervous system of the body, governing functions that happen automatically and don't require conscious awareness. It comprises two wings with opposite functions: the sympathetic (fight or flight) and the parasympathetic (rest and digest). Foreground alarm is a term I created to describe the activating fight-or-flight reaction of the sympathetic nervous system (SNS) that comes with all humans as standard equipment.

I call this fight-or-flight reaction foreground alarm because it is relatively easy to observe inside of us as a predictable response to a perceived danger. The operative word here is "perceived," because this fight-or-flight reaction of foreground alarm is activated in modern times just as it was in our ancestors when they were faced with an unexpected threat. Foreground alarm will suit its original purpose of protection from threats that are real, external, and physical (such as a tiger attack or an impending car accident), but it will also fire up the alarm for threats that are also only imagined, internal, and emotional (such as the speech we fear we may be asked to give at an upcoming business meeting). In other words, the foreground alarm of the sympathetic, fight-or-flight nervous system

THE AUTONOMIC NERVOUS SYSTEM

PARASYMPATHETIC NERVES "Rest and Digest"	SYMPATHETIC NERVES "Fight or Flight"
Constrict pupils	Dilate pupils
Stimulate saliva	Inhibit salivation
Slow heartbeat	Increase heartbeat
Relaxed "belly" breathing	Tense, upper chest breathing
Relaxed muscles	Tensed muscles
Stimulate activity of stomach	Inhibit activity of stomach
Stimulate activity of intestines	Inhibit activity of intestines
	Secrete epinephrine and norepinephrine

responds not only to actual danger but to the perceived danger of our worries as well.

In contrast, background alarm is a chronic energy. It is a remnant of old, unresolved trauma, typically from childhood, that was too much for our young mind to process and became stored away as an energy in the body.

We all experience emotional pain as children—that is just a fact of life, but the critical factor is if you had comfort and support at the time of that pain. If you had a securely attached, attentive parent, that parent's presence and reassurance would have helped you see that you're not alone, and helped you successfully process and metabolize whatever trauma you experienced. However, if you did not have an available and supportive parent, you would have felt alone and that trauma energy would not have been processed and resolved. As energy cannot be created or destroyed, the form of that energy is changed and deposited in the body as background alarm.

Complicating matters, some children are just born more sensitive than others, and what is traumatic to one may not be so to another. I have seen a child with a connected parent work through the loss of a close family member in a matter of weeks, and I have seen another child unravel for many months over the loss of a pet fish. Some traumas are more serious, and some children more sensitive. But, in general, when the trauma involves abuse, abandonment, deep loss, rejection, or neglect, that is very difficult for a young mind to resolve. If you don't have a supportive and reassuring parent—or worse, if the parent is the source of your alarm—the energy is even more likely to overwhelm the mind and spill over and be sequestered into long-term storage in your body.

I call this background alarm for two reasons: 1) because it is unresolved energy from things that happened in our background (usually childhood) that our minds could not metabolize or process, and 2) because it sits in the background of our unconscious. Unlike the foreground alarm that is obvious and easy to attribute to a clear precipitant, background alarm hides in the shadows of our psyche. It took a trip on LSD for me to find where mine was hiding. Finding the source of my alarm in my body was an indispensable insight and an invaluable part of my healing, and I am confident this will be true for you as well.

Although background alarm shows up differently in different people, it has consistent characteristics or an "emotional signature" within the same person. For example, the background alarm that was shown to me on LSD is a fist-sized, hot, sharp, irregular, purple crystalline structure located in my right solar plexus area that exerts pressure up into my heart. I have shown many of my patients how to find their background alarm and they often have exquisite descriptions of it. Soon, I'll show you how to find your background alarm, and you won't have to drop acid to do it.

While everyone has foreground alarm, the normal fight-or-flight aspect of the sympathetic nervous system, background alarm only appears in those of us with deep, unresolved emotional wounds. That being said, if you are reading this book to help yourself heal from chronic nervous system hyperactivation and worry, I can pretty much guarantee you do have background alarm in your system. I can also guarantee I can help you with it, but we first need to find it.

Because you can't change what you don't know is there—and most therapists don't know it's there—most doctors and counselors will, instead, try to treat the obvious worries patients complain of. But the worries you can see and describe are only the tip of the iceberg, and by directing your efforts at the surface, you'll only get superficial results. We must address the alarm underneath the surface, and when we melt that, you'll get long-lasting relief. By the time you finish this book, you will know more about anxiety and its effective treatment than most doctors do.

Again, foreground alarm is normal sympathetic nervous system ("fight or flight") activity that is in everyone; background alarm is abnormal and only found in those of us with significant unresolved trauma. Background and foreground alarm are both processes that activate an energy in the body, and each one tends to energize the other. Panic attacks are one example of how foreground alarm and background alarm can combine to create a massive reaction by escalating each other.

Panic attacks come from background alarm that is bubbling to the surface and activating foreground alarm. Once this happens, the two alarms energize each other synergistically in an explosion of nervous system hyperactivity. Panic attacks are a more extreme example of acute activity, but background and foreground alarm can also activate each other chronically in what doctors call *generalized anxiety disorder*.

foreground alarm + background alarm = chronic alarm

Together, background alarm and foreground alarm resonate together to form a state of chronic alarm. This is often what we feel when we are having a "normal" day with no acute stressors, yet we feel this sense of uncomfortable activation or energy in us. Some of my patients call it a sense of impending doom. This chronic alarm is not present in people who do not have background alarm. Without background alarm, foreground alarm works as it should, the fight-or-flight response arising quickly in the presence of a threat and fading quickly once the threat is gone. But for those of us who do have alarm constantly simmering in the background, this maintains a little chronic alarm in our system at all times, although it may fall below our awareness at points. However, it doesn't take much to fire it up, as anything even remotely reminiscent of our old trauma will trigger it (like a trumpet solo), and once activated, it takes a long time to settle. This is our central amygdala in action as it has many cells devoted to recognizing exactly what has hurt you in the past and is ready to sound the alarm directly in your body when you encounter anything that is reminiscent of your old trauma.

When we learn to separate background alarm from foreground alarm or to decrease them independently, we decrease our general chronic alarm. As chronic alarm decreases, we feel better and calmer at our core. With less alarm in our system, there is less energy to create anxious thoughts, and we are no longer blocked from engaging in both thinking- and feeling-based approaches to prevent the alarm from coming back. It's a win-win.

> **Point to consider:** What are a few of your triggers from childhood? People arguing? Being bullied or rejected? Being abandoned? When you bring those to mind, where do you feel that in your body?

39

The Source of Background Alarm

You may be wondering: If I don't have unresolved trauma from childhood, but I suffer from anxiety, can I still have background alarm? The answer is yes.

Not everyone reading this book will have obvious unresolved trauma. Many of my patients endured trauma that was obvious in the form of abuse, abandonment, neglect, or great loss. As for me personally, growing up with a schizophrenic father was highly traumatic.

However, for some people, their trauma may be subtler, or they may not even view it as trauma. I have seen countless people who claimed to have had wonderful childhoods, but on closer observation had parents that were physically or emotionally abusive. I think children deny the severity of their parental traumas because they are painful and they have repeated the lines "it really wasn't that bad" and "my parents did the best they could" to themselves so often they believed their own fabrications and stop perceiving their parents' actions as harmful. They then claim to have had a "normal" childhood when asked, the self-deception being another result of background alarm. If you have chronic anxiety and it's not from something obvious, your childhood may not have been the securely attached experience you may have told yourself it was.

Some people require less trauma to activate their background alarm because they are highly sensitive and were probably born that way. I see this inherent sensitivity in virtually every anxious patient I've ever seen. Other people are less sensitive by disposition and appear to handle fairly easily what most people would consider traumatic. To be clear, you don't have to have an obvious trauma history to suffer from chronic worry, but if you suffer from chronic anxiety, it has to be coming from somewhere. You almost certainly have background alarm that is feeding your chronic worrying, even if you can't find an obvious source of trauma from your childhood.

I am not one of those people who wants you to go back and find blame for your parents. The truth is, we often parent the way we were parented, and for the most part, our mothers and fathers *did* do the best they could with one of the most difficult undertakings in life—making a human baby into a functional adult. (For the most part, making the baby is considerably easier and more pleasurable than creating the functional adult.)

New information is showing that trauma can be transmitted from parent to child through non-coding genetic material. (In other words, it operates not on the genes themselves but on their packaging, which affects how they are expressed.) Of course, there is another mode of transmission of trauma—namely, behaviors that are repeated from generation to generation without awareness that they're dysfunctional. Even if you can't specifically point to trauma in your childhood, you may very well still carry it. And that means you have an inherent susceptibility to anxiety—which ultimately means you are carrying background alarm in your body that may not have come from your own life experience!

On the topic of childhood experience, I've seen the rate of anxiety in young people skyrocket in the last ten to twenty years, and I think much of their alarm comes from 1) picking up on parental anxiety, 2) a lack of emotional and physical connection (especially touch) from overly busy and stressed parents, and 3) screens (computers, tablets, smartphones, and the like).

We humans are wired for connection through a mind-body system called the social engagement system (SES), also called the human resonance circuitry (HRC). We use our SES to feel truly safe and connected to each other and ourselves. The system uses elements like eye contact, tone of voice, prosody of voice, body language, and facial expressions to relate the experience of one human being to another. In short, our SES soothes and relaxes us when we are engaged and connected with others. If you've had the experience of having an anxious day and then go out with your friends that night and laugh and connect, it is likely your SES activation that saved the day. The SES not only soothed your feeling of alarm but actually helped you feel good by the time you got home.

Whenever I talk of the power of connection of the SES you can equate that with the ventral vagus Dr. Stephen Porges talks about in his polyvagal theory. The vagus nerve is the tenth cranial nerve and the largest nerve of the parasympathetic (rest and digest) nervous system. I'll talk about the ventral and dorsal vagus in more detail in part 3, but to keep it simple here I'll just use SES to combine the functions and nomenclature of the HRC and the ventral vagus, because there is significant overlap in name and function of the SES, HRC, and ventral vagus.

A childhood atmosphere of safety and connection creates an often engaged, high-functioning SES that helps metabolize and resolve our physical and emotional stressors. We need frequent and positive personal connections to engage and mature the system. The SES learns best by engaging with others face-to-face who are happy, sad, excited, loving, hurt, lonely, or frightened. It need not be an interaction with love to mature it, but love is probably the best maturation factor. We engage our own SES to read emotions and connect to other people. And, perhaps more important, this soothing connection with others promotes a soothing connection within ourselves. As a critical example, the SES is highly active in both a mother and her baby, as each soothes the other with eye contact and vocalizations and facial expressions. In contrast, unresolved alarm in childhood impairs the growth and function of the SES, because SES maturation is impaired or shut off when we do not have a sense of basic safety. If our SES development was slowed by unresolved pain in childhood, as adults we often find it hard to be warm and emotionally connected to others (and ourselves!) when we are in alarm.

The most powerful maturation factor of the SES in the developing brain is face-to-face contact. But now, many of our social interactions (especially in our kids) are coming through a screen (and perhaps not even with real people on the other side of the device), impairing our ability to develop this system and to benefit from its connecting and healing power. Face-to-face interactions are being replaced by face-to-screen interactions and anxiety and alarm in our children are increasing, while at the same time, empathy in our children is decreasing. It is no coincidence that the lack of face-to-face activities that mature the SES corresponds to a lack of social connection and a marked jump in anxiety and alarm in our children.

I wrote this book to explain where my own anxiety comes from in the hope that I am not some emotional mutant and that you will find elements of your experience in mine. I hope that my theory—that a separation or lack of connection in childhood (for whatever reason) led to background alarm, which is the real cause of what you have been told to call anxiety by modern medicine—will point you toward your own healing.

When I say that unresolved trauma is the cause of background alarm, know that your trauma could be from something as obvious as being abandoned or abused as a child, or it could come from something as widely accepted as spending much of your life in front of a screen or smartphone. Although it may not seem traumatic in the sense you've understood the word before, know that your system views a lack of connection (whatever the source) as traumatic. In other words, we are hardwired to be socially engaged creatures, and social isolation and loneliness (especially in childhood) is a massive source of background alarm. A common theme in many of my anxiety patients was a subjective feeling of loneliness, even when they were surrounded by others.

Point to consider: How lonely did you feel as a child, and how lonely do you feel now? Note: you're not alone in this feeling.

40

How Background Alarm Takes Root in the Body

Again, it is not so much the specific childhood traumas we experience but how those traumas are handled by our caregivers that determines the long-term effects. In my case, the trauma of my father's illness was both acute and chronic, and there was nobody in my life skilled enough to mediate it for me or help me process and metabolize that alarm. As a result, it was too much for my child mind to handle, so I buried that state of painful energy in my body as an energy you now know as *background alarm*.

My chronic background alarm impaired my SES and significantly affected my ability to form connected relationships. I blamed my disconnection on my busy, hyperactive mind, but my LSD experience showed me that the "engine" of my emotional pain was not my worries per se, but rather the background alarm that stole my safety and blocked my SES from fully maturing, impairing my subsequent ability to truly connect with others, and mostly with my very own self.

Background alarm develops when there is trauma that is not mediated by a secure attachment figure, usually a parent. My brother and I needed loving reassurance, and my mother—while being a very organized and efficient registered nurse, good at caring for other people—had no real idea of how to reassure us over my dad's craziness. (Hmmm, a medical professional good at caring for others externally but not that connected internally, where have I seen that before?)

My mother was a product of her very reserved and emotionally cool Scottish family. I've also often heard from children of British parents that you were expected to know you were loved by default. The fact that you were clothed and fed negates any further responsibility to actually say the words "I love you." There are many other cultures that are resistant to being open and affectionate with their children, and those children hesitate to be open and affectionate with their children. It is hard to give to your children what you didn't get yourself, and that was the certainly the case with my mother.

Since my mother received little in the way of loving reassurance from her own family of origin, I am not surprised she wasn't equipped to give comfort to my brother and me. She was not cold or distant by any means; I just don't think she had an experience of loving closeness so had no template to show it to her sons. Her background alarm is still active to this day, and she is ninety years old!

You can't give what you didn't get, and you can't teach what you never learned. I do believe that background alarm can be ameliorated if you are seen, heard, protected, and loved by a secure attachment figure. As you'll learn in part 3 of this book, one of the ways of neutralizing your own background alarm is creating a real connection with yourself, in essence becoming the attachment figure to yourself now that you so badly needed back then.

As my mother did her best but couldn't give me the attachment and attunement she didn't get herself, the trauma of my father's illness had nothing to ameliorate it, so year after year my background alarm grew, and that fed my worries in the alarm-anxiety cycle.

Traditionally, psychiatry and psychology have attributed the lion's share of chronic worry to the mind, assuming the body has only a passive role. It is only relatively recently, with books like *The Body Keeps the Score*, that traditional disciplines have even begun to consider that something other than the mind may play a significant role in the propagation and treatment of the condition commonly referred to as chronic anxiety.

Prior to my LSD experience, I was of the same mind. For many years, I kept trying talk-type (cognitive) therapies that would address the conscious mind. I know now why these cognitive therapies weren't that effective: remedies that focus on the foreground of the mental, conscious mind are going to be of limited help when the true cause of the problem is background alarm stored in the physical, unconscious body.

With every new trauma that overwhelmed my mind's ability to process (like going through medical school, moving across the country, and getting divorced—twice), the body stored it in my solar plexus reservoir of repressed alarm, throwing it on top of the pile of all the other old, unresolved traumas. (After a divorce or two, it was getting pretty crowded in there.) It was like one of those dated, neon signs that had a flashing arrow pointing to my solar plexus saying, WE NEVER CLOSE! COME ON IN! (Incidentally, I've always thought Come On Inn would be a great name for a brothel.)

Jokes aside, not knowing how to metabolize and release these unresolved traumas from my body, the background alarm grew more and more intense as each new trauma followed the well-worn path into my solar plexus.

Those old traumas weren't resolved by cognitive therapy because they weren't centered in my mind—they were secreted away in my body.

41

Is This Plane Crashing, or Can I Get a Snack?

Have you ever wondered why some people have a more prolonged response to traumatic or anxiety-inducing situations than others? I believe that in many cases, it's because of background alarm.

For example, if you are in an aircraft experiencing severe turbulence, your fight-or-flight foreground alarm will activate. This is natural and normal.

Let's say the plane has two passengers sitting beside each other, Restless

Rusty and Stable Shirley. When the plane starts to bounce around violently, both of them experience activation of their sympathetic nervous systems. Their heart rates and blood pressure increase, their muscles and guts tense up, and their breathing becomes rapid and shallow. This is foreground alarm.

Then the plane stabilizes. The pilot comes on and says, "Sorry about that, folks. We're through the rough air and it should be smooth sailing from here." About ten minutes later, Shirley's foreground alarm has fully resolved and she is enjoying pretzels and a Coke. Rusty, on the other hand, will feel on edge and have no appetite until a few hours after the plane lands. Why?

Rusty is me, with all my old background alarm, and Shirley has no background alarm because she was raised in a securely attached home.

Background alarm can make it difficult for the body to wind down from stressful experiences, or cause worries and anxiety to appear seemingly out of nowhere at times when our physical safety is not in danger.

Perhaps you, too, have been safe and sound in a fancy hotel room, comfortable and peaceful in your bed—when seemingly out of nowhere the worries come. For me, it's usually something like "Your talk at the conference tomorrow is going to go badly." From there I start envisioning all the times I bombed onstage as a comedian, and both my background and foreground alarms flare up until it feels absolutely inevitable that the next day's talk will be a disaster.

In that comfy hotel bed, there is nothing in my environment that is in any way threatening—yet my background alarm is still with me, so my anxious mind needs to invent a story to match. This, in turn, revs up the foreground alarm—the sympathetic, fight-or-flight reaction that was in high gear earlier on my flight to get to the hotel. (Just when I was finally able to eat something!)

This is also what happens with PTSD. A soldier's mind knows he is safely back home, but his body maintains the alarm as if he is still in an active combat zone. His mind knows he is not in danger, but his body doesn't, and the body keeps the score.

Foreground alarm serves a definite purpose. If your house is on fire, you are better off getting out of the house immediately versus waiting until you've calmly finished going through your credit card bill and trying to figure out this strange charge for the Come On Inn.

But when our foreground alarm is being activated by our old background alarm and not by an actual live threat in the environment, we're trapped in the alarm-anxiety cycle. The unresolved pain from the past fires up the future fabrications of worry with no access to the sense that you are actually safe in that present moment. This was my life for many years.

But I now know the way to find safety in the present moment. Read on. And pass the pretzels.

42

Fix the Hole in the Boat

Have you ever had a thought that caused you distress and yet that very same thought hours later seemed like no threat at all, or even seemed laughable? It is very likely that in the first instance, your bodily sense of alarm was active and by the latter, it had eased. Another way of saying this is you will think the way your body feels.

For many years, I was a doctor by day, stand-up comedian by night. I can't tell you the number of times I would wake up in the morning in a panic, knowing I had a show that night and fearing I wouldn't be able to perform because I was too alarmed (although back then I would have told myself I was too anxious). All the way to my clinic and all morning, I would be dreading the evening's event, imagining the worst, and trying to come up with a plausible excuse to get out of it. However, by three that afternoon, I would often start looking forward to doing the show!

What was the difference? In the morning, my sense of alarm was up. I was in survival brain, and everything looked scary. By the afternoon, my alarm had settled and I had my rational brain back. By the time I got to the venue and was ready to go onstage, I was psyched and so grateful I was able to get up there and entertain. It was a true gift.

But the next morning, I would go through the exact same process!

Chances are you've had a similar Jekyll-and-Hyde experience with your thoughts, and it was your feeling state (alarmed or not) that determined your perception. Contrary to popular belief, it wasn't the thought itself that disturbed you; it was the state of your body and nervous system. Simply put, in a state of alarm, thoughts are perceived as painful and dangerous when they are not. You can have the same thought and have two entirely different perceptions of that thought depending on the alarm state in your body. Given this fact, the thought itself cannot be painful. It's the state and degree of alarm in your body that makes it so.

Remember—trying to fix anxious thoughts of the mind without regulating the alarm feeling in the body is both futile and exhausting, like bailing water out of a boat with a hole in the hull. Relentlessly trying to think positively and moderate the anxious thoughts is just bailing water. It may help you stay afloat, but unless you fix the source of the problem, you'll be bailing forever. Furthermore, it's exhausting to think in opposition to how you feel. If you feel alarmed, trying to bail yourself out by forcing yourself to think happy thoughts requires a tremendous amount of energy, attention, and effort, and eventually you're going to sink.

Anxious thoughts are like the water in the boat. They are the obvious sign of danger, but not the ultimate cause of the problem. The cause—the hole in the hull—is the alarm. Fix the hole and you solve the problem at its source, and you can easily stay afloat as long as you like.

It was no wonder the mind-based strategies offered by my therapists had limited effect, as I was trying to fix the problem of the sinking boat by bailing water while the hole in the hull was willfully ignored.

The take-home message is this: a worrisome thought is infinitely more likely to be believed habitually, automatically, and unconsciously when there is alarm in the system. When there is alarm in the system, the mind goes into survival mode, and that shuts down both the SES and the rational brain. It is just how we've been wired for thousands and thousands of years. Through the process of interoception the mind reads the body and makes up scary stories and worries that are perfectly consistent with the scary feeling of alarm in the body. This is the origin of worry.

There is a story about how they train military pilots. They put them in a room and have them sort cards into piles of black and red while the oxygen is withdrawn from the room. As the oxygen drops lower and lower, the pilots experience different symptoms. Some will get a tingling in their hands, others will get a headache, and others will become nauseated. The pilots are trained to be keenly aware of their personal response to hypoxia (low oxygen in the blood), and once they sense that particular symptom they are told to automatically and expressly, without thinking, flip their oxygen mask over their face. Putting on oxygen had to be instantaneous and automatic, because the brain impairment from low oxygen would soon prevent them from realizing they were losing oxygen!

Some pilots, instead of flipping their oxygen masks on, try to figure out what the problem might be and in the process become so hypoxic they fall unconscious. Failing to recognize this hypoxia has led to catastrophe.

In a way, we worriers do an analogous thing. We try to fix our thinking when our brains are impaired by the alarm in the body. Failing to understand that the worries themselves are not the problem, we busily try to fix our thinking while the alarm builds in our system and zaps our ability to see and fix the real underlying problem: the increasing alarm in our body.

When we decrease the alarm in our body, the mind moves out of the surviving/emotional brain and into the thriving/rational brain. When the alarm is removed from the system, we move back into the rational prefrontal cortex and reengage the SES to both increase the mind's ability to critically appraise thoughts and to create a soothing connection with others (and ourselves).

In the morning of my shift at my medical clinic, I was in alarm and my thoughts about the stand-up gig after work mirrored that alarm ("What if I am so anxious I can't think and I blank onstage?"). Once the alarm dissipated, I got my rational mind back. I could see and feel the positive aspects of performing, I knew it would probably be fun, and it (almost) always was!

Imagine I am going to teach you how to ride a unicycle. You'll need a clear, unimpaired mind to learn this new skill. Now imagine I give you five shots of tequila and try to teach you how to ride that unicycle. While you may retain some of the skill of riding the one-wheeler, you would be able to perform much better if your mind were unimpaired by the silver sombrero sauce. You would be better off going home, sobering up, and trying again tomorrow without the alcohol.

In the same way, you are better off clearing the impairment (alarm) from your system first before working on the skill of dealing with your thoughts. When your system is hijacked by alarm (just like with alcohol or low oxygen), you lose the ability to rationally examine your thoughts because the rational part of your brain has been taken offline. The first goal is to clear the impairment in your body (the alarm), and then we can go after the thoughts and worries.

> **Point to consider:** Begin to localize a sense of alarm in your body when you are caught up in the worries of your mind.

43

Alarm Is the New Anxiety

We all know that forty is the new thirty and orange is the new black. Well, I have a new one for you: alarm is the new anxiety.

At that 2015 anxiety conference in Vancouver, British Columbia (a bunch of nervous people in a room, remember?), where I first heard Neufeld say that all anxiety is separation anxiety, it was the first time I heard the term "alarm" used to refer to the state associated with anxiety.

Like that moment where, under the influence of psychedelics, I'd been able to see the separation between thought/feeling and mind/body, this was also a moment that created the "refill on my perception" I mentioned at the start of this book. When I heard the word "alarm" used that way, my mind started to race with excitement.

What if this painful sensation I had in my solar plexus was the manifestation of alarm? What if this alarm held emotional energy that could not be contained upstairs in the mind? What if the anxious thoughts of the mind were adding to or aggravating the alarm in the body? What if the alarm in the body somehow created worrisome thoughts of the mind to be consistent with the uncomfortable feeling of alarm in the body? What if each charged the other? If the anxious thoughts of the mind and the alarm in the body could be separated, would that break the cycle?

I had so many questions—and maybe by now, you can see in that moment how the entire premise of this book began to take shape in my mind. The shift in seeing that my emotional pain could be more a function of my feeling body versus my thinking mind was an absolute revelation that made me start thinking about my condition in a brand-new way.

I've come to understand that alarm and its by-product, anxiety, almost always result from a break in the perception of safety during childhood—from a deep experience of being isolated or separated, usually from our parents or caregivers. When we are separated from our attachment figures, either physically or emotionally, our bodies go into a state of alarm. (As a bit of foreshadowing, when we become critical and judgmental of ourselves that also creates a split from within that also generates alarm.)

Gordon Neufeld has been one of my greatest influences and mentors. While the alarm-anxiety theory is my own, and my view of alarm is different from his, I could not have come up with my path to healing without the information I obtained from his teachings. Since that conference, I have come to see clearly that virtually all mental illness has its roots in childhood, and understanding a child's psychological development (or lack thereof) holds the clues to treatment and recovery.

In those of us without childhood wounding, there is only foreground alarm, the natural reaction of the sympathetic nervous system. In those of us with unresolved trauma from childhood, we have both the regular, acute, fight-or-flight foreground alarm and chronic background alarm. As a result, our alarm reaction is likely to come up twice as fast and resolve twice as slowly. This is why it took Rusty hours to be able to eat anything after the turbulence settled while Shirley was enjoying a Coke and pretzels only ten minutes later.

Remember, foreground alarm is logical and functional in the sense that it responds to an identifiable, justifiable cause. But what if we start feeling a tense gut, dry mouth, muscular tension, and a flushed sensation when there is no obvious danger? What if your body is reacting as if you're facing a dragon when you're just lying in bed or heading out to watch a movie with your partner? The background alarm in your body is the likely culprit, as it can activate the foreground alarm at seemingly random times. This is why we can feel significantly alarmed and anxious for absolutely no apparent reason. This is because we are not living in what is happening *now*, our amygdala and insula have transported us the stress in our bodies we felt back *then*.

Panic attacks are a classic example of background alarm that we are not consciously aware of, suddenly and violently activating the fight-or-flight reaction of foreground alarm. Panic attacks feel exquisitely more frightening and disorienting precisely because there is no obvious reason for the panic. It is excruciating when you are attacked by an extreme state of foreground alarm completely out of the blue.

The mind's response to this acute state of alarm is to make up a story that is consistent with the intensity of the alarm you feel. In a panic attack, your thoughts jump very suddenly from being nervous about going to a party where you won't know anyone, to thoughts like "What if I'm having a heart attack?" or "What if I'm having a stroke?"

But it gets worse.

Because we are in a state of alarm and our brains are in survival mode, we've lost access to our rational mind. Since we can't reassure ourselves that we are probably not having a heart attack or a stroke, we believe the doomsday thoughts, and this plunges our bodies even deeper into alarm. As we lose whatever ability for rational thought we had, the mind creates horror stories that the body defenselessly believes and reacts to. Panic attacks are devastating at the time they occur, and what is almost worse is the fear of having another. Until ayahuasca and LSD, the acute fear of a rising panic attack was the worst fear I had ever experienced.

(As an aside, and this may sound ludicrous to you, I actually enjoy panic attacks now. I embrace the rush and don't get caught in the victim mentality and belief of my thoughts that allows panic attacks to escalate.)

Although I don't have the space in this book to specifically go into how to approach panic attacks, if they are something that afflicts you, I do have a video on my YouTube channel, *The Anxiety MD,* that addresses how to specifically teach yourself how to neutralize panic attacks.

When we have childhood trauma, the mind will minimize uncertainty at all costs. So using the panic attack example, given the choice, the mind will make you believe that you are dying of a heart attack or stroke rather than just leaving the reason for the extreme reaction in your body uncertain. Said another way, the mind creates (and needs) worry to explain alarm and decrease the pain of uncertainty.

Everyone's mind makes up stories to make sense of feelings. But we worriers have scaring the sh** out of ourselves down to an art form.

Although we typically describe foreground alarm as a fight-or-flight reaction (i.e., the impulse to run away), I return to Neufeld's concept of pursuit. I believe the sympathetic nervous system's activation of foreground alarm is to provide energy for a state of pursuit to reconnect to a safe attachment figure. If we look back to early childhood, any type of danger that would have caused foreground alarm would cause us to retreat not just away from the barking dog or the hot stove but toward our caregiver in search of protection and comfort. Recall how my alarm in childhood stemmed from a desire to reconnect with my dad when he was lost in his illness—it was motivated by pursuit. And when that pursuit failed to create a connection, a great deal of alarm got created and stuffed down into my little body.

Alarm-based pursuit, as a reaction to real or perceived separation, is an automatic human response that seeks to reconnect us with our attachment figures. The example of a child who loses his parents in a store illustrates this principle. Rather than fight or flight, the child directs his foreground alarm energy into pursuit, desperately trying to find his parents and reconnect to his secure attachment figures. If the pursuit fails and despite best efforts the child remains separate from their source of security, the child eventually gives up and will often lapse into a freeze state. The longer the child stays in freeze with no resolution, the more alarm is created and stored in that child's body.

When I was young, this pursuit scenario played out in a less direct way between my father and me. Up until age twelve, I was very close to my father. Through my early teens, he became mentally ill and I would experience threats that would trigger my foreground alarm. But instead of fight or flight, I would move into pursuit in an attempt to connect with him. As his episodes of mental instability were time-limited, once he started to become more lucid and we reattached, my pursuit would eventually be rewarded. I would reconnect with him, my foreground alarm would fade, I would come out of freeze, and stop stockpiling alarm in my body.

However, as I got into my middle- to late-teen years, he would plunge deeper into mental illness and stay there longer. My pursuit would still activate, but as my father became more incapacitated and the episodes lasted longer, he would stay unreachable and there came a point when I felt pursuit was futile and I would stay frozen without resolution for longer. Without connection, my foreground alarm would not resolve and then turn into freeze, and in the freeze state the energy would be dumped into my solar plexus as background alarm.

I understand now that when pursuit did not end up in reattachment— when my efforts to reconnect were thwarted—without a way to resolve this uncertainty and disconnection, my mind became overwhelmed and my acute foreground alarm morphed into chronic background alarm. When the connection was lost and I could find no way of getting it back, it became too much for my mind to bear, and I went into freeze (or dorsal vagal shutdown in polyvagal theory terms; more on PVT in part 3), so the energy was packaged up and shipped off to my body, where it was stored "out of sight, out of mind" as background alarm.

My father was ill, off and on, from the time I was a teen until he died when I was twenty-six. As I got older and more jaded, with every bipolar or schizophrenic episode he would have, my system would abandon the futile pursuit more quickly and just pour the trauma directly into my body, adding to the reservoir of background alarm that I already held in my solar plexus.

You too may have tried to connect with your parent when your foreground alarm was activated until you saw it was futile, as I did. As children, if our foreground alarm was activated and our pursuit reaction failed to resolve the disconnection, the emotional trauma would likely spill over into our body and get stored as a background alarm. The more times pursuit was futile, the more background alarm was added.

Returning to Freud's concept of repression, the pain of the trauma of being unable to connect to a pursued parent would be too much for the child's mind to bear. As a result, the energy would be exiled from the mind and buried in the body as background alarm.

Remember Jane, my patient who repeatedly picked abusive alcoholics as partners? I can't know for sure, of course, but it is very likely that when Jane was a little girl she felt pursuit energy and tried to connect with her alcoholic father when he was drunk. There probably came a point when Jane felt that pursuing him was futile and stored the pain of that disconnection as background alarm. As an adult, Jane's choice of partners helped her mind make sense of her body's background alarm by replicating the familiar dynamics from her childhood—including the pursuit energy of trying and failing to connect with her alcoholic father.

Perhaps you had a similar story with one or both of your parents? A perception that you were no longer connected? Perhaps your parent was the cause of your feeling that you weren't safe?

Maybe your parent was an addict and you would "lose" them to alcohol or workaholism or some other addiction, or maybe your parent neglected or abandoned or abused you. In any of these events your inability to gain their comfort and safety would create a considerable amount of background alarm in your body.

If you struggle with anxiety, it is highly likely that you have a version of this background alarm state smoldering in your system—and it's likely to be from a time in your life when you were frozen in emotional pain and separated from your attachment figures and you weren't able to close the gap.

Unresolved trauma does not have to be chronic or repeated to generate background alarm. Acute episodes of overwhelm, especially in childhood, can most certainly create significant background alarm. I have had many patients ask me if a discrete incident can create background alarm, and the answer is an emphatic yes!

Acute trauma that is too much for the mind to bear, like an episode of emotional, physical, or sexual abuse; the death of someone important to us; or an episode of abandonment or rejection by someone we love can also overwhelm the mind and deposit background alarm in the body. My own experience of unresolvable trauma was chronic, but any childhood trauma, acute or chronic, that isn't resolved with love and attention from a caregiver will overwhelm the mind and deposit as background alarm in the body.

> **Point to consider:** It may be that females secrete more oxytocin during the stress response than males do, and this oxytocin may be responsible for females trying to pursue and attach to the alarming person more tenaciously than males. This may be why females stay in relationship with challenging or abusive people more than males do.

44

The Tuna Lady

When I was a med student on my psych rotation, circa 1990, I had a patient I called the Tuna Lady. She was a little older than me, at the time about thirty-five, and she reminded me of a young Sally Field. She was admitted to the hospital for severe anxiety. She was experiencing mild swelling around her ankles and had read (there was no Google back then) that ankle swelling was a sign of protein deficiency. She had decided that protein deficiency was also the cause of her anxiety, and it became all she could talk about. In a five-minute conversation, she used the word "protein" about a hundred times. Every time I saw her, she asked me how she could get more protein.

She was not psychotic, but she was fixated and clearly alarmed.

In an attempt to reassure her, I did a blood test that showed her serum protein (albumin) was actually in the high end of the normal range. I showed her the results, but it made no difference to her. She insisted that before her blood was drawn for the test, she had just finished eating a full can of tuna, and that is why the level had come out okay. I told her that protein levels are stable over days to weeks and do not change quickly, and that she could eat twelve cans of tuna and it wouldn't alter the results of the test.

In hindsight, this was the exact wrong thing to say to the Tuna Lady. She had been having her friends bring in cans of tuna and she was eating about three cans a day, so saying she could up the ante to twelve cans a day and it still wouldn't make much difference was probably one of the dumbest things I have ever said to a patient. She even asked the nurses if they could mix the tuna with cream in a blender, if her friends brought one in for her. (Incidentally, the blender request is when I gave her the official designation as the Tuna Lady.)

She was alarmed, and her mind looked for why. Since nothing was obviously wrong with her, other than some very mild ankle swelling, she drew the false conclusion that she was protein deficient and the lack of protein was making her anxious. With this conclusion, her mind had a "good" reason to explain her emotional state. But the more she worried about her protein intake, the more alarmed she got, which made her eat tuna in quantities comparable to an open-ocean barracuda. She was caught in a loop of creating a story in her mind to explain the alarm she felt in her body. It may seem like an extreme example, but I can relate. My own mind, on multiple occasions, has come up with its own hypochondriacal and irrational fixations that would rival the Tuna Lady's obsession with her protein levels. How about you?

Why are we so irrational? Why couldn't the Tuna Lady understand her protein level was completely normal and not in any way responsible for her alarm and anxiety?

Because worry has a purpose. When people say worry is useless, I disagree. Worry distracts us up into our heads and specifically away from the background alarm we store in our bodies.

If you have unresolved emotional traumas you probably have chronic (background) alarm, although you may not be consciously aware of an alarm reaction in your body. What you may be more aware of is fatigue, brain fog, or worry. I know that for many years, I wasn't aware of the background alarm in my chest and solar plexus, but I was definitely aware of the chronically anxious thoughts.

Because the activation in my youth was chronic and perpetually anticipatory (I worried about my father going crazy much more than he actually was crazy), I created a general feeling of always being unsafe, and this both added to my background alarm and made it impossible to resolve.

One of the favorite tricks of background alarm is to hide behind worry. If the worry is powerful enough, we don't even consider looking anywhere else for the source of our pain.

To illustrate how background alarm works, I like to tell the story about the smoke detector in the kitchen of my condo in Vancouver. That smoke detector was hyperreactive. Even the tiniest amount of smoke when I was cooking would set it off. In fact, it would also be set off by steam or by dust I stirred up—for example, while sanding my wooden countertops or even just dusting the tops of the cupboards. Sometimes it would give a quick blast in the middle of the night for no reason at all.

My background alarm in my solar plexus is like my jumpy smoke detector. It is always ready to react with a blast at the slightest provocation.

Perhaps the worst part of background alarm is that it creates an environment where we don't feel safe, even though in reality we *are* safe. The message of background alarm comes from childhood: "Stay vigilant; danger is always present." My background alarm kept me in a state of readiness, taut at the starting line for a race that wouldn't begin for another year or two.

I had unconsciously begun to equate this familiar state of activation or hypervigilance (aka my background alarm) with keeping me safe. Actually, nothing could be further from the truth—but in my child mind, I associated this feeling of vigilance with protection. Now I was really screwed, because I'd become afraid *not* to be alarmed.

In other words, I had stopped trusting safety.

I'll talk about victim mentality in more detail later, but perhaps you're starting to see how this constant vigilance and looking out for trouble puts us in victim mode. In a self-fulfilling prophecy, we victimize ourselves by constantly seeking out confirmation that our fears are valid by worrying, while at the very same time ignoring cues of safety. If this sounds like a bad deal, it is. This is yet another example of accepting the certainty of misery over the misery of uncertainty.

It's like the old joke about a twenty-year-old woman who goes to her doctor every year convinced she has cancer. Every year, for forty-nine years, the doctor reassures her that she is perfectly healthy. When she goes in for her annual checkup at seventy, her doctor says, "I have some bad news. It looks like you have cancer," and she shouts, "*I told you so!*"

Like foreground alarm, background alarm does carry a physiological and emotional signature (mine is in my solar plexus). With foreground alarm—in the presence of an acute threat—there is an intense, all-over reaction. Heart rate and blood pressure increase, blood flow is directed to the extremities and away from the gut, the muscles tense up.

With foreground alarm, the cause is obvious and the reaction is supposed to be acute and short-lived. If another car cuts you off in traffic and you narrowly avoid an accident, there is no need to ruminate about the other driver's lack of skills or manners; you should breathe a sigh of relief and just move on with your day.

As I got into my late teens and early twenties, whenever my alarm faded and I moved into a period where I felt calmer and let down my guard and stopped worrying so much, the old fear of being blindsided came up and snapped me right back into alarm. This is why it's common to have an anxiety attack just when we start to feel safe—because feeling safe in childhood was often demolished by the next household upheaval. Feeling relaxed reminds us of a time before when we felt safe but it turned out we weren't. It leaves us vulnerable. When I let down my guard in October and my dad got sick in November, I would feel blindsided. So I stayed with the certainty of maintaining my background alarm, because part of me perceived it was protecting me. Like the woman who shouted "I told you so!" to her doctor, I used my father's (anticipated) illness as a reason to maintain my constant alarm.

In a similar fashion, the Tuna Lady was in a deep state of background alarm stored in her body from her own (many) childhood traumas. The bottom line was she was not consciously aware of her background alarm in her body, but she sure felt it. Further, the painful energy and uncertainty of the background alarm feeling that she could not define made her seek certainty and definition in the story that she had a protein deficiency. The irrational story got even more irrational when her impaired rational mind convinced her that tuna milkshakes were the answer to her problems, when the true source of her pain was the background alarm stored in her body some thirty years earlier.

This is a classic example of the alarm-anxiety cycle in action. We worriers believe the worry is the reason for our current pain, when those fearful stories are just smoke screens that prevent us from seeing the true source, the deeper background alarm stored in us decades ago. Further, one of the most damaging parts of worry is that we need to make those worries so scary to keep us up in our minds today, because otherwise we might fall down into the background alarm stored in our bodies from yesterday. Returning for a moment to my hyperreactive smoke detector, you might wonder why I didn't just replace it. 1) I am lazy, and 2) I grew attached to my little smoke detector. I had a kinship with it. I understood it. I knew what it was like to have a hair trigger and to react to little things like they were big things. I also knew what it was like to wake up in a panic in the middle of the night. I saw my little misfiring smoke detector as myself. I wasn't going to toss it away; I was going to care for it.

There's a reason I'm telling you this. Taking care of the smoke detector instead of tossing it is a metaphor for how to relate to our background alarm. You'll soon see that it's much better to care for your alarm than to try to get rid of it!

> **Point to consider:** I wish I could have shown the smoke detector the "I Am Safe in this Moment" tool in the Anxiety Toolkit, so it didn't have to blast me in the middle of the night for no reason!

45

When Making Sense Doesn't Make Sense

When I tell people I'm a doctor and anxiety specialist, just about everyone tells me they have a child, partner, parent, close friend, relative, or tuna lady who struggles with it. They will often tell me they don't know how to support them, and they have a hard time understanding what they are going through.

I remember my dentist, Angela, asking me about her daughter, Jenny, as Jenny had recently shown signs of what Angela called anxiety. Angela had very amicably divorced from Jenny's father three years earlier, and Jenny seemed okay for the first couple of years. Angela and her ex had agreed to have Jenny and her brother stay at the family home while the parents would take turns looking after the kids, with each parent spending one week living at the house and then one week staying elsewhere. It seemed to be going okay until, about two years into this arrangement, Jenny, then sixteen, began having panic attacks, issues with eating, insomnia, and mood swings. Angela had never really experienced anxiety herself and said she wanted to understand what Jenny was going through but felt completely lost.

I asked Angela if she had ever been frightened for her life. She confided in me: years earlier she had undergone a biopsy for cancer. Her family doctor had told her that the tissue he could palpate was suspicious for cancer, and the biopsy results would take five days to come back.

She told me for those five days she couldn't eat or sleep and was "full of anxiety."

I told her, instead of calling it anxiety, she should more correctly say she was full of *alarm* for those five days. Angela told me that referring to what she felt as alarm felt more resonant to her. (Indeed, people generally tell me when they start calling their emotional pain alarm instead of anxiety, it feels much more resonant and authentic.) Angela asked me if the alarmed feeling she had experienced in those five days could be what her daughter was experiencing now.

It was a light-bulb moment for Angela, as for the first time she had a real sense of what her daughter was going through. For the first time, Angela wasn't dealing with the concept of anxiety as a label with little resonance or meaning. She could relate to the feeling sense of the alarmed state she had experienced in her own body while waiting for her biopsy results. As I told Angela, although many people don't experience anxiety regularly, everyone has experienced alarm.

Once Angela could relate her daughter's experience to her own, she had a better understanding, but there were some specific differences. Using the terms we've gone over in this book, we can say that Angela was experiencing foreground alarm because she had a distinct and direct cause for that alarm—the biopsy results. In contrast, what her daughter was experiencing was likely originating from background alarm because Jenny had trouble pinpointing the source of her pain. Jenny had convinced herself that she was fine with her week-on, week-off parents. She was even proud of the way the family was "staying connected," but clearly the divorce of her parents was traumatic for her, and because she resisted dealing with it consciously, the energy got buried in her as background alarm. It was this background alarm that was feeding Jenny's anxieties, disordered eating, and panic attacks.

One of the most alarming (forgive the pun) things about background alarm is that we are clearly in fight or flight in our body without an obvious reason in our mind. We feel distinctly unsafe, but there is nothing we can put our finger on that supports that threat in our surroundings. I have heard this anxiety described as "fear without eyes," and that makes sense to me. This is why panic attacks can be so difficult. If we were looking over the rail of a balcony on the forty-ninth floor of a high-rise and our body went into alarm, that would make sense, and it would be an appropriate reaction. Our body and our mind would be in sync at the potential threat of falling, so there would be no confusion as to why our body was so activated.

But with anxiety and panic attacks, our bodies are acting like we are about to bungee jump when we are just sitting in a coffee shop, watching a movie in a theater, or waiting in line at the bank. (Except if you're waiting in line at the bank with the intention to rob it. Then you would have a good reason for the alarm in your body. But most of you reading this book aren't likely to be bank robbers. And if you are a bank robber, that's probably because you experienced trauma as a child that is still alive in you and creating background alarm—so please keep reading this book, and maybe once you get out of prison you can live a productive life without chronic worry.)

The Tuna Lady, whom you met in the last chapter, existed in this state of dissonance where her internal state was out of sync with the external environment. In her admission history, she told me her parents had split when she was eight years old. Her father disappeared and she had to live with her abusive mother. It is no wonder, with that degree of childhood trauma, that she had significant bouts of becoming alarmed and irrationally fixated on elaborate worries, with some episodes requiring hospitalization. I saw a woman in her prime with mental illness robbing her of her life. But because her body was held frozen in the alarm of a traumatized eight-year-old, her mind believed that consuming tuna like a great white shark was going to cure a protein deficiency she did not have.

When people experience a similar environment to what created their background alarm, their amygdala lights up like a Christmas tree (holiday trauma, anyone?), and they often dissociate and regress to a confused and irrational younger state. When triggered, we regress to the emotional age and coping skills we had at the time of the original trauma. This is why the holidays can age-regress us back into a scared six-year-old, with all the emotional volatility and coping skills of a scared six-year-old (more in part 3).

When our background alarm is feeding into worries that then feed into more alarm, we can say that "making sense doesn't make sense." There's a mismatch between our internal state and what we see around us. Irrational worries and panic attacks are our mind's attempt to match our inner world with our outer world.

When we have alarm in our system, if our minds cannot find a rational reason for that alarm, they will simply make one up, and the younger we were when the original trauma(s) occurred, the more irrational those worries tend to be. It is amazing what we can convince ourselves to believe, but we can understand our irrationality a little better when we see it is coming from our six-year-old self and not the present-day adult. More on this later, but we should not judge ourselves as irrational adults when we are deep in alarm, because in many respects we have regressed back to our childhood pain, we just aren't aware of it. And when you can't see it you will be it.

When we focus on resolving the alarm in the body, we don't need to create elaborate fears of protein deficiencies that can only be resolved with three tuna milkshakes per day. A bit of foreshadowing here, but when we heal the alarmed child in us, we regain our rational brain so we can return to a capable and resilient adult. At the end of her three-week stay on the psych ward, with her alarm significantly calmed, the Tuna Lady told me she was embarrassed by her tuna fixation and by her invention of the tuna milkshake, which hasn't seemed to have caught on. If I could talk to the Tuna Lady today, I'd tell her not to be embarrassed, as her mind was profoundly impaired by revisiting a deep state of background alarm that began when she was an abandoned and frightened eight-year-old. So, dear Tuna Lady, if you are reading this book, thirty-five years after your admission to St. Joseph's Hospital in London, know that you made a profound impression on me, and I sincerely hope you're okay.

Point to consider: What is the "tuna" in your life? What irrational fear did the child in you create?

46

Foreground and Background Alarm

Foreground alarm and background alarm are man-made inventions (made by me, a man) and as such, they cannot explain everything perfectly, especially since feelings, by their very nature, are difficult to capture in words.

Still, the two alarms explain quite a lot about anxiety and how to heal it, and thus it's worth understanding them in more depth.

A few key points in review:

- Background alarm can be localized in one area, while foreground alarm is a body-wide activation.
- Background alarm isn't in everyone, but it is in those of us with unresolved trauma.
- Foreground alarm often responds to an observable (new) event, but can also be activated by our thoughts and worries.
- Background alarm and foreground alarm form a feedback loop. The more the two systems are activated together, the more likely they are to "wire" together and continue activating together in

the future—and if you had a particularly traumatic childhood, your foreground alarm and your background alarm were frequent table tennis opponents.

- Think of two tuning forks that vibrate at the same frequency. If you hit one and put it beside the other, both will start to vibrate, even though one wasn't physically touched.
- Background alarm can be triggered by experiences similar to the ones that first created it, which often then trigger foreground alarm, which retriggers background alarm in a feedback loop.
- Background alarm generates a survival state in the mind via interoception and foreground alarm, and that state creates worries, which activates background alarm. This is the alarm-anxiety cycle.

As I've said before, if you've read any of Eckhart Tolle's books, he refers to something called the *pain body*, a kind of amalgamation of pain and trauma that human beings carry within them, both from their own life experiences and from the traumas of their close and distant ancestors. What I call background alarm is directly analogous to what Tolle calls the pain body, but my definition is more personal. While we all carry trauma from our ancestors, background alarm is more unique to our own personal experience. This is not to say that we can't absorb some background alarm from our parents and ancestors (I believe I carry alarm from both my mother and my father and further back), but the more trauma we do not neutralize as children in this lifetime, the more it accumulates in our (pain) body, and subsequently, the more worries it creates in our mind.

One thing to note about background alarm is that individual levels vary not just based on one's experiences but based on one's temperament or personality. Some children seem to experience trauma and metabolize it without moving it into long-term storage in the body as background alarm. This has to do with the severity and frequency of trauma and with the presence (or absence) of adults to help them process it, but also with the child's own disposition—sensitive or less sensitive. This is one of the reasons we shouldn't compare our trauma to others' and assume because we had it "easier" we should be less affected. Your feelings are real and valid. There is not some arbitrary amount of background alarm you should have based on what you have experienced. The amount you have is what is there—and it can be healed.

I once had a patient, Brian, who was what we sometimes call an alpha male, an athletic and muscular lawyer in his late thirties. On vacation, he met Marta, a vivacious and beautiful redhead who was almost fifteen years his junior. It was love at first sight. They had a long-distance relationship for about a year, and then she moved to be with him and they got married. Marta became a patient of mine as well, and I envied their relationship in a way.

But things are not always as they seem.

When I asked Brian at one of his yearly physicals, "How's married life?" I expected a glowing response, but instead, his face became pained. Brian told me all was well when they were traveling to see each other, but once she moved in with him and they got married, things started to change. Brian was very active in the law society and would often have responsibilities that kept him away from home. He said Marta would often become angry when he had to go out at night, and that would escalate into fits of rage if he had to travel without her. I found this a little hard to believe. Marta was smart, funny, and appeared very self-assured. I couldn't picture her flying off the handle with rage. But Brian told me of many times that Marta would completely "lose it" and throw things at him and even physically hit him when he would need to go somewhere without her. This didn't happen every time he had to leave, but often enough that he needed to "walk on eggshells" when he approached the subject of going out.

During an appointment with Marta, I didn't ask about the rage specifically, but I did ask her about her childhood. She told me that both her parents were alcoholics. She said she and her younger brother were always clothed and fed, their physical needs looked after, but after 6 P.M., "the booze came first."

Knowing this, I could clearly see why Marta would revert back to the attitude of an irate six-year-old when Brian left. It triggered her amygdala and evoked the same feelings in her body (likely via the insula) that she felt when her parents abandoned her in favor of alcohol.

So it wasn't what Brian was doing now that was the cause of her alarm and rage; it was what her parents had done when she was young. She was regressing back to the little girl who had no idea why her parents left her every night. She had needed her parents to reassure her and diffuse her alarm, but they were the ones causing the alarm by choosing the rye whiskey over her and her brother. Marta had transferred the childhood rage at her parents to present-day Brian. This is a classic example of background alarm in action.

Remember that a response driven by background alarm is not about what is happening in this moment; it is an age regression, and you will not fix the root of the problem by only addressing the foreground alarm of today. Brian trying to reason with Marta about how he had to travel to keep his job would have been a useless strategy because his rational story could not penetrate her irrational, alarm-driven mind. Again, the root cause of Marta's reaction was not what Brian was doing now, but what Marta's parents did back *then*. It had nothing to do with the underlying problem. Similarly, taking deep breaths, doing qigong or yoga, or inhaling essential oils will calm your foreground alarm—and that does reduce the intensity of background alarm and help to break the feedback loop—but for a lasting solution, you must address the true source of the problem, your background alarm. You must stop bailing water out of the boat and instead focus on patching the hole in the hull. More on healing background alarm in part 3.

47

The Autonomic Nervous System: The Engine of the Unconscious Power of Alarm

I've touched briefly on the sympathetic (fight or flight) and parasympathetic (rest and digest) nervous systems, but now I want to go deeper. When I talk to patients about the autonomic nervous system, I often substitute the word "automatic" for "autonomic." This is an easy way to

THE AUTONOMIC NERVOUS SYSTEM

PARASYMPATHETIC NERVES	SYMPATHETIC NERVES
"Rest and Digest"	"Fight or Flight"

Constrict pupils

Dilate pupils

Stimulate saliva

Inhibit salivation

Slow heartbeat

Increase heartbeat

Relaxed "belly" breathing

Tense, upper chest breathing

Relaxed muscles

Tensed muscles

Stimulate activity of stomach

Inhibit activity of stomach

Stimulate activity of intestines

Inhibit activity of intestines

Secrete epinephrine and norepinephrine

remember what this system does using a word we all know. To review, the autonomic nervous system controls heart rate, blood pressure, gut motility and digestion, and many other functions of the body that aren't under our conscious control—and therefore seem to happen automatically.

In the diagram above, the autonomic nervous system (ANS) has two components: the sympathetic nervous system, often referred to as the accelerator because it revs us up, and the parasympathetic nervous system, which we can call the brake because it calms us down. As a review, sympathetic = fight or flight, and parasympathetic = rest and digest.

When one side is activated, the other side is deactivated but never completely "off." One is up at any given time and the other down, like a seesaw. For example, if you've just finished a big meal and you're at home watching a movie, you're probably feeling safe and relaxed, with your parasympathetic rest-and-digest nervous system dominant. But then your daughter runs into the house and tells you your son has fallen out of a tree in the yard and may have broken his arm. (Aren't you glad I didn't say bitten by a dog?)

When this happens, you quickly flip into sympathetic activity. Your heart rate and blood pressure increase, your muscles tense up, and your breathing gets faster. You rush outside and assess the situation. As you talk with him and comfort him, you conclude that his bone probably isn't broken and he seems to be more emotionally stunned than physically injured. After about twenty minutes, as you become more certain he'll be okay, your body's sympathetic response fades. Parasympathetic activity takes over again, and you move back into rest and digest as you return to your movie, and you and Shirley go back to your Cokes and pretzels.

A normally calibrated ANS rises quickly to a challenge and then calms down quickly when the challenge resolves. This on/off regulation is mediated by our experiences—and when we generally feel safe and connected during childhood, our autonomic nervous system develops with proper seesaw-type on/off calibration. Fight-or-flight foreground alarm activates in the presence of a threat, and this smoothly moves into parasympathetic activity once the threat resolves.

That's how it's supposed to work, anyway. But remember Restless Rusty and Stable Shirley. When traumatic experiences in our youth have taught us that it's best to stay on high alert, we have a hard time settling down. In those of us with background alarm, the sympathetic nervous system (foreground alarm) stays activated for much longer than is necessary or healthy. In a way to think about it, background alarm never really completely takes its foot off the accelerator part of our automatic nervous system, and it's also ready to floor it at any inkling of real or imagined danger.

This reminds me of a story. Two monks accidentally walk into the Come On Inn and see Jackhammer Johnson . . . no, sorry, wrong story. Two monks were walking together, returning to the monastery after a long day of monking. It was the rainy season, and they saw a woman having trouble crossing a creek. One of the monks approached her, gently picked her up, and transferred her safely to the other side. The monks continued their journey in silence. They had taken a vow never to touch a woman and after hours of walking in silence, one angrily said to the other, "You know we are not to touch women. Why did you pick that woman up?" The other monk said, "Oh, I put her down hours ago. Clearly, you are still carrying her."

I was still carrying the foreground alarm from the turbulence. Shirley had put it down well before the plane even landed. Those of us carrying background alarm have a slower resolution of foreground alarm as they stubbornly potentiate each other.

I've never really been good at resting or digesting. I've rarely felt grounded enough to move deeply into parasympathetic mode. Even when I did make conscious attempts at relaxation, it was like trying to offer a large, frightened dog a piece of meat. (Again with the dogs, can you tell I live with three of them?) You want the dog to relax and take the meat, but it could turn bad in an instant, so you need to stay vigilant. This kind of acute and prolonged sympathetic nervous system activation, with slow resolution, is a very common pattern for people with old, unresolved trauma stored in the body as background alarm. For those of us with unresolved trauma, our foreground alarm is like a coiled spring, suspended in limbo by background alarm and constantly ready to stomp on the gas of our sympathetic nervous system.

Have you ever had the experience of anxiety making you lose your appetite? This is your sympathetic nervous system in action. As blood flow is diverted from your digestive system to your tensed-up muscles, the intestines grind to a halt—and your body rejects food when it senses it can't move through.

Another hallmark of sympathetic nervous system activation is adrenaline, also known as epinephrine. This is what primes your muscles with energy to fire and carry you away from whatever is threatening your survival. From an evolutionary perspective, for this system to be activated quickly and easily was lifesaving. When in doubt, it was better to assume danger than assume safety. If you assumed the crack in the reeds behind you was a predator and you ran, you had a better chance of survival than if you just assumed it was nothing and stayed obliviously munching on your berries and grubs. A hair-trigger adrenaline fight-or-flight response may have saved many of our ancestors from perishing—but in the process, natural selection was favoring nervous and paranoid humans to pass a sensitive (or even hyperreactive) temperament down the genetic line.

(As a little aside, in my informal polling of my hypervigilant patients, I've found that the vast majority hate scary movies. I know I do. I already have an oversensitive nervous system that makes me jump—I don't need more of that!)

One of the reasons exercise is so helpful to calm us is that muscular activity helps metabolize the adrenaline that would otherwise stay circulating in our systems, maintaining a sense of agitation and hypervigilance. Adrenaline feeds both foreground and background alarm. Since we chronic worriers can fire up our whole system with only the thought of danger (aka worry), we often have too much adrenaline running around for no viable reason. Thousands of years ago, when humans faced a physical threat, the sympathetic nervous system would fire up and help them fight or flee. This physical activity would metabolize the adrenaline, leaving them ready to stand down in parasympathetic mode once the threat was gone. Today, since we aren't running off our adrenaline like we did thousands of years ago, it stays in our system and maintains both foreground and background alarm. Further, we can become addicted to the adrenaline and dopamine we get from worrying and compulsively make more of it! Remember when I said addiction is when you can't get enough of what you don't want? We get a dopamine hit from worry when we believe we are on the right track of making the uncertain more certain, and that can become addictive. Neurochemically, dopamine, adrenaline, and noradrenaline are in the same chemical family called the catecholamines and they are highly tuned to the sympathetic nervous system that runs our foreground alarm.

In addition, there is evidence that the brain's natural painkillers, endorphins and enkephalins, are released from the periaqueductal gray matter in the brainstem during worry and panic, potentially increasing our attraction to worry. There are good neurological reasons why it's so hard to stop worrying!

48

Game Drive: How the Alarm System Works in Real Life

I remember being on a game drive in South Africa in 2003. On these safaris, you go out twice a day, dawn and dusk, in an open-air Land Rover. There is a guide who drives the vehicle, and he has a rifle in a sun-bleached leather sling that appears to be glued onto the hood. I imagine this rifle is to protect the tourists from the animals, but this particular gun looked like it was from the Boer War of 1902 and had yet to be fired in the current millennium. The Land Rover we were in was more modern, maybe from the Korean War of 1953.

On the day of our excursion, a pride of lions had been spotted by some other guides, and we were driving to the lions' last seen location, about five kilometers away. I had never seen lions in the wild before, and Restless Rusty was nervous. Dawn was just breaking and the six of us tourists were in the Land Rover. Even in Africa, it's still very cold in the morning before the sun rises, so we all had wool blankets that kept us warm-ish. I reassured myself that we had the rifle and now the blankets to protect us from the lions. My alarm was certainly up, and I was looking for reassurance. I went back to the gun. It was a bolt-action rifle that looked like it had seen better days firing blanks on the set of a black-and-white Tarzan movie. It did not inspire much confidence.

Did I mention this vehicle was an open-air Land Rover?

But that didn't matter because we couldn't find the lions. Apparently, they had moved on from their last seen location. If you don't know by now, I can be more than a bit of a chicken, and I was torn. On one hand, I wanted to see the lions, and on the other, I felt more than a little uneasy being in an open-air Land Rover with only a pop gun and a protective blanket. As I mentioned, I had never seen a real lion in the wild before. The sun was coming up, and it was getting noticeably warmer, and I started to feel calmer.

As my alarm came down, my irrational fear of being plucked from the Land Rover and disemboweled abating, I now wanted to see the damn lions. Before my disappointment set in too much, the guide got a message on the radio in a language I didn't understand. The guide swiveled around and said the lions were about one kilometer away.

Remember when I said the body goes into foreground alarm in response to a real or perceived threat? Just the anticipation of the lions revved up my alarm. Back in 2003, I had a full-blown anxiety (or should I say alarm) disorder, and while my conscious mind knew I was safe, my body wasn't taking any chances. My body had grown so used to always being in some form of fight or flight that it didn't take much to activate the familiar body state of alarm. My gut started to get queasy, my heart would race, and I could feel my breath getting shallower and shallower. I was already halfway down the hill on my toboggan, with the runners cutting the familiar grooves of anxiety and alarm ever deeper.

At this point, the reaction I was experiencing wasn't about the lions. Yes, they are dangerous predators, but they were actually still one kilometer away. I couldn't see them yet, and therefore what I was experiencing was actually excitement that my overly sensitive nervous system was misperceiving as the presence of a threat.

The way alarm impairs the mind is actually not that different from what happens when we drink alcohol. With alcohol, it's in a different direction—sedative instead of stimulant—but it's impairment nevertheless. Imagine you go to the bar with your friends after work. As you're parking your car and heading inside to meet your friends, you wonder to yourself how long you're going to be there and how many drinks you can have and still be able to drive home safely. Skip forward to 11 P.M., and you've had a great time. You've had five drinks (give or take—at this point you're not quite sure) over the four hours you've been there. You have to work tomorrow, so you tell yourself you can drink a bunch of water and in half an hour you should be okay to drive.

If you'd asked yourself when you'd gotten there, "How many drinks can I have over four hours and still be okay to drive?" your rational mind would have said three, max. But now you've had five-ish and that same mind (or so it seems) is telling you just to drink some water and you'll be good to go—and you believe it!

Both alcohol and alarm impair the mind, and both do so in a way that makes you think you're still using your rational capabilities. It's still *your* mind, after all!

Believing the mind to be a homogeneous, consistent, and reliable source of information is a fundamental misconception that makes us humans prone to believing everything we think. It is a profound problem if you tend to worry, as a part of you will believe the worry simply because your own mind conjured it up. Your mind gives you the impression that it is a unique and reliable tool that operates independently and consistently, no matter what is happening in the body—but that is simply not true. Sometimes our mind is operated by a rational adult, and other times, by a freaked-out five-year-old. Even though you see the mind as yours, it's not the same mind! Here's an interesting analogy: as cell biologist Dr. Bruce Lipton asserts, a cell's environment is in many ways more influential than its genes. A cell's environment determines whether it goes into growth or protection mode—and a similar dynamic exists between the mind and the body. The environment of the body also determines whether the mind goes into growth or protection mode. Do not make the mistake of believing that the mind operates consistently, independently, and objectively from the influence of the body it resides above.

Once I started to see the same thought could lead me to two completely different reactions, everything started to change for me. Here's an example from that same South Africa trip. During that trip, I had a total of fifteen flights in twenty-four days. I was uneasy with flying back then (understatement) and there were points on the trip when all I could think about was what might go wrong in the air—like turbulence, a midair collision, or running out of pretzels. Yet, there were other times I would think about an upcoming flight and feel elated by the sense of how much I was fascinated by flying. I was aware of this inconsistency at the time, but I didn't yet understand it, until I understood that the state of my body determined the state of my mind.

But back to the lions. My brain had misread excitement over seeing the lions and pushed me down into my old groove—perceiving a threat where there wasn't one and moving me deeper into survival brain, where everything looks more damn dangerous than it really is. If I'd taken a few breaths and made an effort to truly connect to myself, my body would have likely calmed down and I could have reframed the experience as excitement. A grounded body would have allowed me to keep blood flowing to my rational brain, and I could have enjoyed the situation more, but I didn't know that back then. I was in survival brain, and the idea of lions jumping into the Land Rover and ripping me clear of my safety blanket seemed plausible. There I was, in the same place I'd been so many times in my life, having an amazing experience absolutely ruined by the background and foreground alarms in my body. I'll bet you can relate.

Our guide slowed the Land Rover down as we got closer to the sighting area. We turned a corner in the bush and saw two full-grown lions beginning to mate about ten gun-lengths away. The guide kept inching closer until we were about fifteen feet away.

I didn't know this then, but when lions mate, they do it for forty-eight hours straight. Each coupling lasts for eight to fifteen seconds, and this is repeated day and night every thirty to forty-five minutes for two days. The female was getting pretty angry and growling very loudly and aggressively at the male during and after coupling. I can't say I blamed her. I believe if someone mounted me for ten seconds every half hour, I'd be irate as well.

Initially, being so close to those lions and having them in a state of high activation put me in a state of high activation—and not in a good way. But after about ten minutes, without me understanding yet what was happening and why, my foreground alarm started to resolve (which eased my background alarm), and I could better experience this awe-inspiring scene as I moved slowly out of my survival brain.

This story illustrates a pattern that was so familiar to me. When my body was in alarm, my mind was tainted, and I perceived a threat when no real threat was present. I wish I'd known then what I know now. Back then, I just assumed my worries were the problem. I had no idea how to break the alarm-anxiety cycle because I wouldn't know it was there for fifteen more years. Back then when my body was worn out by being in alarm all day, the alarm wore itself out and I would get some relief as evening crept in, only to restart the cycle the moment I awoke the next day. Maybe you have that diurnal variation in your anxiety and alarm and they're worse in the morning and ease at night, or vice versa. In any event, I'll show you how to break the cycle so you're the master of your body and no longer the servant to your worries.

The take-home message is this: you can have the exact same thought at different times and your perception of threat will be determined by the state of your body when the thought occurs.

49

Potentiation: Deepening the Groove

Typically, in a well-calibrated autonomic nervous system, the degree of activation is proportional to the threat. Hearing a mosquito buzzing around you would elicit less of a response than realizing someone is trying to break into your home. But in those of us prone to the alarm-anxiety cycle, the sympathetic nervous system becomes both hyperactive and hypervigilant and often responds well in excess of the actual level of threat.

To understand how this works, imagine a fresh snowfall on a hill. You get your toboggan and climb to the top of the hill, put the toboggan in the snow, and have a fun ride to the bottom. Then you do this three more times. Now a groove is formed in the snow and each time you ride down the hill you go a little bit faster as the groove gets a little bit deeper and smoother.

In neuroscience, *potentiation* (also called *long-term potentiation*) is the term we use to refer to the process that shows increasing strength and speed of nerve impulses along pathways the more they are used. Learning in the brain incorporates this process of potentiation. When we learn something, the more we practice it, the more adept we are at repeating or remembering it. The less we practice it, the more likely we are to lose the skill or forget the concept.

Connected to potentiation, virtually every book on neuroscience includes some version of this concept (attributed to fellow Canadian neuropsychologist Donald Hebb): the neurons that fire together, wire together.

Although our nervous systems learn protective habits very easily, remember that potentiation applies to habits that serve us as well as those that hurt us. When you were first learning to ride a bike you had to pay close attention to every detail, but after years of practice, the program has been repeated so often (potentiated) that you don't have to consciously think about it. It gets recreated rapidly and unconsciously and as Dr. Joe Dispenza says, the body learns to do it better than the mind.

So, potentiation isn't inherently harmful—in fact, we couldn't do anything skillfully without it. Instead of being able to brush our teeth by mindlessly going through the motions while our mind is already on tomorrow's to-do list, we would be using up all of our brainpower on "First, I squeeze the toothpaste. No, first I unscrew the cap. No, first I pick up the tube of toothpaste." Potentiation helps us a lot—and we can consciously leverage its power to learn new habits that serve us.

Once we recognize that we have Stone Age brains in a digital world, we can work to bring back sympathetic/parasympathetic balance. We can know that we're here today because our ancestors were hyperreactive and cautious and passed down that tendency to us. We can thank our nervous systems for being hardwired to keep us safe, while at the same time create awareness that not every activation in our body needs to be attached to a worry or threat. We can choose to pick up our toboggan out of those well-worn potentiated grooves and start constructing a different path down the hill.

As Viktor Frankl pointed out (and I am paraphrasing), awareness creates a space between stimulus and response, and in that space we can choose a new path (in the snow).

Just because we feel alarmed (the stimulus) we do not need to reflexively ride our toboggan down the well-worn groove straight into Worrytown (the response). We have the freedom to choose our own way, and that is what part 3 is all about. Stay tuned!

50

Sea Monster

I used to play this game with my daughter, Leandra, when she was about four. The game was called Sea Monster. Leandra would run into the room and yell, "Sea monster!" I, being the aforementioned sea monster, would jump up and chase the damsel around the house. She would squeal with a combination of fear and delight. After about three minutes, the sea monster would get tired. (Sea monsters need to do more cardio.) The little lass would invariably want to continue the game, but the sea monster would agree to throw the damsel into his ocean lair (the sofa) only one more time. The sea monster and his captive would then have a cuddle until the sea monster had to go back to learning about the fasciculations he was dying from.

I didn't know it back then, but I was calibrating my little daughter's autonomic nervous system. I would get her all riled up for a dangerous sea monster attack, with high-tone foreground alarm and fight-or-flight activation of her sympathetic nervous system, and then calm her back down into parasympathetic mode with some safe, connected snuggles on the couch. I was teaching her body that she could get all fired up into sympathetic fight or flight and then, in a safe and loving environment, the seesaw would move to parasympathetic rest and digest. In other words, her body learned to quickly and smoothly go from fight or flight (mostly flight) to rest and digest.

For many of us with anxiety and alarm issues, calming down is not that simple. Ideally, we should be able to press on either the gas or the brake. But if you grew up with uncertainty, abandonment, or abuse, your system never feels safe enough to take your foot completely off the accelerator and place it fully on the brake. Your background alarm is never completely off (that's why I call it "background"), although there are times you may not be consciously aware of it. But like your startle reflex, the alarm is always ready to jump into action at the slightest provocation. (I also believe this is the case with PTSD. The body stays in a state of fight-or-flight foreground alarm, in relentless readiness to jump back into action in pursuit of safety.) We worriers always feel we have to maintain a little fight-or-flight energy to be ready to deal with a trauma that could arise at any moment. We might be consciously trying to brake hard to stop and relax but are still unconsciously keeping one foot on the accelerator and revving the engine—which causes our shell-shocked nervous system to become even more confused, perceiving danger where there is none.

When we don't feel safe and connected as children, our autonomic nervous systems never adopt that beneficial "when one is on, the other is off" cooperation. We never feel safe letting our guard down because in the past when we relaxed and let the parasympathetic wing take over, we often got blindsided. The longer my dad was well, the more painful the crash was, so eventually I stopped allowing myself to let my guard down and rest.

The neuropsychologist Rick Hanson says we have minds that are like Teflon for the good stuff and Velcro for the bad. This goes double for those of us who carry alarm in our systems. I took that innate fear bias programmed into the nervous system of every human—telling me the sound in the reeds is a crouching tiger and not the wind—and I amplified it by telling myself it wasn't safe to feel safe. If we had intermittent chaos in our family home, this "waiting for the other shoe to drop" mentality significantly impairs our ability to feel safe as adults.

It still happens sometimes that I'll be driving on a beautiful, sunny day, feeling good, and then my mind will suddenly conjure up a worry to snap me back into vigilance. I recognize what I am doing to myself now, but those old toboggan tracks of hair-trigger activation are deep. Now I just laugh at my mind trying to trick me into creating worry on a beautiful, sunny day, and I take a moment to reassure Rusty that he is perfectly okay. (More on creating this internal self-reassurance later.)

When we don't recognize our "it's not safe to feel safe" program, it's like the old story of the artist who paints a picture of a tiger that appears so realistic they scare themselves to death. Our bodies create the alarm, and then we react as if our self-created illusions (our worries) are real. We create our own painted tigers in our mind, but the alarm in our body impairs the mind's ability to see those tigers aren't real.

We are not scaring ourselves on purpose, although it sure feels that way sometimes. This "it's not safe to feel safe" program hides in the darkness of our unconscious and is a feeling more than a thinking. Once we see it in awareness and bring it into the light, we can use the feeling of danger as a focus for change. We can see that our painted tigers are only made of brain droppings.

51

Heart First, Brain Second

Imagine you were just a brain, kept alive by artificially bathing in cerebrospinal fluid and receiving blood and nutrients via the cerebral arteries and veins. Would you *feel* anything? It is ironic that the brain has no pain sensors itself (you can cut right into a living brain and it will perceive no pain), but if that brain is attached to a body, it reads that body (interoception, remember?) and creates an interpretation of pain that it doesn't actually experience itself. If there is pain in the physical body (like stubbing your toe), the brain is very good at identifying the location and extent of the pain via its interpretation. But if we experience emotional pain, the brain's interpretations are ill-defined and often completely inaccurate.

The brain does not feel on its own. For perception of physical and emotional sensations, you need a body. So, if feeling emotional pain requires a body, why are traditional therapies fixated on the mind and not doing anything to treat the body? Why aren't we directing the lion's share of our treatments to the sleeping tiger in our bodies? (Couldn't resist— lions and tigers and dogs, oh my!)

Why indeed are we spending so much time treating the anxious thinking of the mind and paying so little attention to the alarm feeling in the body—especially when that is the most painful part?

I know I have alluded to this already, but it's such a critical point that I'm going to flog it again. The body has just as much (if not more) to do with healing from suffering as the mind. In our development as embryos, there was a body and a heart before there was a mind or nervous system. Heart first, brain second.

In this way, the source of alarm (the body) was present before the source of anxiety (the mind). It was key in my own recovery to give reverence to the body, to create a new paradigm where the locus of emotional pain was more in the body than the mind and to direct attention to healing with that in mind (or should I say, in body).

After my decades-long search for relief, which included taking trips on psychedelics that took me far, far away from my years of academic training and experience as a medical doctor, I arrived at a new paradigm that I never would have seen had I stuck to Dr. Russell Kennedy's view of conventional medicine. Under the influence of LSD, ayahuasca, psilocybin, and MDMA, my scientifically trained mind was shown that emotional pain is rooted in the body and *only interpreted by the mind*. Seeing the source of emotional pain as alarm stored in the body, with the mind playing only a supporting role, has been invaluable as a healing construct for my own recovery, and I am confident it will greatly benefit you in yours.

Point to consider: Are you beginning to see that the feeling stored in your body is a much bigger player in your discomfort than the worries created by your mind?

52

The Purpose of the Alarm

If I had to sum up the purpose of alarm in one word, I'd have to say protection. We activate alarm to protect ourselves from actual or perceived danger, which can be physical or emotional. When we are young and our minds are overwhelmed by trauma or separation that is too much for us, initially we create a foreground alarm energy to activate our sympathetic nervous system, maybe not so much for adrenaline-based fighting or fleeing, but oxytocin-based pursuit of a lost connection. If that boost of sympathetic nervous system energy does not resolve the situation (and this high-energy activation can only be maintained for so long), eventually part of us just gives up. Like a cornered animal, we stop the fight and go into freeze.

When I saw my father first start to lose his mind, my sympathetic nervous system would activate and I would go into an activated pursuit phase, using the classic fight-or-flight activation energy in an attempt to reduce my separation from him. When I saw that my pursuit was futile, as my dad was not able to connect with me no matter what I did, I would freeze. Remember Mitch, the guy I met at a retreat who had been physically abused by his father? It is likely he experienced the same freeze reaction, but he would have been in flight trying to escape from his abusive father. The difference was that Mitch's experience of futility was trying to flee from his father, and my futility was in trying to get closer to mine. In both cases, our sympathetic nervous systems would be highly engaged but would meet with futility as our goals were blocked. The response to that sense of futility would be to freeze, and it is often in the freeze state where the alarm is transferred into the body.

Point to consider: Were you trying to get closer to your parent or get further away? Was it different with different parents or caregivers?

My sense is that the freeze state is a sign of complete overwhelm and is the immediate precursor to dissociation. Like when you hear people speak of being attacked or when escape from peril was impossible, they often say they "just froze." At a conscious level, they may have felt and looked immobilized, but at an unconscious level, the trauma was very active, overwhelming the mind's ability to cope and then shunting that energy into background alarm to be stored in the body.

Although Mitch and I both felt frozen, albeit for different reasons, our energy sure wasn't. Remember the scientific law of conservation of energy? Energy can't be created or destroyed, only changed in form. This is a great analogy for how trauma initially overwhelms our system and is stored in the body as background alarm in the long term. In my communications with Mitch over the years since we met, we have been able to isolate where he feels his background alarm in his body (upper chest and throat), and he has been able to use that sense of alarm as a point of connection to his younger, wounded self. I'll talk specifically about using the felt sense of alarm as a conduit to your younger, wounded self in part 3.

One of my relatives is a retired pilot for a major airline. I am always fascinated by his stories. Every six to twelve months, he was required to get certified on a flight simulator that would simulate an emergency on his Airbus A320. In one of these tests, he was given a scenario of severe wind shear on takeoff. The correct response was to push the throttles up to 100 percent to escape, and that was exactly what he did. This is where the story gets interesting.

Apparently, modern jet engines are almost never used to even 75 percent of their capacity, and they are so powerful they don't even come close to that in regular use. He told me that if this scenario had occurred in the real world and he had used max power, both engines would have had to be scrapped. The reason being maximum thrust can cause a groove or score on the metal that may lead to future malfunction. He did what he needed to do to keep the passengers safe, but if the scenario had occurred in real life instead of the flight simulator, it would have meant throwing two multimillion-dollar engines in the trash!

When I heard this story, my imagination took hold of it. Our nervous systems are like those jet engines—if they are too strongly activated, they are never the same. This is what happens when we experience chronic and repetitive trauma that forces our sympathetic nervous system to maximum output. If no resolution occurs, we freeze and dissociate, and the thwarted energy creates a pathway or shunt that stores, or grooves, the trauma in the body. The more the system is pushed to overwhelm and futility, the more that pathway becomes a deeper groove that additional trauma can more easily flow down, adding to the increasing reservoir of background alarm in the body.

Like the jet engines, our nervous systems are not cut out to be used too intensely too often. They have tremendous capacity, but they're meant to be used in the presence of actual threats to our lives—the kind we are supposed to encounter only rarely, not every day at home where we are supposed to be safe. In case of emergency, we can rev up our engines, but the system will experience some changes due to excessive demand. When that happens chronically, we are like the car at a standstill, one foot on the gas and one on the brake—the engine spinning high RPMs, frozen in place externally but creating a lot of energy internally.

Fortunately, when we overwhelm our nervous systems in this way, we don't have to throw the whole thing out. When we apply the tools of love and compassion to our protection instincts and background alarm, each of us can become skilled jet engine repairmen and -women.

53
Dark Night of the Soul

When I met my now wife, Cynthia, in June 2013 at a personal development retreat, I was both mentally and physically debilitated. I had left medicine after my Achilles rupture in February and was still in a boot cast recovering from surgery. Strangely, a month before, I had a premonition I was going to meet my future wife at this retreat and I knew immediately when I saw her. I don't want to weird you out, but I have some clairsentient ability, and I've had it since I was a child. It makes me a good doctor in that I can read people and the energy around them, and it especially helps me clearly see where my patients' alarm is coming from. Much of the material from this book comes from my ability to see things most people do not, both in myself and others. This clairsentient ability is not that strong however; I've never been able to intuit the Powerball numbers or correctly predict the winner of the Super Bowl.

When I met Cynthia, it was one of those meetings you just know is going to be life-changing. She was beautiful and vulnerable. I could see her energy was kind and giving, but I also saw her pain. Cyn-Cyn (as our granddaughter Avielle calls her) and I have created a tremendous bond in healing ourselves and others. Since our meeting in 2013 she has become a somatic trauma therapist and we have learned so much from each other, both personally and professionally. She has shown me it is actually safe to be in my body and it's safe to trust love. The primary thing that's really kept me going over the years since leaving the official practice of medicine is my relationship with Cynthia (along with pups Buddha, Riley, and Ellie).

My early days with Cynthia had tremendous joy and pain. I still don't know why she stuck it out with me and my constant and crushing worries. Many days I was so alarmed I wouldn't get up until one or two in the afternoon (Cynthia would walk Buddha). I was desperate for some kind of relief and told her of my plans to take psychedelics. Cynthia is a very conservative person in many ways, and I knew this idea of taking a powerful substance scared her, but buoyed by my fellow comics' stories of miraculous relief from mental suffering and addiction, I was desperate and optimistic to try something that might actually work. I found a shaman who would, for a significant amount of money, guide me through a private two-night ayahuasca experience in a remote area. I expected to find a shaman with a name like Arechron or Dorhuk or Norbundo. (These are real shamans' names.) But do you know what this eternal, divine mystic's name was?

Dave.

Yes, Dave. The name Dave didn't inspire a lot of mysticism or confidence, but again, I was desperate.

In October 2014, I had two successive nights dancing with the snake called ayahuasca. The first night I sat in front of Dave while he mixed the medicine, and I was about twenty-two times as scared as I was of flying—and I was pretty scared of flying (understatement).

Dave and his assistant, Paul, did some incantations. Cynthia was there with me, but she did not want to take the medicine. Buddha was there, too, for canine support, but he didn't want to take the medicine either, probably because he was an enlightened being already.

I took the cup from Dave and swallowed in one gulp. It tasted like bitter seaweed. I went back to my place across from Dave and waited. And waited. In a way, I was less scared than before because now I was committed. The long wait to do this was over.

I probably don't have to tell you that much of the pain of anxiety is in the uncertainty of the waiting. Once the roller coaster crests the summit and starts to plunge downward, it becomes fear, not anxiety. Fearful experiences always have an end point, but anxiety is always anticipatory and therefore has no end, which reminds us of the childhood pain that seemingly had no ending, with the constant anticipation of the other shoe dropping . . . I closed my eyes and started to see the most intense purple, blue, and pink geometric figures and shapes. Then everything seemed to disappear but the vivid colors. I was in a new world I couldn't even begin to explain. Even as I write this, I can feel my alarm come up in my body.

I had the sense I was falling, which was very disturbing. More disturbing was that I was trying to understand what the word "falling" meant. I was trying to make sense of what was happening, but I had no cognitive function that I could understand. I felt I did understand and I could explain what was happening, but when I tried, there were no concepts I could grasp to explain it. My mind wouldn't "catch," kind of like a car engine that would turn over but not start up.

Apparently, I kept repeating out loud—and I don't remember this—"There's nothing to hold on to."

I have no memory of saying this, but I have often felt, in times of deep alarm and anxiety, that there truly was nothing to hold on to. I think this is the same way I felt as a child when I was grasping for something, anything, to support me or give me a reference for what was happening. At the mercy of the serpentine mother ayahuasca, I was being shown the well-grooved pattern my mind and body had defaulted to—and it was terrifying. At least when I am going through anxiety and alarm in my daily life, I can do some yoga, focus on my breath, or even just distract myself. Now I was faced with my alarm and anxiety full force, and I had no defense—at all.

As I write this now, it makes perfect sense to me why this was so terrifying. I have decades of background alarm repressed and stored in my body. To get away from this pain in my body, I escaped into my head and from childhood became an elite-level worrier and overthinker. I even went into a profession that required a massive intellectual investment and became even better at using my mind. I know now that I used thinking as a way of escaping feeling, as most worriers do. Thinking and worrying in my head became my coping strategy to avoid feeling in my body.

And then I ingested a substance that removed any ability to think. Without my familiar coping strategy of thinking and worrying, all those decades of pain I had avoided hit me full force. In the open-air Land Rover that is life, ayahuasca took away my protective blanket of overthinking and I was now face-to-face with the lions of my past—and they were ripping me apart. I have never experienced anything as ghastly, grim, hideous, and horrifying as that experience on ayahuasca.

If I got anything out of ayahuasca, it is that in life there is truly nothing to hold on to, especially thoughts. There is no "thing" to hold on to. Ayahuasca showed me the only thing to hold on to is something that is not "hold on to-able," and that is faith.

More on faith in its own chapter later, but faith is not a tangible thing. You can't pick faith up and move it from one place to another. My scientifically based doctor world loved concrete concepts, but faith is ethereal. Faith is not a thinking of the mind as much as it is a feeling of the body.

With my ability to think removed, I could still have faith that this human experience is its own illusion and that we are truly connected to something that has no resemblance to our human body.

In that experience, I was shown there is a universal wisdom that has order, and death is sometimes a part of that order. Your human form may die, but the essence of you will always be a part of the fabric of consciousness. Energy cannot be created nor destroyed, only changed in form.

I was shown on psychedelics the more I try to make sense of things with my rational scientifically trained mind, the more man-made and ultimately wrong I was. I was shown that I am the grape-colored Kool-Aid (there's the purple solar plexus color again) in the eternal water of existence and that my human form borrows the suspension of the water but is not it, but is all of it.

This sentence still makes sense to me, and it likely won't make sense to you but it will give you a sense of the chaos that was created in my mind on ayahuasca.

Here's another ayahuasca-ism: I was shown that I don't know and trying to know is different from knowing. I know that sounds vague and nonsensical, but that's another little taste of what psychedelics did to scatter my mind's constructs into a million little pieces. . . .

I was also given a sense that I overthink (there's a big surprise!) but, more directly, that my mind-based perceptions were subjective, filled with protection, and very often dead wrong. What I saw as bad may well be one of the best things that has happened and vice versa. For example, something I assumed was bad—my anxiety—has pointed me toward becoming more connected to myself and others than I've ever been. In contrast, something I viewed as good—getting into medical school and becoming a medical doctor—may actually have been one of the worst things for me. In many ways, becoming a doctor took me further away from my real self by forcing me to look after others before myself, going deeper into my cognitive mind and away from my feeling body. In addition, being a doctor put me in a chronic environment of illness (and more important, mental illness), which is where my background alarm originated as I watched my father become sicker and sicker. I had to realize that my perception of good and bad was a story I became locked into by my mind. In my compulsion to reduce uncertainty and make sense of my life by using my thoughts, that very thinking stood firmly in the way of the feeling messages that would allow me to heal.

As Dr. Wayne Dyer put it, "If you change the way you look at things, the things you look at change." But if you never question (or renew) your perceptions, you'll never see the deeper meaning in your suffering.

My perception was that being a doctor was saving me, when in reality it was sinking me. What I perceived as my anchor and a force keeping me grounded was an anchor all right—but it was dragging me to the bottom! Psychedelics and more somatic approaches to healing have allowed me to renew, or at least revisit, the perception that I had to think my way out of everything.

With that experience, I saw I was like the tree surgeon who had to give it up because he realized he couldn't stand the sight of sap. I had to give up thinking for feeling, and in light of my belief that my thinking was the only thing keeping me safe, moving to feeling was terrifying.

My psychedelic dance with the snake was both horrifying and enlightening. Ayahuasca showed me faith in a higher order that my simple mind-based interpretations, thoughts, and mental constructs of good and bad simply could not see. Because as a child I had not received the support I needed to resolve my alarm, I had concluded that I was solely responsible for protecting myself from the vicissitudes of life. Becoming a doctor furthered that illusion and kept me trapped in my belief that my anxiety could be "figured out" if I only tried hard enough.

Being a doctor hadn't helped with my chronic alarm. In fact, it reinforced my mind-based story that I had the power to go at life alone. Here's the kicker. I had adopted the unconscious assumption that I needed to look after myself (and my parents) around thirteen years old and had been carrying it around ever since. How accurate and complete do you think any thirteen-year-old boy's understanding of life is? I had built a house of cards based on my own intellect and pseudo-independence. Ayahuasca knocked it down.

Point to consider: Did you become the caregiver for your family well before you were ready? How old were you?

There was tremendous, excruciating, confusing pain in my ayahuasca experience, but I'll share with you some realizations: 1) having faith (not necessarily religious faith) means you can allow something you can't see to look after you; 2) you don't have to do it all by yourself; 3) your perceptions of what is good or bad for you may be entirely inaccurate; 4) there is wisdom in life that goes far beyond our own personal subjective experience, even in death.

After my disappointments in India and then ayahuasca, I was at an extremely low point. I'd had such high hopes for relief, and once again they'd been dashed. In the days after ayahuasca, my psyche was fractured like the proverbial broken mirror. There was no consistency I could rely on in my mind or my body. The thoughts I had relied on since childhood to keep me sequestered in my thinking mind no longer buffered me from the alarm in my body. Leaning on my worried thoughts was an illusion I used as a child to give me a sense of certainty and security, but now I could not even hold on to them because they were fractured too.

A quote from Eckhart Tolle's book *A New Earth* kept showing up at the entrance to my mind: "Danger. All structures are unstable." In the days following ayahuasca, I was a ghost, as disconnected from life and as close to suicide as I have ever been. The background alarm in my body had reached nuclear proportions due to the destabilizing psychedelic experience, and my mind had been dis-integrated by that same psychedelic. That period gave me a sense as to why people commit suicide. I looked in every direction and found nothing to hold on to. In my past, even in my most intense anxiety and panic there was this sense that there were pros and cons to a certain action, but in the days following ayahuasca there was a terrifying sense that there was no place that was different from the one I was in. I was on thin ice, unable to get traction from my thoughts or my mind, with the feeling I might fall through at any moment. There was no escape from ubiquitous pain in all directions. I wonder if that is exactly what my father felt before he ended his life.

That emptiness post-ayahuasca lasted two days, and it was the longest and most painful forty-eight hours of my life. If you've been in the dark night of the soul, you know the seconds pass slowly and each minute that clicks by is a victory. You tell yourself to just make it through the next minute, (and sometimes the next second) and the next, and the next, and after what seems like an eternity, the sun starts to come up.

Thank goodness for one last thing I did see on aya: slowly, I began to sense that I was somehow protected—by what, I did not know, but I could develop faith in the feeling I didn't have to do it all by myself anymore. I didn't have to be that thirteen-year-old who pretended he had it all under control when deep down he knew he was just a kid, woefully unprepared for guiding his own life, let alone being a physician to guide others.

With this realization I understood why, during my whole career as a doctor, I had felt like an imposter. I was just "playing doctor"—not in the way that Jackhammer Johnson played doctor in the film *Genital Hospital,* but I did feel like a child in a doctor costume. Even though I did a good job as a physician and had an exemplary record, part of me felt I was a thirteen-year-old boy in an oversized white lab coat with a stethoscope around my neck still looking after others over myself. Ayahuasca (eventually) showed me I did not have to only rely on that persona, in fact I could leave it behind and have faith in a new path—the path of belief that I am protected and guided, and I can, and do, have faith in that.

As a child who took it upon himself to look after his parents and himself, I had given up on someone looking after me. Now I knew there was something that looks after me and that it comes from faith inside my body and has nothing to do with the machinations of my mind. I saw the paradox that to keep me safe, something inside of me had to gain faith in something outside of me that would watch over me. That paradox is consistent with my ayahuasca and LSD experiences, showing everything is connected, and the separation from inside and outside is a premise of the anxious mind. The security of knowing that there is no true separation, only imagined separation, is what brought me on the path to write this book. As "all anxiety is separation anxiety," anxiety relies on believing the lie that you are separate from yourself.

You are not (see part 3).

At the time, I felt ayahuasca was a total bust, and I would never recommend anyone with anxiety or control issues put themselves through it. It took away the anchors I had put in place to feel in control. And, in many ways, it retraumatized me, as I wasn't quite right for eighteen months after and I've never been closer to suicide than following those two nights on ayahuasca. When people with anxiety ask me if they should do it to heal, I ask them: "How much do you need to feel you need to be in control to be safe?" Typically, I find that when people feel a need to be in control, they depend on their mind to do that. Anxiety is an attempt to keep control of the uncontrollable and predict the unpredictable, so ingesting a substance that removes control by separating you from your mind may be your life's biggest challenge, as it was for me.

That being said, for some people, that may be exactly what they need to heal. Seeing your world without any control may be a "reset" that gives you the ability to accept uncertainty and unpredictability. At points, ayahuasca showed me I had to face my fears of uncertainty if I was to overcome them. It also showed me I was infinitely connected to the universe, whether I was alive in this human form or not. In a way, it showed me that there is no death—so what was I afraid of?

I have found that we worriers are most afraid of being afraid, which is an endless circle. In Scandinavian cultures and folklore, a dragon is often pictured on top of a treasure chest signifying we must slay the dragon (fear) to access the treasure (love). It took me a long time to really see that I had to face the fear before I could access the treasure of love for myself and for my child self, Rusty. Faith and courage allowed that return to love, and I'll show you how you can find that same healing connection to the child that lives in you.

Ayahuasca was the undisputed heavyweight champion of terror for me. Dave said I must do at least two nights to get the benefit, so I went back for a second night. Since the time ten years ago I faced the dark night of the soul and danced with the snake for not one night but two, I learned that I am infinitely stronger than I give myself credit for. Going back for a repeat performance after that horrendous (understatement!) first experience showed me I would not allow myself to be a victim. If I could have the most terrifying experience of my life and go back the next night, I could go through anything. It also showed me how much I used my thinking and worry as a way of controlling and predicting, and how excruciatingly painful it could be when my ability to control and predict was removed. My experience with ayahuasca also showed me that control was an illusion of the mind and faith in the feeling of the heart was critical to my healing. Faith allowed me to see that it wasn't all up to me. There are, and always will be, uncertainties beyond my control, and accepting and loving uncertainty with an open sense of feeling and faith gave me the key to healing my anxiety and alarm. Feeling in my body was a far superior way to live than being limited by the endless false promises of finding security in my mind.

Feeling cannot readily be vanquished by thinking, and there is a good reason for that. Feelings are where life is. Faith in something bigger than me gives me a felt sense that I can focus on looking after myself, while knowing even that isn't completely up to me. It took months after the experience, but the snake did visit me and show me I was a spirit in human form and I was divinely protected in both life and death. That knowing precipitated my next journey, the one I am still on—that of creating a feeling connection to my thinking self, bringing these disparate parts into a functional whole.

Before I leave this chapter, I want to say that despite what I kept saying on ayahuasca, there *is* something to hold on to and that is faith. Not necessarily religious faith, but faith in consciousness itself, in the inherent order of the universe. I just couldn't reach out and touch faith because my overprotective, worried mind was too distracted to see it, or rather, feel it. As I'll show you in part 3, faith in the universe is one of the most powerful antidotes to worry.

54

Feel It to Heal It

If I've shown you anything by now, it's that our worries aren't the root of the problem. Thoughts make the problem feel worse, no question, but they are more of an effect than a cause. The feeling of alarm is the real source of our pain and the energy source for our worrisome thoughts. The root of the problem is the emotional energy that is trapped in the body. We are just less aware of it because it's harder to describe a feeling than it is to describe a thought.

Thoughts are already in our home language, the words we use to communicate with ourselves every single day. Feelings, however, are in a language of the body, and that is considerably less readily understood. When you see people having a peak experience, like a professional athlete winning their championship or a mother describing the birth of her child, they often say that they can't describe it in words. The same is true for healing from anxiety. Words are not enough. We need to delve into the feeling for our healing.

In fact, words and thoughts often function as a distraction from the feeling. If we detour into our worries, we never actually access the feeling, and for a long time that was just fine with me. I didn't want to access all that old feeling. That's why my system pushed it out of my conscious awareness in the first place. But I've learned the hard way that you can't think your way out of a feeling. If that worked, cognitively saying "Just forget about her/him!" would immediately absolve you of the pain of a breakup.

Now, if you know on some level a relationship isn't good for you or you need to get over it, you might purposely call to mind the bad in the relationship and all the ways the person hurt you in an effort to try to ease the pain. Although it may feel like it's working, by trying to think your way out of a feeling, you are bypassing true healing and resolution. Hey, I'm all for doing what you need to do to get through the emotional pain at the beginning when it's at its rawest, but just know, if you don't eventually face the feeling, there won't be any true healing or learning for the next time, and you may well pick the same person with a different haircut. Remember Jane's alcoholic boyfriends?

We need direct access to the root of the problem—i.e., the alarm feeling—before we can change it. Again, you need to feel it to heal it. You can temporarily make it easier by manipulating your thoughts, but this doesn't fix the root of the problem.

If I ask you "What are you thinking about right now?" you can probably tell me easily that you're thinking about what you're going to make for dinner or the errand you need to run this evening or your plans for the weekend. If I ask you "What are you feeling right now?" that takes an order of magnitude more attention, self-awareness, and introspection. If it takes you a minute to come up with an answer or if you maybe even draw a blank, you're not alone. It's actually pretty rare for us to stop and pay attention to our feelings in everyday life, especially if you are male. Humans are a left-brained, linear, logical, analytical, thinking species that tends to look down on the right-brained feeling state as self-indulgent and nonproductive. On top of that, we are conditioned to push away negative feelings and pretend they aren't a part of life. (Retail therapy, anyone?)

In general, we are much more well-versed in describing thinking processes than feeling, emotional ones. And that focus on thinking is dangerous, as we condition ourselves to believe life is a thinking process rather than a feeling one—and in times of crisis, we are much more inclined to go for what we know (thinking) and bypass the true source of the problem (feeling).

It is the feeling moments that give life its meaning. It is feelings that have the most important messages for us. And yet, especially in North America, we live in a society that denies feelings, especially uncomfortable ones. We are encouraged to live life from the neck up and not pay much attention to emotion, and even urge people to discount or disown feelings that are unpleasant. Feeling sad after a breakup? Just forget about your former love! Dive in to retail therapy: buy a new car or binge-watch Netflix! I call this the cognitive bypass, where we distract ourselves and dissociate into thinking precisely to avoid feeling. This cognitive bypass can relieve some emotional pain in the short term, but if we don't eventually make an effort to cycle back and feel it (to heal it), the bypassed energy just gets pushed down and added to our alarm.

In addition to it not working—because even if we manage to change our thinking, the feeling still has to go somewhere—I believe positive psychology's focus to "think positive" actually creates harm by locking us out of right brained sensation and into more left-brained explanation. When we distract ourselves, gloss over, or dissociate from uncomfortable emotions, 1) we lose the message the feeling is trying to give us; 2) we lose the ability to process that painful emotion so it no longer drives our worries; 3) when that emotion invariably comes up again we have gained no confidence in metabolizing it so we need to compulsively escape back into our worries to avoid it; 4) the unresolved emotional energy piles back into our reservoir of alarm.

In contrast, when we sit with the alarm-based feelings instead of resisting them (sensation without explanation), we train ourselves to see that those uncomfortable feelings are transient and can be resolved, instead of compulsively distracted from by worrying. As an example, I firmly believe at the root of much of alarm and anxiety is unresolved childhood grief from losses that were never addressed, and if the anxiety and alarm are to be uncovered and resolved, the underlying grief must be consciously moved into, processed, and moved through. Feelings, both comfortable and uncomfortable, are woven into the tapestry of life. If we try to think our way out of every feeling, aka positive psychology, those feelings will not be processed and stay in a form of limbo as background alarm. This accumulating emotional "slush fund" of alarm will grow stronger and more alarming as we bypass feeling with worrisome thinking.

If your beloved pet has just died, forcing yourself to redirect your energy into happy thoughts of your wedding day every time you feel sad never allows you the opportunity to metabolize and integrate the experience. We are a highly intelligent culture in many ways. We greatly value technology and science. But when it comes to emotional intelligence, I'm not sure if we would even be given a passing grade. Our society is fixated on the idea that uncomfortable emotion is bad and must be avoided at all costs. Less explicit but omnipresent is the belief that we can buy our way out of negativity, that money heals painful emotions. I'm not saying that thinking strategies are not helpful for initial coping, but we worriers are so skilled at overthinking we get trapped there and never allow the feeling to be felt and resolved. Said another way, *overthinking is a way of underfeeling.*

I valued thinking over feeling for decades. In diverting my energies into my thinking mind, where I felt more comfortable in my intellect, I increasingly lost touch with the feeling in my body. For many years, I didn't know I was doing this as a protective measure, I just accepted that I was a worrier. Many of us with childhood trauma lost touch with our bodies because that was where our background alarm lived and we didn't want to visit that part of us. I lived in my head, not my body, not sensing I was hungry until I was ravenous or that I had to go to the bathroom until it was urgent.

I had to learn the hard way that staying in my head was a precarious place to live. Sure, for a lot of us worriers the by-product of living in your head is accomplishment and productivity. Becoming fixated on thinking makes us "good" at thinking and it did make me a doctor, clinical neuroscientist, and author, but preferentially living in my head came at the cost of losing touch with my body and the feeling of life that lives in it. That progressive separation as my thinking took precedence over (and split from) my feeling created a great deal of accomplishment, *and a greater deal of alarm*. I know many people who are very accomplished and very unhappy and anxious!

I know now that to heal from anxiety and alarm, you must go back to the childhood body you've been avoiding and make that place as safe as you possibly can. If you get trapped in your thoughts, you can learn the body is your escape route, not your torturer. Once the body is grounded, then, and only then, does thinking actually help you feel better. It took me years to figure out changing or controlling my thoughts was not the answer. I was already an expert-level thinker (as you probably are), and it was killing me. I had to direct my energy and attention away from the trap of the thinking mind and toward the feeling body. It was living in my feeling body that had to become my preference and my grounding, because healing the old, unresolved pain of my past stored in my body was the answer to resolving my incessant worries for the future.

But my ego mind did everything in its power to convince me my salvation lies in thinking. (Notice the word "lies" there.) I had to escape that trap, and my goal with this book is to show you the way out too!

Point to consider: What never got resolved when you were a child? How much of your anxiety and alarm stems from unresolved grief that has never been addressed?

55

The Body Keeps the Score

If I hear about someone struggling with psychosis, schizophrenia, or bipolar disorder, a little alarm tripwire gets activated in my mind and body. Although I have done a tremendous amount of emotional work in integrating the story of my father, I'll feel my background alarm perk up and I'll put my hand on my lower chest, take a few breaths, and focus on the gratitude I have for my dad. I'll recall how he was there to teach me to throw a ball and get me my first job cleaning up the pool hall he ran. He was a great teacher when he wasn't incapacitated by the vagaries of his mind.

Hearing of someone struggling with mental illness is a trigger for me and, if I'm sleep-deprived or emotionally stressed, can easily send me into an alarm state, but in general, I have integrated much of the trigger of seeing or hearing of someone in emotional distress. (Oh, and by the way, my job is helping people in emotional distress.)

Let me tell you about grocery stores and me. My wife knows I hate grocery shopping, but I still almost always go with her because I know she enjoys the company and appreciates the help.

Sometimes I am funny and silly and I have a good time with her at the store, but most times we go, I dissociate. I often become fixated on my phone and not very interactive with her.

Zoning out is a big clue that I am heading into alarm, and I've trained myself to use that as a signal to reconnect with myself—and her too. (You'll learn in part 3 how to recognize your own clues and what to do with them.)

My mind and body associate grocery stores with emotional pain. I never knew the exact reason, but shopping with my mother for groceries is a painful memory for me. I have the distinct impression that it started when I was a younger child—perhaps about six—but I don't recall any episodes of food-based trauma, other than Cap'n Crunch cereal shredding the skin on the roof of my mouth. (And like a child with Stockholm syndrome, I always went back for another bowl. Cap'n Crunch is the most masochistic cereal I know.)

Anyway, I was never attacked by a head of lettuce or insulted by a chicken, but I was curious about my resistance to grocery stores, so I recently asked my mother about it. "Did I have any traumatic events happen to me in a grocery store that I might not remember?" She thought for just a moment and said, "Well, we lost you in the grocery store in Ogdensburg once."

I was indeed six at the time. She remembers because at the time Canada was celebrating its centennial, so the year would have been 1967. She told me that in my usual style with stores, I was hyperactive, relentlessly exploring and running through the aisles. This was not unusual behavior for me, and I would always find my way back to her. But on this occasion, we had gone for a quick trip across the international bridge at Prescott, Ontario, and entered Ogdensburg, New York. We were in the United States, and grocery stores are different there.

The layout of this particular Yankee store was different from my usual, normal Canadian grocery store, eh? As my mother described it to me, my usual custom was to be wary of new things, as most sensitive children are. But as I said earlier, I have another distinct side to me that does stand-up comedy and challenges wild lions on the savannah armed with nothing but a blanket, and that side runs counter to my scaredy-squirrel nature, and that more hyperactive side was often described by my dad as "Rusty's got more balls than brains (MBTB) today."

This particular day, the MBTB version of Rusty had accompanied my parents to the store. Not that I would have had much of a choice at six years old. As soon as we got there, I wanted to explore, and it didn't take me long to get lost. According to my mother, another mother of the American variety found me in tears after my foreground alarm pursuit energy failed to track down my parents. She took me to the store manager, who announced over the intercom that a child with more balls than brains had been lost and found and could be claimed by the frozen fish section at the back of the store.

To my point—and I do have one—this may be the reason I don't like grocery stores. It also may not be. I enjoy department stores that do not have food, and I love sporting goods stores. I only seem to react adversely to grocery stores. How I would know the difference as a six-year-old, I'm not sure—but the amygdala is odd and sometimes things trigger our alarm and we have no idea why.

These triggers are implicit memories, also called body memories. (You may recall we talked about them in part 1. Remember how much I love hearing someone practice the trumpet?) Implicit memories can trigger a fight-or-flight reaction in our bodies and we may have no idea what caused it. When triggered, it feels exactly the same way each time. I believe many panic attacks start when these implicit/body memories are triggered by stimuli we are not consciously aware of.

Over time, I've learned that the alarm in my body has its own emotional signature, meaning it feels the same way each time it is triggered. While the intensity can vary, the quality of it is the same, and it's the exact same background alarm I was first able to visualize in my solar plexus during my LSD trip.

The feeling of being triggered becomes its own implicit memory over time. The more the body has the experience of being alarmed, the stronger the memory becomes. This potentiated body memory of alarm, then, is not just the memory of the initial traumatic experience but also the memory of all the other times we've been triggered layered on top.

There is a theory that when you experience significant wounding as a child, like parental divorce or death, abuse, or abandonment, a part of you stays frozen in the trauma at the age you experienced it. This is consistent with my concept of background alarm, the concept of body memory, as well as what I believe is Eckhart Tolle's concept of the pain body.

Our background alarm is flared by any experience or even a memory that is reminiscent of the original wound. A significant flare of background alarm often results in an age regression, our amygdala freezing us in the time of the original wound, although as I've said we often don't notice we have turned into a scared six-year-old. In any event, our present-day adult self becomes split from our wounded child self and the child in us gets stuck in the trauma and time of the original wound. This regression happens because the amygdala has no sense of time, so when it activates, along with the insular cortex it can create the felt sense we are right back in the time of our original wounding. Much more in part 3, but when we learn to feel our background alarm, soothe ourselves in the present moment, and then go back and reconnect and rescue that younger version of ourselves (perhaps by the frozen fish section), we find a path to recovery from anxiety and alarm.

Yep, a medical doctor just said alarm is frozen into your body and fused with your wounded inner child. All that official-sounding amygdala/insula–based neuroscience and then this!

Still with me?

While it's sequestered in our body, our stored background alarm protects us from our direct experience of it, like mementos or photographs of a painful relationship that are stored in a box in the basement. In a way, it's like *hiding a trauma from the mind in the body*. When we experience trauma that is too much for our minds to bear (especially when we are children), we may repress it to a place that is "safer," where it is out of mindsight—but always simmering in the body in hindsight, like the chronic-level activation of the fight-or-flight nervous system I talked about in chapter 49. The old trauma may not be directly available to the conscious mind, but that energy and information had to go somewhere, so it finds a place in the more unconscious body. This is why people sometimes cannot actively or consciously remember the details of their overwhelming trauma, but there is always a remnant of it stored in the unconscious body. Once again, the body keeps the score.

I have seen many adults, when reminded of their childhood trauma, age-regress back to the time that it happened. One of my patients, Jamie, had just had a baby with her husband, Ward, and things in their life and relationship seemed bright and connected. But in the first few weeks of her new baby's life, Jamie started to display some tendency to self-injure. She locked herself in the bathroom and superficially cut her wrist with a knife and threatened to kill herself. This was a complete shock to Ward. Up until that time, Jamie had shown no signs of significant mental illness other than some OCD, but even in her OCD, she had never been suicidal and certainly never anything that appeared as fragmented as this. I asked Ward about Jamie's own infancy and found out that Jamie's mother had been hospitalized for three weeks right after Jamie's birth and that Jamie had had limited contact with her mother for her first few months of life as her mother recovered. I suspect that in addition to feeling stressed by the demands of caring for a newborn, Jamie was also triggered by implicit memory of her own isolated experience of infancy. The amygdala never forgets, and can send us back to an earlier time in an instant. Jamie's alarm was activated and she may well have regressed back to the time when she herself felt abandoned by her mother as a newborn.

More times than I can count, I've seen the body keep the score and reactivate old body memories that the mind has long forgotten.

Point to consider: I don't want you to feel you have to force yourself into your old alarm and stay there in an effort to "feel it to heal it," like you must grit your teeth through five solid minutes of "sensation without explanation, dammit!" In working with Jamie, it was important to touch in to the trauma sensation around her own birth and then come back out into a safe place in her body. In somatic therapies this back-and-forth between pain and peace is called pendulation or oscillation. More on this in part 3, but we must titrate the duration and intensity of our old emotional traumas so as to resolve them. Early on we may only be able to stay with our old alarm for a matter of seconds and then gradually increase our tolerance. With severe traumas we will often need a therapist who is skilled in this titration procedure.

56

What ALARMS Us

I know I have mentioned the word "alarm" more than a thousand times in this book. Believe me, I'm a little sick of it too, but I am getting into your implicit memory, and this "felt sense" will really help you understand and treat the anxiety that sits above the alarm.

When I say alarm, I know what might come to mind is a fire alarm or an alarm clock—something that gets your attention and lets you know you need to do something. The alarm in my body was doing the same thing. But here's the problem: I didn't know the alarm was my messenger. Because it hurt, I unconsciously assumed it was my enemy. As I perceived it was hurting me, I either tried to push it away or distract myself from it using the bypass of chronic thinking and worrying. It took me a long time to realize that these alarms had long ago been pushed out of my child mind into my body so that my mind would have room to cope. Then I was lucky enough to discover a way I could revisit those alarms with the intention to resolve them, and then write this book to show you how to resolve your alarms too! I truly believe that in showing you how to heal I can be the doctor that I was meant to be, so be prepared to open wide and say ahh-ha!

Learning acronyms got me through medical school. I loved making them. So, of course, I had to come up with one for alarm! Well, actually, ALARMS.

These ALARMS that are not metabolized by your parents or caregivers are pushed out of your conscious mind and stored deep in your unconscious body. Those traumas are still in you, frozen in time at the age they occurred.

Abuse: Any physical, emotional, verbal, or sexual abuse is over-whelming for a child and will be stored in the body as alarm.

Loss: We all experience loss as children. We lose toys, friends, dignity, and we lose control. Some losses like divorce of our parents, the loss of our health or having surgery, the loss of a parent or family member to illness, addiction, or death are overwhelming and become stored in the body as alarm.

Abandonment: When a child feels their caregiver has left them it is completely overwhelming. Children know intuitively that they are not prepared to face the world on their own and are completely dependent on their caregivers to look after them and keep them safe. Remember that all anxiety is separation anxiety (thank you, once again, Gordon Neufeld). Any sense of being abandoned or being separated from our protectors creates a tremendous amount of alarm in our systems. Abandonment can be physical, but it can also be emotional if our protectors are physically present but show little to no emotional connection.

Rejection: Being rejected by peers or family, as with bullying or ridiculing, can be completely overwhelming for a child. School is a very common source of rejection and alarm for a child.

Mature too early: Becoming a caregiver for parents, having sex too young, using drugs or alcohol—anything that puts the burden of responsibility on the child before they are ready—will create and store alarm in the body.

Shame: Anything the child perceives as shameful will create alarm in the body.

Point to consider: How many of these ALARMS did you have in your childhood? Don't spend too much time on this. I'm hoping this will give you a sense of why you create so much anxiety.

57

Shooting the Messenger

If you had ALARMS in childhood and they weren't resolved, they are likely driving your anxious thoughts and worries today.

The alarm in your body is the root problem we need to heal if we're going to resolve the worries of your mind. I would suggest that knowing your ALARMS points you back to the critical points in your life when you started to accumulate background alarm. Knowing these entry points, we can go back and give our younger self the support now we so badly needed but didn't get back then (see part 3).

In the ten years since my LSD revelation that my anxiety was actually a state of alarm in my body, I have made other observations, especially in meditation. I've seen that there is a part of me, around thirteen years old, that never had a chance to grow past that point. As my father became more seriously ill and I began stockpiling trauma in my solar plexus, I became my reactive thirteen-year-old self and part of me got stuck there.

Maybe you can relate to an age or event (or events) where you became frozen and then became a reactive version of yourself instead of the authentic you that you'd be today if those traumas never happened. In my case I was overwhelmed by my father's illness, and part of me decided I had to step up and take on responsibilities far beyond the abilities of my age. I saw this not as a conscious choice but as a necessity. Like many of my patients (maybe you too?) I lost the freedom of my child self that could relinquish control to adults and just be nurtured and sheltered. Again, like many of my patients who also had to mature too early (the *M* in ALARMS) I flipped the responsibilities on myself and became the nurturer and shelterer far before I was ready.

As I juxtaposed myself from the role of eldest child to parent, switching places with my dad, I was rewarded with praise from my mother, who appreciated the help. That inflated my ego and gave me a sense of control in a world that felt distinctly out of control, so I decided this caregiver role wasn't so bad and ran with it (all the way through medical school). But part of me knew I was in over my head, all the while ratcheting up my background alarm.

When children experience trauma in their family, they often blame themselves. Perhaps this is because to blame the parents would be a threat to that child's survival—that is, the child can't see a parent as fallible because the child needs to see the parent as competent and reliable for their own survival. Because a problem cannot be seen as a parent's fault, the child assumes the blame (and shame), which gets poured directly into their background alarm.

There is a sad saying about this: when a parent neglects, mistreats, or abandons a child, the child doesn't stop loving the parent, they stop loving themselves. When you stop loving yourself, you split from yourself, and this internal separation deposits a tremendous amount of background alarm in your body. Much of healing is bringing this internal split back into your awareness, realizing it truly was not your fault, and reprocessing, metabolizing, and integrating that alarm so as to love the scared child in you that stopped loving themselves so long ago.

In another bit of foreshadowing of part 3, when you see, hear, understand, love, and protect that alarmed child in you, you resolve the split that created that alarm in the first place. When the separation is resolved, so is the alarm, and as the alarm feeds the anxious thoughts, the worries resolve as well.

What do you think would happen if you had a child come up to you crying in pain from ALARMS and you distracted away from them, withdrew into an addiction, or otherwise pushed them away? That child would likely get louder and pursue you more. Over time, that's what alarm does too: it gets louder and pursues you more. Here is a critical message of this book: *The alarm is your younger self asking for your attention and support.*

With this awareness, we can see that asking "How do I get rid of my anxiety?" is the wrong question. Instead, I would encourage you to ask what inside of you—the emotional pain you could not metabolize or integrate back then—is asking for your love and attention now?

Just as we once engaged in sympathetic activation of pursuit to get back a secure attachment to our parents, your child self is now trying to close the gap with your adult self and get the nurturing it needs—and this pursuit energy is expressed as alarm. It is one of the unfortunate parts of alarm that it causes an automatic and unconscious rejection of the painful sensation (and the child in us that carries it), beginning a vicious cycle that keeps that child feeling isolated and alone.

If you deny and reject your younger self's attempts to connect, the alarm energy gets diverted into worry. You may temporarily be able to ignore, distract, dissociate, or addict your way into suppressing that background alarm, but know that it will rise up again. I can't tell you how many times I had to increase a patient's antidepressant medication because it failed to contain their emotional pain. The wounded, alarmed child comes back because that wounded, alarmed part of your younger self has not been connected with and healed—only drugged so it's not as loud.

When you start to see that the alarm you feel is not an enemy to be defeated but a younger version of you that deserves compassion, the whole game changes.

Instead of interpreting the alarm as the enemy that you need to get MADD at (that is, treat with medications, addiction, distraction, and dissociation—see, I told you I love acronyms), you can channel the sympathetic nervous system energy of pursuit created by the alarm into a pursuit of your younger self! My goal is to show you how to use the energy of alarm in your body as a direct conduit to your younger, wounded self.

The alarm is not your enemy, it is actually your wounded child self, so trying to get rid of the alarm is only going to cause the wounded version of you to get more alarmed! Instead of trying to rid ourselves of the child in us and their pain, we need to learn to embrace that child, even if it is at first a monumental task to learn to love what we perceive as tormenting us. The good news is you are an adult now and you have the information and resources to address those old wounds now in a way you did not back then.

When you welcome the alarm, you welcome the wounded child in you and start the process of metabolizing and healing the old wounds in your background. There is a process called *integration* in which disparate parts are united to heal into a functional whole. When integration happens, the energy of your alarm can be embraced as contributing to a constructive, functional whole you instead of energizing a destructive and disparate part of you that perpetuates your alarm.

When you view the alarm as some sort of weakness or punishment, you are likely to further separate from that wounded child by medicating it, overpowering it with addictions, dissociating, or using distraction. But when you distract, dissociate, reject, or worry, that alarmed child feels the same abandonment and separation it did years earlier—which only creates more background alarm. As the alarm ramps up and becomes potentiated, we become less and less rational, like a lost child at the grocery store, freaking out with more worry each minute that goes by without connecting with our parents.

I need you to see the alarm is actually not a threat but a messenger showing you the path to healing. For as long as you've been trying to get rid of your anxiety, you've been shooting the messenger—but the messenger is you, so you've been shooting your child self (often manifesting as biting your own tail with worry).

Your background alarm is your younger, reactive, vulnerable self—not your enemy but a beacon for a closer connection to the real, authentic you that you were supposed to be before your trauma(s). It's time to stop hurting yourself and start helping yourself.

58

On Integration

When you neutralize and integrate your old wounds, they leave the body and go back into the mind in an organized state where the energy can promote wholeness and growth. It is the reverse of what happened when you were young when the energy was too much and you became disintegrated as a form of protection.

This integration is what happens during childhood in families with a strong sense of attachment that can fully support children through the trauma so that the negative emotional energy is metabolized, digested, and neutralized instead of overflowing into background alarm.

The story of my patient Alanna illustrates this concept of integration.

Alanna came to me when she was fifteen, just after her parents divorced. Alanna had yellow-blond hair and intense blue eyes and an athletic, muscular frame. Unfortunately she had also developed a significant issue with OCD. (I've often joked it should be called compulsive obsessive disorder, because shouldn't we put it in alphabetical order?) Alanna would perform elaborate physical movements like tapping her chest five times before getting in the car or turning around in a clockwise circle three times before entering a room. She also exercised a lot and developed disordered eating (though stopping short of any clinical diagnosis).

Alanna's parents had an amicable divorce, but Alanna felt very polarized—compelled to be close to her physically distant father and resenting her mother, even though her mom was the one who provided most of the connection and support.

Over the six years we spent working together, Alanna did therapy that focused on her body, called somatic experiencing therapy, along with traditional psychotherapy. Somatic experiencing is a form of therapy created by Peter Levine, PhD, that tunes into the trauma stored in the body.

My wife is a certified somatic experiencing practitioner (SEP), and she has taught me a great deal about the process of healing trauma using the body. I have completed the three-year SEP training as well. Working with this modality has confirmed what I first saw during my LSD experience—that my pain had more to do with the alarm stored in my body than the machinations of my mind. Healing trauma, it has become clear to me, is less about talking through it and more about *feeling* through it. When I say you can't think your way out of a feeling problem, this is exactly what I mean. I believe that in the very near future we are going to see the field of psychotherapy as a whole move in the direction of using more of this type of body-based therapy, along with other therapies like internal family systems therapy and psychedelics.

When I met Alanna, she had a very rigid posture and her voice was tense and muted. In therapy, she was encouraged (slowly) to tune into her body and become aware of how tightly she held herself. Alanna had been unable to feel (and therefore metabolize) the grief of the dissolution of her family. She would tell me that because the divorce of her parents never got "ugly" and because her mom and dad were amicable toward each other, she couldn't understand why they needed to separate in the first place. It was like she didn't believe the divorce was happening, and therefore she couldn't grieve (and therefore integrate) a loss she didn't expressly feel. That changed once her father found another partner, and the reality that her family wasn't coming back began to sink in and she started to access her grief. When I asked her why she didn't eat, she told me she didn't feel hungry. When I asked her if she had hunger pains she said there was a "frozen numbness" around her stomach. I'm shortening this quite a bit, but once she allowed herself to feel, and specifically more into her body sensations, especially the numb and frozen parts, Alanna came to accept and even see the positives in her parents' divorce. In addition, Alanna's parents developed a friendship as they became committed to emotionally and physically supporting Alanna together.

Alanna's issues and obsessions with food and exercising resolved, and she became less muscular. Today she would probably say that although the divorce caused her great pain at the time, she could see why it had to happen and that it led to a connection with both her parents that is actually closer in many ways than before the divorce. She also came to feel that talking about the divorce, although still not her favorite topic, did not trigger her anymore. (When you are no longer triggered by an event, this is solid evidence that integration has taken place.) Finally, she said she felt more connected to herself as she connected with her body.

Initially, the divorce of Alanna's parents had created a vulnerability that was too much for her mind to tolerate and which, therefore, was stored in her body as that background alarm in her stomach, driving her disordered eating and obsessive movement rituals. The old trauma was integrated once she understood how to feel and listen to the alarm in her body, and once her mind fully accepted the divorce and even grew to see the positives that came from it. Alanna no longer felt so alarmed when the old wound was touched, and her obsessions and compulsions no longer cropped up as a coping mechanism.

To reinforce the point of integration, the trauma energy is felt, metabolized, and neutralized in a supportive environment and no longer stays a trigger with the power to reignite alarm. Alanna had plenty of emotional support throughout her healing and learned how to connect with both her parents—and, probably more important, with herself. Her background alarm was brought to the surface, metabolized, and integrated. Her OCD behaviors and disordered eating were signs she was dissociating because her mind was overwhelmed; once she was able to feel the loving association and connection with her parents and herself, she was able to come back into an associated and integrated state.

59

The Dissociation Association

Remember Jane, my patient who picked one alcoholic boyfriend after another like they were bourbon-glazed doughnuts at a New Orleans bakery? I once had a session with her the same day one of her boyfriends had emotionally abused her. She was not physically harmed or touched in anger, but her boyfriend had berated her verbally for simply talking to another man.

When I saw her in my office later that day, she could not meet my eye. Her facial muscles drooped, and she talked with a weak, monotone voice. There were episodes where her voice just trailed off. As I looked at her, with her shoulders hunched and her head hanging down, it seemed to me I was looking at a chastised eight-year-old girl.

And I probably was.

When Jane was being verbally abused by her boyfriend, the similarity to her father's tongue lashings would have certainly fired up her background alarm. Remember the amygdala, the structure in the brain that never forgets? If there is a situation that shares any similarity to your original wounding, the amygdala will flare up and fire both background and foreground alarms in an effort to protect you from what it perceives as the very same wounding happening again. The amygdala is very much like the hypersensitive smoke detector in my old condo, firing off not just at smoke but also at things that only vaguely resembled smoke. Jane's amygdala would have fired up her background alarm, which would then have started the game of ping-pong with her foreground alarm, and she would be in a full-body reaction. If the situation carried on and the abuse from her boyfriend kept going, her rational circuits would shut down and her survival circuits would engage, activating a maximal response in her alarm—like pushing those airplane engines up to 100 percent capacity in an emergency.

Because the mind cannot handle energy like that for long, a protective reaction called dissociation steps in. Dissociation is a type of escape when the present moment becomes too intense for the mind to stay engaged, so the mind leaves the present moment. When faced with an acute state that reminded her amygdala of severe trauma from her past, the "shutdown" of dissociation would occur to prevent the system from staying at the maximal response.

So why did Alanna's dissociation look different from Jane's? My theory is that Alanna's dissociation was slower because her trauma was not as acute. Alanna's trauma, although very intense and painful for a teenager, occurred when she was older, was never life-threatening, and she knew that. In contrast, Jane, being a young child when her trauma began, likely did fear for her survival on some level because of the abusive nature of her father's behavior. When Jane was faced with similar abuse from her boy-friend, her amygdala sensed the similarity and fired her into full-throttle foreground and background alarm in a matter of seconds, so her disso-ciation looked more like the freeze response that animals go into when cornered. If they've already expended too much energy fighting and/or know they have no chance of escaping, the animal feigns death in hopes their attacker will lose interest. This *dorsal vagal shutdown* (more later) frequently happens in humans that carry a lot of alarm and old trauma. When faced with a reminder of our old trauma many of us will adopt this severe dissociation and widespread system shutdown and age regression, as I witnessed firsthand with Jane.

When we get knocked off balance and are acting from a disconnected, disorganized, and volatile place of alarm, our responses will also be prim-itive and disorganized. Although we may appear withdrawn to an outside observer, there is plenty of volatility happening inside.

Maybe your parent or caregiver "cornered" you with emotional or physical demands that overwhelmed you? You may have attacked back or just gave up into dissociation and shutdown when you saw your attempts at protecting yourself were futile. Had your parent recognized your ac-tivation and made an overture of connection at the time, you may have been able to resolve the issue and avoid dumping a bunch of alarm down into your body.

Or maybe your parent was also in shutdown, so they couldn't connect with you because they were also dissociated. My mother was like this, she loved me but lapsed into shutdown and dissociation, often because she was overwhelmed with the reactivation of background alarm from her own childhood.

Many of my patients with anxiety often had parents that had anxiety themselves and were not able to make connections with their children, so background alarm flows from generation to generation. Anxious parents, anxious children.

Over the course of our office visit, child Jane began to come out of her dissociated state once she got some reassurance from me and started to feel safe. She started the visit as her eight-year-old self in full collapse but, by the end of the visit, adult Jane was able to make eye contact, gain some strength in her voice, and even laugh with me about the fact that she had "picked another one!" in her recurring cast of questionable boyfriends.

Remember the social engagement system (SES), the innate part of our nervous system that allows us to connect with ourselves and others? This system is also sometimes referred to as human resonance circuitry because we literally use it to resonate in safety with another person. I used Jane's familiarity with and trust in me to engage her SES and help her emerge from her dissociated state. Jane also had a counselor she felt safe with, and over the course of multiple sessions with her trusted therapist, Jane was able to become acutely aware of her compulsion to pick alcoholics like her father. She came to see that she would dissociate and, in her words, "leave herself" when she accepted the advances of a man who fit the abusive or alcoholic profile of her father. In a moment I still vividly remember to this day, she even used the term "repetition compulsion" in describing her attraction to these guys. Jane is a great example of the power of bringing her alarm to awareness and the power of simple social interaction in helping us heal and calm our alarm.

Point to consider: I asked this question in part 1, but it's so important I'll share it again: What patterns from your childhood are you unconsciously recreating in your adulthood? Hint: look for places of pain in your life today.

60
Alarm's Association with Dissociation

Dissociation is a protective mechanism. It is a daydreaming-type state where we zone out, go into freeze, and shut off our social engagement system. People dissociate in different ways, up to and including becoming fully unconscious (either falling asleep or fainting), but mostly it involves withdrawing from interaction with other people. Eye contact is lost, our face loses expression, our voice becomes monotone, and our body movements are minimal.

Alarm is almost always the precursor to dissociation. The more intense the state of alarm, the more likely we will distract into dissociation. Alarm also opens the door to our addictions (shopping, trips to the Come On Inn, alcohol, etc.) and to the desire to take legal and illegal substances to soothe ourselves. But this chapter is all about dissociation and I won't get distracted from that.

"From what?"

Dissociation.

Oh, right. Sorry, I dissociated there for a second.

Maybe you notice periods when you are anxious and alarmed and you can't connect to others. Perhaps more insidiously, you've dissociated to the point that you've lost the ability to see you've lost connection with yourself, too. This dissociation can also show up as absent-mindedness, and this is often a place where ADD and anxiety overlap.

My wife used to see me moving into this dissociated state on a very regular basis. I often didn't notice it because I was in it. An early telltale sign for her was when I would begin to lose my sense of humor. Normally, I'm always doing silly things around the house to make her laugh, but that would disappear as my mind and body headed into alarm and I began to withdraw. I would lose the warmth and play in my voice, and it would become more flat and monotone. My body would turn inward, my head and shoulders slumping forward. Often, I would withdraw into the bedroom. Maybe you can take a moment and see if you can notice your particular dissociation association, a pattern that you fall into when you feel alarmed and withdraw from the people closest to you.

If you can begin to see it, you don't have to be it.

Have you ever forced yourself to go to a social engagement and just felt frozen and out of place? You get stuck in a corner or having awkward conversations, and you just can't shake the urge to escape? Chances are your alarm was triggered and paralyzed your SES, and when you can't connect (to others or yourself), you can't soothe yourself. In a vicious cycle the alarm magnifies, deepening your sense of disconnection and dissociation which intensifies your alarm . . . you get the picture.

We simply can't be socially connected and engaged when we are in alarm. From an evolutionary perspective, when we are alarmed and in survival physiology, our brain will prioritize threats and activate the more emotional parts of our nervous system. We saw in the last chapter the healing power of the SES, but when we are in alarm and move toward a dissociated state, we lose access to this powerful tool for self-soothing. Without our SES we can't find the soothing connection with others or, more critically, ourselves.

There were days when just getting out of bed to have a shower or take Buddha out for a walk seemed like a monumental task. While I know this narrow focus on life-sustaining functions was my nervous system's way of protecting me, it cut me off from nurturing, caring interactions with other people. In dissociation, there is a perverse sense of comfort in staying frozen and still, and this is why it's so hard to get out of the house, or exercise, or phone a friend, even though you know it would help you! For many of us as children, this sense of freeze, withdrawal, and dissociation was perceived as a familiar and protective state. As I've said before, humans couple what is familiar with what is secure ("family" and "liar," remember?), so we still fall into dissociation and withdrawal as adults when we feel overwhelmed.

If we can understand this seduction into the dissociative state as our primitive brain's way of trying to protect us and not some personal failing, we can see it, accept it, and neutralize it. Once again, awareness is the key. If you know your pattern of dissociation you can see it early and make a conscious choice not to be it. I want to show you how to gradually introduce a new relationship with your SES that will help you ease into connection with yourself and others when you need it the most. Practicing self-compassion and using sensation to bring you into the present moment are great ways of pulling yourself out of dissociation. I'll show you more of this in part 3 (unless I dissociate into my ADD and forget).

Point to consider: Some people find that ADD meds that activate the system paradoxically ease anxiety, and that may be because the medications keep us focused and out of painful dissociation.

61

Insights from MDMA

From the time I was a teenager, I had started to feel uneasy in my love for my dad. To see someone I loved in deep pain—to see someone I loved literally losing his mind—and not have a damn thing I could do about it was devastating in a way that defies description. To an extent, part of me was beginning to feel that to love him was not safe, and because there is only love and fear, as you push out love, you gradually begin to fill with fear and alarm.

You might ask whether another option might be indifference toward a parent who has abused, neglected, or otherwise failed you. Here's my more ethereal side coming out, but I do not believe we can truly be indifferent to a parent. We may tell ourselves we are, and we may even convince ourselves that we feel nothing, but there is an undeniable, unconscious, spiritual linkage we have to a parent, regardless of what they have or haven't done.

Perhaps the biggest sin of an unworthy parent is that they engender a mistrust of love in their child. When your ability to trust love is compromised, fear quickly takes over the empty space and pushes you into survival brain, further limiting your ability to mature your SES. As your SES is compromised, your ability to connect to love diminishes as well, and in a vicious cycle, the fear and alarm slowly block your ability to trust the love you will need to heal the alarm!

Early on in my teen years, when my dad would return from the mental hospital, I was quick to pursue and connect with him again, each time hoping that he was cured. But every single time, with sometimes as much as a year of relative normalcy in between, he would return to madness, and after a while, out of self-preservation, I started to withhold my connection with him. I wasn't aware of this of course, but fear and alarm were slowly taking me over.

My experiences with loving my father and seeing him in excruciating pain made me withdraw in self-defense. But when we withdraw love from a parent, we compromise our SES and limit the ability to love anyone else fully, including ourselves. When we withhold love from ourselves, fear takes up the dead space and we are unable to find solid ground and are left defenseless to the ravages of increasing alarm and the anxiety it creates. So allowing and accepting the feeling of love again is key to bringing the SES back online so we are open to loving connection. The more connected we feel to others, the more connected we will feel to ourselves, and this self-connection is the best route to integrating and dissolving our old background alarm. Just as when love is excluded fear rushes in to fill the void, when love is allowed back in, the fear is pushed out. As we make the intention to accept loving connection to ourselves and others the SES comes back to do the job it's been designed to do for thousands of years of human social evolution: connect us to ourselves and to others.

I had shielded myself from love for many years, and while I still felt it, there was always a little "once bitten, twice shy" element to it. My trusted LSD guide suggested that I could try MDMA to really feel the unbridled sense of love I'd disconnected from after being disappointed so many times by my father. Once again, I was scared, but as I knew MDMA was not a psychedelic, I felt confident I was not going to go back into the science project from hell—and it turned out to be quite the opposite.

So, in the summer of 2015, at the ripe old age of fifty-four, I took my first hit of ecstasy. (At this point I want to point out that I am not some kind hallucinogen-crazed psychonaut. I have taken ayahuasca twice, psilocybin once, LSD once, and MDMA once, the last experience with any being in 2015.) All in all, MDMA was a wonderful experience that showed me that when my brain had a healthy dose of love running through it, anxiety was impossible to conjure up. I could still academically bring up worrisome thoughts (even those of sickness and death), but they seemed trivial and did not disturb me in the least. My mind was full of love for everything and everyone, and my body felt a lightness and peace I had never remembered experiencing before. MDMA didn't fracture my mind into a million pieces the way the psychedelics did. On MDMA, I had much more control of my mind, and I felt a sense of unity with my environment more so than I had with psychedelics. Even if it was drug-induced, I saw that love vanquished all anxiety in my mind and alarm in my body. MDMA showed me that I was repeatedly trying to mistrust something that I was at my essence—love.

As it began to wear off, MDMA also helped me to see that I was very quick to sidestep positive emotions like love and joy. I found myself looking for reasons to jerk back into protection mode. I was still feeling this sense of love for everything and everyone, but my familiar pattern of recoiling from love and blocking joy started to creep back in as the drug wore off. A benevolent part of me wanted to ride on in the loving experience, but another part (a part I was all too familiar with) started to mistrust feeling good. Perhaps fifteen minutes earlier I'd had nothing but love in my heart, but as the drug's effect faded I felt my old pattern of discomfort in feeling "too good" creeping back in. In real time I observed how my pattern of familiar worry slowly but steadily began squeezing the unfamiliar good feeling from my experience.

Curiously, I saw my worries in a new light. As I was still feeling warm and loving, I could watch those worries start to line up like excited children outside the gate at a swimming pool that was about to open. I realized I was seeing my worries in a way I'd never been able to before—objectively. Thanks to MDMA, I was not in alarm, so my mind stayed out of the typical muddy survival brain that had been inextricably coupled with my worries before. For once, I could stay in my rational brain and really see the worries in a dispassionate, non-alarmed way that gave me the objective choice to believe them or not.

As I noticed my old protective habit starting to give the worries credibility, I wondered why I was "ruining" the experience and proposed to myself that I should just stay in love. In a moment of introspection, I asked myself why I felt the need to destroy this feeling. My answer was clear: "Don't enjoy it, because it's just going to be taken away from you." I was afraid those emotions would be ripped from me, just as I perceived my dad was ripped from me by mental illness. I saw that I didn't let myself stay in positive emotion for very long without sabotaging it by thinking of something scary or uncomfortable or discounting my own abilities. In short, I was learning how to remain separate and separated from myself, and since all anxiety is separation anxiety, when you are separate from yourself, you have no chance of healing from chronic anxiety and alarm.

My unconscious self-talk had told me, "Good things don't last" and "Don't get too comfortable, for this will all be taken from you" because that was exactly my childhood experience. Those thoughts were repeated so often that they became an unconscious program, like the implicit memory or body memory I talked about in my unconscious aversion to grocery stores. The "don't get too comfortable for all this will be taken away" program had been just as deeply ingrained in me. My system had adopted the implicit program that I should not enjoy positive emotion because it was going to be taken away anyway, and the pleasure wasn't worth the potential pain of losing it. This is exactly the "foreboding joy" Brené Brown talks about when she says, "When we lose our tolerance for vulnerability, joy becomes foreboding." To me, this means that when we block our access to love out of a sense of protection, we block our access to joy as well. It's like never allowing yourself to enjoy a piece of chocolate cake because you know you'll ruminate on getting fat the whole time it's in your mouth.

There's the old fear bias in action. Even the most emotionally healthy human child is still programmed to use fear for protection, so it doesn't take much in the way of experience to make that fear response a preferential groove in the snow, especially if that human child is very sensitive. I needed something powerful to bump my toboggan out of the deep groove of believing that love was too big of a risk to take.

To cut a long story short, MDMA showed me *I could feel love without fear.* This was a revelation to me. It also showed me how disconnected I was from myself and that I should make an effort to allow the positive emotions to stay as long as they liked. MDMA also gave me the inkling that a compassionate connection to myself would go a long way in reducing my alarm and the anxiety that followed it.

I'd like to note that my MDMA trip wasn't without pain. Although it was a positive experience overall, the two to three days following it were difficult, as I experienced a big rebound in my anxiety. So, like psilocybin, LSD, and ayahuasca, it had a significant downside for me, and I am in no way recommending someone with alarm experiment with these "medicines." I won't ever use them again, but in hindsight I'm glad I did. They gave me insight into how the mind and body handle trauma (and the path to healing it) that most doctors will never know. I've come to know it's not so much the trauma as the way that trauma was handled that determines the outcome—so I could have blamed my mother for her inability to fully look after my emotional needs, but I don't. She had her hands more than full. I love my mom dearly. She did remarkably well given all the demands on her. She was simply spread too thin. She is remarkably strong and resilient, and the family needed those qualities to survive as well as we did.

There was a time I actually did blame my parents, until I came to see that holding contempt for them locked me in contempt—and my psyche could not afford the cost of any more negative thoughts or emotions, since that just kept me out of my own SES, and while I stayed in that state of contempt and blame, I had nothing to pull me out of the turbulent sea of alarm.

On MDMA I saw clearly that I needed to provide the connection to myself that my parents were unable to give me. I have come to see that what both parents went through in their own childhoods made it virtually impossible for them to give me what they didn't get themselves. The connection that I refused to give them would be the connection I refused to give myself. As a result, in maintaining my split from my parents, even if it was unconscious, I maintained my split from myself. That, in turn, maintained the alarm in my system, which kept me in survival mode and out of touch with my own SES, which prevented me from healing my alarm. Simple, huh?

For many years, I was in an almost perpetual state of either alarm or dissociation/shutdown. In that withdrawn state, I was unable to connect with myself or others. I was trapped in a catch-22—in a constant state of alarm/pursuit yet unable to trust the connection I was so desperately pursuing. I repeated this in all my romantic relationships, and they didn't go well. In the initial stages of my relationships, idealization and infatuation kept me in an oxytocin-like, MDMA-type pursuit state where love could flow readily. But my own "this is all going to be taken away from you" program always popped up as the oxytocin naturally began to drop down, and slowly I became more dissociated from each partner—and then I would resent them for not keeping me in love! In some respects, I did the same thing with my parents, resenting them for my own feelings of dissociation.

It's been said many times that holding on to resentment is like drinking poison and expecting the other person to die. The bottom line is that maintaining resentment for my parents maintained my alarm, and maintaining my alarm maintained my anxious thoughts. You can see where this is going: as long as I maintained separation from my parents, I continued to recharge the alarm-anxiety cycle because separation is exactly what set off my alarm in the first place.

"All anxiety is separation anxiety."

—DR. GORDON NEUFELD

"All alarm is separation alarm."

—DR. RUSSELL KENNEDY

In my own case, separating from the feelings in my body started early. I began to split from the very thing I needed to connect to the most—my own self. As I became more numb and separate from myself as my inner critic judged, abandoned, blamed, and shamed me (much more on JABS soon), I became more alarmed, causing me to separate further from my body and to move away from my source of stability and grounding. As I numbed out my body in an attempt not to feel the alarm that lived there, I retreated into the worries in my head. As a young adult, I went along with traditional dogma that I could think my way out of a feeling problem, so I did all sorts of head-based talk therapy, but none ever really got me back into my body, where I could reconnect with myself and my SES. I was trapped in alarm with no way out until I started doing body-based therapies like somatic experiencing. I was chasing (and biting) my tail up in my head. There's no tail up there, as far as I know—and neither was there a solution up there to my alarm and anxiety.

So let me ask you: When did you start to separate from the love you had for yourself? Was there a point when you separated from your care-givers? When did you experience ALARMS: abuse, loss, abandonment, rejection (or bullying), maturing too early because of the demands placed on you, or shame?

As I go through the list, I can see the loss of my father to his illness, the abandonment I felt from both parents due to their own overwhelm, and being forced to mature too early—all of which I've already discussed at some length. But I also recall being bullied by kids in school and feeling rejected. I remember being ashamed of myself at times when I felt weak or wasn't effectively carrying out my father's role in taking care of the family. I say all of this not to garner sympathy but to show you how many ALARMS one person might have. Don't minimize your own experiences and tell yourself they weren't that bad. This list of ALARMS shows us all the places we lost or abandoned ourselves along the way. Knowing where you split from yourself allows you to find yourself again. Just as the child lost in the store can feel safe again when their parents are found, you can find yourself in your own ability to feel and create your own sense of safety.

But first and foremost, we need to trust that we can be safe.

62

When It's Not Safe to Feel Safe

I love getting massages, because it's one of the rare times my body completely lets go. It used to happen to me often that I would fall asleep during a massage and then awaken with a jolt of alarm.

Remember, for me it didn't feel safe to feel safe. I came to understand this was causing my reactions during my massages. I would get so relaxed, and then I would feel a jolt of alarm, like a milder version of a panic attack. This was my body falling into the old groove: "Don't get too comfortable because this will all be taken from you."

I realized this was a throwback to when things were going okay, even good, with my dad, and then it would all collapse, sometimes completely unexpectedly. In essence, if my dad collapsed, I felt everything would be taken away from me, so I could never let myself relax—either my father was falling apart or I was worried he was going to. I felt no other option.

Normally, I had worries in my mind at all times. If a medical test came back normal, I'd immediately start to worry about the next thing. I invented all kinds of worries, and the more horrible they were, the more effective they were at keeping me in my head and out of my body. Of course I never felt safe—I made sure of it!

When the emotion held in the body is not expressed, this trapped energy wreaks havoc in our system. In medicine, the prefix "dys-" means abnormal, as in dysfunctional. The alarm-anxiety cycle is a dysfunctional relationship between the mind and the body. It's not so much they're cut off from each other as the relationship is skewed toward surviving rather than thriving.

For a long time, I had a relationship with myself that did not have the luxury of rest. In that hypervigilant state, it was very easy for my mind to focus on the negative, or to tell myself I should be doing something productive. It was almost like there was a gate where the negative was let in without question but the positive had to be overwhelmingly positive before it was allowed admission. As a result of this negativity bias, my mind and body remained dys-connected and dysfunctional and never learned to trust each other. Therefore, it was second nature for me not to trust positive feelings, to trust myself, or to trust in the general safety of life.

During a massage now, I actually allow myself to stop thinking and just settle into feeling. This had always been a recipe for disaster before, but now I know that my body may still snap me back into vigilance and worry when I feel "too safe." But I am fully aware of what is happening, and I can consciously return to the sensation in my body and enjoy the feeling of safety. This ability to settle in and realize that it is safe to feel safe took a long time to cultivate, but I will show you exactly how to do it in part 3.

Point to consider: How do you make sure you never allow yourself to feel safe?

63

Waiting for the Other Shoe to Drop

There are a few different origin stories for the phrase "waiting for the other shoe to drop," but the most common one seems to be that it originated in the nineteenth century, when people lived in wooden buildings with limited soundproofing. At night, someone above you would drop their shoe to the ground while getting into bed, which would make a loud sound. The person below would know there was no point in trying to fall back asleep until they heard that inevitable second shoe hit the floor.

That time spent in limbo, literally waiting for the other shoe to drop, was often a throwback to our childhood where we knew something bad was likely to happen but we didn't know exactly when. This familiar state of vigilance is not unlike the hypervigilance I've observed in myself and many of my patients who suffer from alarm and anxiety. We don't allow ourselves to feel calm and peaceful because of the fear of the inevitable loss that is coming, as that was the pattern when we were kids. In addition, we worriers think that if we keep ourselves in constant readiness for trouble, we will be more prepared to handle it when it arises.

But we are wrong on both counts. One of my favorite stand-up comedians, the late, great Norm Macdonald, has a line I love: "What doesn't kill you only acts to make you very, very weak." Allowing ourselves to be calm and peaceful is actually what allows us to better handle pain when it arises. Your vigilance does nothing but tire you out so that you lose twice. First, you lose from the pain of keeping yourself in a constant state of worry and alarm. And second, you lose when you lack the resources to handle the pain that does come up because you've exhausted your mind with hypervigilant worry and your body with chronic alarm.

I mentioned her in passing when I talked about foreboding joy, but renowned shame and vulnerability researcher Brené Brown talks about this. No matter how many times you rehearse that phone call from the school saying your child has been seriously injured, it does not help or empower you to deal with the situation. No matter how many times you worry about something terrible happening, the "practice" does not help you deal with it any better in the very unlikely event that it does happen.

Remember, worry is an illusion we use to trick ourselves into believing we are reducing uncertainty, when in truth worry actually does the opposite. When we worry about something, we are not reducing the chances of it happening. If anything, we are creating more focus on uncertainty by chronically raising the worry (and the inevitable internal defense and reassurance), which by its very nature implies more uncertainty, since you can only worry about something that by definition is not happening.

I have seen that many of my patients dealt with painful uncertainty during childhood: "Am I going to run into my bully today?" "Will my mother/father be drunk when I get home from school?" "Is there going to be anyone there when I get home?" "When are my parents going to have another huge fight and bring up divorce again?" "When's the next time I'm going to have to protect my mother from my father?" The list goes on.

In all these questions, notice the uncertainty—the waiting for the other shoe to drop. This uncertainty was especially apparent in my patients who grew up with alcoholic parents. There would be a period of relative calm before the inevitable blowup, binge, and chaos. When the binge ended, the chaos would resolve and often the drinker would apologize and there would be a period of relative calm again—until the next binge.

That cycle repeated itself countless times in many families I looked after as a doctor. As a child growing up with plenty of uncertainty around my father's mental state, I could relate.

When you grow up constantly waiting for the other shoe to drop, background alarm continues to accumulate, and with its accumulation, it brings a level of reflexive hypervigilance and hyperactivation of your foreground alarm in your sympathetic nervous system. Background alarm carries a perpetual activation of the nervous system—a preparatory, protective level of fight-or-flight readiness that keeps the system primed and ready for action. But the true need for action rarely comes, and we exhaust our resources in a constant preparedness, so if and when there is a real threat, we are too tired to be able to effectively react to it (which creates more alarm!). The more unresolved trauma gets added to background alarm, the higher the level of readiness for threat becomes ingrained over time—and the more we deplete ourselves by operating under the illusion that worry and hypervigilance are protective, when they never allow our bodies to fully rest.

I experienced a version of this (with less emotional charge than the hypervigilance related to my father) being on call overnight when I was a resident in the hospital. I would often fall asleep, but was still ready for the call. As an intern, if there was a cardiac arrest or other emergency, we were expected to get to the patient within two minutes. I would sleep in my scrubs so if the emergency pager sounded, I was ready. During these shifts, I never slept deeply, as my body was always waiting for the call.

When I was resting in the doctors' lounge, my parasympathetic rest-and-digest response was impaired by low-grade activation of the sympathetic fight-or-flight response because part of me knew that I may need to spring into action at a moment's notice. I'm sure every doctor has this to some extent, but because of the background alarm already in me, I suspect my inability to rest when on call was more pronounced than that of my colleagues who grew up in more securely attached and less traumatic homes.

When background alarm is active, even if you don't feel it consciously, at an unconscious level it is working to make your body feel unsafe. As an example, if I hear that someone died by suicide, my amygdala (because it recognizes the salience of suicide in my past) will fire up my old background alarm, which touches off a foreground alarm response. As this happens I'm not feeling overtly anxious, but when I check in with my breathing, it is shallow and superficial, evidence that my body is reacting to a perceived threat with an element of foreground alarm.

If you have chronic background alarm from unresolved pain in your past, it is likely your autonomic nervous system never properly calibrated the balancing act between the sympathetic nervous system and parasympathetic nervous system. The rest-and-digest part of the seesaw was never fully settled on the ground, as the chronic fight-or-flight activation held it suspended in the air. You never knew when someone would charge into the room and yell, "Sea monster!" You just had to be ready.

In those of us with chronic alarm (more commonly known as chronic anxiety, of course—but now we know the *real* truth), both foreground alarm and background alarm have been fired up so often that they've made their own grooves in the snow and take our toboggan from zero to sixty very quickly.

The good news is that you can recalibrate your autonomic nervous system. With time and practice, you can learn to feel safe feeling safe. But this recalibration must be done through the body—quieting the mind alone is not enough.

64

Am I Safe in This Moment?

Have you ever been ziplining? You clip yourself into a moving carriage that slides on a steel cable suspended above tall trees. Safely clipped in and secured, you can slide at a high speed at a terrifying height above a ravine or river.

This experience activates a bit of primal fear in our Stone Age brains. But for some worriers, ziplining can actually feel refreshingly safe, since we are focused on only one scary thing, and we have specific protection. This solitary fear of heights makes sense to us in the moment, and pales in comparison to the sheer number of ill-defined uncertainties and fears we stacked up in our childhood homes.

I've alluded to this earlier when I talked about "family and liar" but it bears repeating here. Human children equate familiarity with security. What was familiar in childhood we often unconsciously repeat in adulthood, for a deep, unconscious part of us equates security with what was imprinted on us as children.

A part of Jane had falsely equated her alcoholic father, as perverse as this sounds, with the "security" of familiarity. Equating familiarity with security works fine if you grew up in a healthy, securely attached family, but not so much if your family was dysfunctional or traumatic. Freud was right in that we will often repeat the circumstances of our childhoods in our adulthoods, as we unconsciously and compulsively recreate old pain in an attempt to recreate the security in our childhood that wasn't actually there.

In addition to placing ourselves in unhealthy relationships that replicate our trauma bonds, another way we enact the repetition compulsion is by staying disconnected from ourselves. This is another way of saying we unconsciously stay in our minds with our worries, not consciously realizing the worries are keeping us out of our bodies where the path to healing lies. When we are used to spending all our time in our minds because the feelings in our body are too painful, we gain a sense of familiarity with the worry, and we choose the devil we know (the worries of the mind) instead of the *uncertainty* of the devil we don't (the alarm in the body). Unfortunately for us, if we stay away from our alarm we can never tame it. When we make the unconscious conscious, as Jung says, we can take our unconscious compulsion to stay with our worries and turn it into an adult, conscious decision to go back into the body of the child and resolve the pain by connecting with that child.

When I was young, I never had a chance to connect with my feeling self because all my attention went to reading my father and mother and trying to make sure they were okay. Typically, in families with trauma, the children don't get the luxury of being able to see how they themselves really feel inside because their focus is outside—on one or both parents. Many children who grow up to be alarmed adults had to look after one or both of their parents in some way. Their survival brain told them, "If my parent is not okay, then I am not okay." As a result, they made their parents' needs a priority over their own, and they lost touch with their own inner world to be responsible for controlling the outer world of their parent. As adults, many of them resonate with the term "empath" and are still adept at reading and looking after others but struggle to read and look after themselves. Dr. Gabor Maté talks about this in his book *The Myth of Normal,* and I am paraphrasing a little. Specifically, Dr. Maté talks about how a child gives up their *authentic self* by capitulating to the needs of their parent, relinquishing their authentic nature and needs in order to not threaten the attachment to the parent. This people pleasing becomes a lifelong compulsive habit that reinforces itself over time, and prevents the child from truly knowing themselves because they have always needed to focus on someone else.

Since your relationship with others can be no better than your relationship with yourself, to break your repetition compulsion and stop finding yourself in people-pleasing relationships where your needs finish last (if at all), you must first foster a closer relationship with yourself than you've ever had before. Once you have a compassionate relationship with yourself, only then are you able to create truly compassionate relationships with other people in your life.

If you compulsively gave to others, it's no wonder you weren't able to integrate your trauma during childhood. You can't break the alarm-anxiety cycle until you feel safe and your needs are a priority. During my own childhood, conditions were never safe enough to give my background alarm a chance to calm down, and this may well be the case with you, too. Many of my patients had a similar soul-crushing, alarming dynamic of looking for safety in a parent who was also the source of their alarm.

My dad could be quite caring and lucid for months at a time, and there were some truly wonderful times in my family. But there was also a profound sense that both my father and the foundation of the family could crack at any moment. This kept my family perpetually off balance and never allowed us to truly connect to each other because the focus was always on my father and his state of mind. My mother, my brother, and I also could not engage each other's social engagement systems with more positive interactions because there was never a big enough foundation of safety to allow our social engagement systems to come out and play.

A common question I get in relation to self-connection is this: How do you connect with yourself when the connection has been broken for so long, or was never really there in the first place?

Good question. You have likely been in a chronic state of self-disconnection and future-based worry for so long you haven't even been aware there is a child in you that is deep in alarm. That child needs a sense of safety, a knowingness that you are going to be the caregiver for them now that they so badly needed back then. (Stay tuned.)

We can start resolving the separation of your mind and body right now with one simple question that has transformed many lives, and that is "Am I safe in this moment?" I know this is part of the Anxiety Toolkit, but it's such a critical component to engage that I repeat it here.

> In this moment, right here, right now, reading or listening to this book, are you safe? Can you take a deep breath in and out and really sense that you are safe? Can you see how you are chronically looking for danger that actually is only present in the imagined future of your mind? Can you close your eyes, put your hand on your chest, and just sit in the experience of being safe, even if it is only for the next fifteen seconds?

This leads me to a truth that most worriers do not want to acknowledge. If you are safe in this moment, then you are safe because *the moment you are in is all you ever have.*

Maybe, in the time it took to keep reading, that sense of safety is gone. Maybe your mind has jumped ahead to one of your automatic "frequent flyer" worries about your health or your credit card bill (and the strange charges that may be on it). That's okay. Just observe what your mind has done—congruently created a story in your mind to support a feeling of danger in your body.

Then ask yourself again: "At this moment, sitting here reading this book, am I safe?" Really feel it, don't just say it. And know you can stop and ask this question 24/7/365 anytime you are stressed or ruminating on your worries. Personally, I get the best use out of "I am safe in this moment" when I wake up in the middle of the night with alarm. You can relish your safety in the moment by adding a focus on your breath or by putting your hand on your chest to connect with yourself while you assert that in this moment you are indeed safe. This adds sensation in the present moment (you can only feel sensation in the moment you are in), and pulls your attention away from the past pain in your body or future-based thoughts your mind is trying to get you to believe. You don't have to believe everything you think, and you don't have think everything you feel.

65

Find Your (Background) Alarm

The biggest gift of my LSD experience was showing me that my alarm is a hot, irregular, sharp, oval-shaped purple crystalline density located just to the right of my solar plexus in my *body*. Before I knew this, I was chasing and biting my own tail erroneously believing the source of my emotional pain was the worries of my *mind*. So, let's help you find your alarm.

When you get stressed and overcome by worry, where do you feel it in your body? Have you ever thought to look for it? Most of my anxious patients are so entangled in the imagined sharks in their mind it never crosses that mind to look a little lower for the true source of their pain.

Go ahead, right here, right now, close your eyes and bring to mind one of your most common "frequent flyer" worries. Really focus on how scary this worry would be if it came true. Keep that worry alive in your mind and intentionally leave that mind space and see if there is an intense sensation in your body. Get really quiet and focused as you go back and forth between the worry in your mind and the sensation in your body. Look for a place that is more intense and stands out. Finding the alarm in your body is a critical skill and it can be hard to locate from a description in a book, so if this book has resonated with you so far, consider getting my online program, Your Mind-Body Prescription for Permanent Anxiety Healing (MBRX). I made the program very affordable and accessible because it is my life's work to help everyone find their alarm and heal it so they don't have to suffer with anxiety for decades as I did.

When finding the alarm in your body, most people will find it somewhere between their chin and their pubic bone, most often close to the midline (or center of the body). For some, it's a pressure or ache in the throat or solar plexus. For others, it feels like nausea or a punch in the gut. It may feel like the heartache after a bad breakup or a feeling of fullness like a balloon. It can be superficial or deep, hot or cold (or both—we are dealing with the dreamlike state of the unconscious where feelings represent complex patterns that don't often make logical sense).

Once you've found where it is, see how much you can observe about it and how specific you can get. This alarm doesn't have to make sense, and it often doesn't. Does it have a shape? A color? Does it have a sharp border or is it fuzzy at its edges? Is it a pressure sensation or a pain? If it feels painful, is it sharp or dull (or both)?

As you feel it and connect with it more, it can often reveal different sensations in more detail. Be patient, for this might be the first time you have looked for the source for your anxiety outside of your mind.

Localizing the sensation and characteristics of my alarm has been invaluable in my healing. Finding my alarm in my solar plexus showed me that my ayahuasca-based sense that there was "nothing to hold on to" was completely false. This alarm in the body is a remnant of your younger, scared self and you can absolutely hold on to them.

But don't worry (ha!) if you can't find your alarm right away. I've had many patients who had to search for a while and just had to stay open and curious until eventually it came into sensation for them. Be patient with yourself. Finding your alarm is probably a brand-new concept to you, and it may seem more than a little strange. But I assure you, finding the source of your alarm in your body is a critical component to your healing.

Sometimes patients who initially can't find their alarm can do so as they repeatedly practice holding a fearful scenario or old grief in their mind while focusing intently on their body. I had one patient who was finally able to locate her alarm during a huge argument with her ex-husband over where their children were going to spend Christmas. ('Tis the season! "Alarm bells ring, are you list'ning?")

Seriously, painful Christmas or holiday memories are an absolute goldmine when you are looking to find your alarm. Holiday season family get-togethers usually light up alarm like a Christmas tree, or a menorah, or whatever symbol your family uses.

Some people feel safer trying to find their alarm in the presence of a trusted person or therapist. Sometimes alarm is difficult to locate because your unconscious doesn't want you to see it, as that's the reason the alarm was buried in your body in the first place! Alarm can be buried deeply and surrounded by a lot of protective emotion—not to mention the hypervigilant, overprotective ego mind whose job it has been to keep you out of this area in your body by keeping you up in your head with worries. If you are having a hard time locating your alarm, I highly recommend enlisting the support of a trusted friend or counselor. (Again, the MBRX program has detailed videos and meditations that are designed specifically to help you isolate your alarm in your body.)

Helping people find their alarm as a version of their younger selves is exactly what my wife does. Cynthia's job as a somatic experiencing practitioner is to take people close to their past wounding while at the same time helping them feel safe and supported, keeping them oriented to the safety of the present moment.

This is where the previous chapter and this one come together. If you have trouble fully believing that you are safe, it may feel scary (even if the fear is beneath your conscious awareness) to get acquainted with your alarm and face something head-on that you've been avoiding since you were a child. Specifically, we cannot heal our alarm without a sense of deep physical safety in the body, and this is where cognitive/talk therapies often fall short. Practitioners like Cynthia are experts at noticing when their clients start to zone out or dissociate because their old alarm has been triggered. She uses, among other things, her own SES to engage her clients' SES using warm eye contact, tone of voice, body language, touch, and facial expressions to connect and create an environment of safety. Using the ancient human resonance circuitry that dwells in each of us, she creates the environment of safety that didn't exist for her clients when they were children and helps them stay present through the tremendous urge to dissociate when their alarm intensifies. With support in developing what Dr. Dan Siegel calls a window of tolerance (see glossary) for their old emotional wounding, her clients are able to create a new path to integrate the trauma and stop following the familiar toboggan track of worry or dissociation. If in this exercise you are finding it triggering to isolate your old alarm, or if there is a powerful urge to numb or withdraw and you keep finding yourself back in your mind with your worries, consider seeing a therapist who uses somatic (body-based) practices to help you stay present with the sensation of alarm.

We worriers needed our worries to distract us from this alarm, so as we go straight into it, 1) the urge to worry can intensify considerably, and 2) the protective ego can try to block or distract us from accessing the old pain. Don't be surprised if you get the MADD urge as you approach your alarm (medication, addiction, distraction, dissociation).

Above all, be patient with yourself.

If you can't seem to access your alarm, don't worry! You can use the heart space to represent your alarm temporarily until the real location becomes apparent. Know that the more you look for it the more it will come to meet you, and make a point to look for it when you are upset, like my patient did when she was arguing with her ex. In the meantime, if you can't find your alarm right away, when you feel anxious, put your hand over your heart and breathe into the space below your hand. You'll be surprised at how grounding this feels, and it's an infinitely more beneficial action than worrying!

Your alarm is where your younger, wounded self lives, so when you touch your alarm, you are also touching that scared child as well. That child wants desperately to come and meet you, but they are afraid. Once you find your alarm, you can use it as a primary focus for healing, along with the techniques you'll learn in part 3.

> **Point to consider:** How do you feel when you know that the cause of your emotional pain is the scared child in you? Can you give that younger version of yourself a loving invitation to exist in your presence?

66

Feeling Your Anxiety in Your Body

When I asked my patient Jane (the woman who kept picking alcoholic boyfriends) where specifically she felt her anxiety in her body, she seemed stunned by the question. She insisted that she felt confused and scared in her mind, waving her hands around her head.

I asked her another question: "What stops you from eating?" To which she replied, "I'm just not hungry anymore."

Next question. "Most people get hunger pangs in their gut area when they don't eat. Do you have any uncomfortable sensations in your stomach when you don't eat?" Jane answered, "No, but my tummy does get upset when I get anxious." Aha!

I asked her to describe this sensation. She said it felt like a rock (she squeezed her fist over her upper abdomen to illustrate) and that it would also feel like pins and needles. Then she said, "It feels cold and hollow and alone."

Wow.

Delving into it more, over time Jane found the feeling in her gut was the focus of her alarm—the residue of unresolved childhood trauma that still lived in her body—and the alarm represented the scared little girl with the drunken father. I'm sure that little girl did feel cold and hollow and alone.

Until I specifically got Jane to focus on her body, she assumed her issues were all in her head. But in truth, the traumas she had experienced as a child were too intense for her conscious mind to bear, and as you know by now, offloaded into her body as background alarm. With the pain taken out of her conscious mind and into her unconscious body, her mind had more "space" to function.

Children often face emotional wounds that are too much for their minds to bear. If that wounding is not resolved by the adults in their lives at the time, the overwhelm energy is repressed/suppressed (pick your Freudian term) into their bodies where it gets buried as alarm. You know that scene at the end of the movie *Raiders of the Lost Ark* where the Ark of the Covenant is buried deep, deep, deep in the warehouse? It's like that. Except we need to find the alarm, bring it to the surface, and open it up slowly and carefully with reverence and love so it doesn't melt our faces off.

67

You Can't Change What You Can't See: Watching for the Hook

When I feel a sense of alarm in my body, I've developed a practice of watching for the "hook," my mind's attempt at solving the cause of the alarm by getting seduced into worry. After all this time and work and study, I've become very aware of my mind's compulsive desire to reduce the painful uncertainty I feel by developing an alarming story (aka worry) to explain it. Since I know the worry is coming, I make the intention to use the energy previously expended on worrying to instead focus on getting grounded in my body.

Have you ever had an itch and scratched it, but that just caused the itching sensation to intensify? This happens with allergic reactions to things like poison ivy. Scratching feels good for a moment but ultimately just makes us want to scratch more. And worrying is exactly the same. The more you worry the more you're going to want to worry.

Recognizing your worries aren't helping you is a great first step in shifting your focus. Remember, although worrying may seem to create a sense of certainty and control, it's actually increasing your alarm and forcing your mind to come up with ever scarier worries to "scratch."

Instead of obsessing about painting a more and more realistic-looking tiger that will ultimately just scare you more, you can decide to put down the brush by doing a few rounds of the physiological sigh.

It's not possible to stop brain droppings—it's just what the mind does. But what you can do is make the conscious intention to pull your energy and attention away from believing your thoughts and consciously redirect that energy to sensations in your body.

When you catch yourself in worry, put your hand on your chest, take a few breaths, and move out of the worrisome explanations in your mind, and instead seek the sensations in your body. You can also consult the Anxiety Toolkit to help you with the acute discomfort of your alarm.

Practice saying "I am safe in this moment," or do some EFT or tapping (see the glossary if you're not familiar with this) as that brings us into the sensation in our body and out of the snowballing worries in our mind.

Anything that pulls your attention away from the hook of compulsive, worrisome thoughts and into the sensation of your body is helpful. The hook is often a common worry or intrusive thought (health, financial, relationship worries, etc.) that is so seductive you are back up into your mind before your body knows you're gone. Going into your body brings you back into the present moment and away from negative future-based thoughts and worries.

Once you've gotten better at noticing the emotional signature of your alarm (how exactly it feels in your body), you can look out for the hook. Or you might first notice the hook—the irrational horror story your mind is telling you—and then look for the alarm. I guarantee that you will get better at this as you practice going into your body when you see the hook of your worries trying to pull you up into your head.

Just remember that you can't beat thoughts on their own turf. That hook may appear very seductive and lead you down the old familiar path, but you know it doesn't lead anywhere good. As soon as you notice you're in alarm, do not pass go—go directly into your body. Easier said than done, of course, but I will show you exactly how in part 3.

68

Sensation Without Explanation

In November 2014, I attended an eight-day residential personal development retreat close to Whistler, British Columbia. Four times during the retreat, every other day, we did a three-and-a-half-hour process called Holotropic Breathwork®. This technique was popularized by Dr. Stan Grof, a psychiatrist who used to do LSD-assisted psychotherapy. Interesting story: when LSD became illegal, Grof remembered that many of his patients who'd had transformative experiences engaged in breathing patterns similar to hyperventilation. He wondered if this rapid breathing alone could produce transformative experiences—and indeed, he found that was the case.

In Holotropic Breathwork®, you inhale intentionally and forcefully, then exhale more passively. The inhalation lasts around one second, and the exhalation two to three times that. This is often accompanied by loud trance music. Usually there is a breather (the person engaging in the breathwork) and a sitter (the person charged with helping them get to the bathroom and generally watching over them to make sure they don't die and continue the rhythm and don't stop the process). Just jokes, nobody dies, don't *worry*! Sometimes people will fall asleep (even with the trance music blaring), and the sleep is usually allowed to continue, for many old emotions can be processed during this kind of sleep. I have seen people jump up, dance, laugh, scream, cry, punch, and kick as part of this practice. It is said to induce a "non-ordinary" state that bypasses the protective ego, allowing the breather to get in touch with old, re-pressed stories, thoughts, and emotions. If this sounds like accessing the unconscious, it is.

Some people have profound revelations about their lives that change them forever; for others, they do not perceive much of a differ-ence, but that is not to say there is no difference. Something may have shifted in their unconscious even if they don't see much in the way of conscious change.

Around the fourth day of the retreat, I was having a particularly un-comfortable day. We were going into many of Restless Rusty's childhood fears and traumas, and I had listened to many triggering stories from my fellow participants about abuse, loss, abandonment, rejection, be-ing forced to mature too soon, and lots and lots of shame. I could dis-tinctly feel that familiar and intense sense of background alarm in my solar plexus. It wasn't even in the background at that time—it was in full "Purple Haze" mode with a tip of the hat to Jimi Hendrix.

The retreat facility was in this beautiful area in Whistler, right beside a rushing river at the time the salmon were spawning. I tried to sit by the river in meditation but could not settle my mind. I felt distinctly lonely and agitated and wanted to leave, and then a very pleasant experience I had had fifteen months earlier on my temple rooftop in India came to mind. For ninety minutes at dawn in the middle of August 2013 on that temple roof, I was as close as I have ever been to enlightenment. I didn't know it back then, but that drug-free experience in India was similar to what I had felt during my MDMA experience where I felt completely light, loved, and connected to everything. By that river in Whistler, I conjured up as much of that enlightenment scene as I could and found it to be easier than I thought. My foreground and background alarms started to be washed away by the presence of the rushing water, and it crossed my mind that my mind and body were being cleansed. In this state, akin to the "out of nowhere" message about anxiety being more in my body than my mind while I was on LSD, the phrase "sensation without explanation" came to me. It was another example of being able to sit with pleasure, pain, whatever, and just feel it without giving in to my usual compulsion to dissociate and distract by automatically adding worrisome thoughts to it.

In that peaceful moment, I turned to the familiar sensation of alarm in my solar plexus. "Just feel it," I said to myself. This suggestion was met with considerable resistance. My mind started the "hook" in its compulsive, knee-jerk reaction to make sense of the uncomfortable feeling by hooking me into negative thoughts, like explaining to me that I was lonely, this wasn't going to help, and why had I spent all this money on yet another self-help retreat. And: Was the loneliness I felt there easier, the same, or harder than my time alone in India? And what was I trying to accomplish anyway? Nothing was helping, and I was going to stay in this anxious state forever since I had been like this for decades and nothing had helped, and I was a lost cause and should just get up and go home, blah, blah, blah.

I felt that for the first time I was observing my mind. I had seen my distinct alarm in my solar plexus, but I had never thought to isolate my mind in the same way. Sitting there by that river, I could watch my mind try to distract me back into my head. I repeated "Just feel it" in a way that reminded me of Nike's "Just do it." With more resolve, I made an intention to stay with the feeling without words or explanations—just the feeling. Just feel the alarm. Don't try to explain it. Explaining it was not going to make it feel better. In fact, trying to explain it only seemed to make it worse. I did a little experiment on myself. I would set the intention to feel the alarm and go into it as deep as I could and feel around.

I'd love to tell you the pain of alarm in my body seemed to fade away completely when I isolated it. Although it didn't fade away, it did fade. Then I started to add thoughts in, and the pain increased noticeably.

When I was on MDMA, I was overwhelmed by the sensations of love, and any worrisome thought seemed to have no foundation, to the point it bordered on ridiculous. But here in my "right" mind, my thoughts had tremendous power to amplify my alarm. When I consciously directed my attention away from thinking and into feeling, I had a sense I had stumbled onto something momentous. I had finally found something that gave me a sense of agency over the previously overwhelming feeling of alarm. Each time I tested it again by committing to the uncomfortable sensation without trying to resist it or explain it, the discomfort faded. Then I allowed and added negative thoughts, and the alarm sensation intensified. I was really on to something.

The background alarm in my solar plexus still hurt. But for the first time, I had something that gave me a sense of control. Many people have told me the worst thing about alarm and anxiety is that they feel at its mercy and have no idea when it's going to end. Although I could not relieve it completely, I was curiously optimistic. Although feeling it was unavoidable, I had discovered that adding thoughts to it was optional. I found I could take the energy that I had previously used to fuel the worries of my mind and redirect it into the focus of sensation of my body, and in so doing I felt a real sense of relief.

By allowing—dare I say, embracing—the uncomfortable sensation of alarm, I was dealing with it on *my* terms. I was no longer a hostage to my mind's compulsive need to overreact by compulsively explaining and worrying. When I took control and divorced myself from the previously overwhelming need to unconsciously and automatically follow the well-worn groove in the snow of relentless thinking, I could let the worry snowstorm calm and pick up my toboggan and forge a new path—one of feeling, of embracing sensation, of cleanly grasping the issue at its root without the muddying influence of my thoughts and worries.

In that moment, I saw a distinct change in my usual process of compulsively trying to use worries to make sense of the pain. I saw there was a space I had not been aware of before—a spot where I could be with the pain of the alarm but not automatically and compulsively fill in the perceived blank with an explanation. For the first time, I could say to myself the phrase "sensation without explanation" and see that I did not have to incessantly add thoughts to a feeling. I had the option of just feeling the alarm but leaving it devoid of thoughts. And in that emptiness arose a fullness I had never been aware of.

When I taught myself to just feel the alarm as sensation alone with no attempt to reason with it, or reason it out, or reason out of it, it got much easier. If I just sat with the sensation itself, although it was still uncomfortable, it seemed to be contained. I don't know if you'll understand this (because I don't know if I understand it either), but for the first time I seemed to be able to get all the way around the pain. Perhaps because I left the alarm in my body and always took the baited hook and got pulled into worry in my mind, I never stayed with the pain long enough to travel around it. I stopped throwing matches on the fire. Sometimes you can make something much better just by stopping what was making it worse. I found a way to stop hitting myself with the hammer of my worries, and it felt good indeed!

When we can't sit with our alarm, we never see the messages it may have for us. We don't learn that we can develop a relationship with it, even—dare I say—become friends with it. Picture a pool of clear water with a layer of silt at the bottom. When we muddy the water (our alarm) with the silt (our thoughts), the water becomes cloudy and obscures the message. We need to learn to let enough alone and let the thoughts settle to the bottom, and then we can see and feel our alarm for exactly what it is without being clouded by our worries.

I love this quote from *The Untethered Soul* by Michael Singer: "The mind is a place where the soul goes to hide from the heart." This is exactly why we overthink. Rumination and worry are a way of cognitively bypassing the old feeling of alarm.

In an effort to do more feeling and less thinking, I suggest to you to "just feel it" by repeating to yourself the phrase "sensation without explanation" and staying in the feeling.

This simple phrase allowed me a space between my feeling of alarm and my relentless need to add a corresponding story. I found that if I just stayed with the alarm sensation, although it was uncomfortable, I could breathe into it and just stay with it. Once I consciously stopped adding worrisome thinking to the alarm feeling, I gained a sense of control I had never felt before.

One thing that may help as you work with this is to give your mind something productive to do while you stay attuned to sensation.

> When you feel alarm, make a conscious intention to inhale the pain. That's right, as much as this sounds counterintuitive, I want you to focus deeply on savoring and relishing the pain as you breathe in. When you run from the pain or resist the pain, it just gets worse. It is often your resistance to pain that causes the pain to snowball. When you make a conscious intention to inhale the pain (combined with a reassuring hand on your chest) the pain simply cannot expand. Try it!

Personally, I find this practice of embracing and taking the pain in quite empowering. The truth is, I am feeling the pain—so why deny it or run from it? When I deny or run away, I become a victim, and that changes my physiology so my brain actually perceives more pain. When I consciously embrace the pain and breathe into it, there is a congruence—it "makes sense." Instead of trying to escape from the pain by denying it, I am facing it and embracing it, and by breathing it in and embracing it, I take a measure of control and move out of victim mentality. I'm saying, "This hurts, but I trust I can deal with it," and as long as I stay in sensation and don't add thoughts to the pain, I find it much more manageable. Essentially, I am proving to myself that I am strong enough to handle it.

Neurologically, I believe when we embrace the pain like this, our brains secrete dopamine and endorphins and enkephalins (the brain's natural painkillers) in response, and adding a loving hand on our chest releases the connection hormone oxytocin, so there is neuroscience behind this process!

For me, there was a sense when I was a child that I was unable to handle the pain, so I pushed it away or ran from it. I avoided my pain for many years under that same childlike assumption.

This may sound melodramatic, but when I acknowledge and embrace the pain by consciously breathing it in, I gain my power back because I am not running away anymore. I face and embrace it as a victorious adult rather than a victimized child who did not have the support to deal with it back then.

> You aren't a child anymore, and seeing you are no longer powerless, you are fully able to embrace the pain of your alarm and face it. Just stay with the pain and the pain alone; do not let your thoughts hijack you. Breathe the pain in and stay in sensation, even if it hurts, actually, *especially* if it hurts.
>
> This is *sensation without explanation* and it is one of the most effective ways to break the alarm-anxiety cycle.

We are constantly encouraged to push pain away in our society. This process of breathing in the pain is adapted from the practice of Tonglen I learned from the Buddhist nun Pema Chödrön. It facilitates facing the pain and even welcoming it by bringing it in with the breath. When we stop running and distracting ourselves from alarm by compulsive thinking and worrying and, instead, willingly accept and encourage the pain to be present, we can begin to digest and metabolize it. Willingly breathing in the pain and savoring the sensation allows us to feel it and even puts us in control of it. When we feel more in control by willingly breathing in the pain, we don't feel we need to run from it—and because you've got to feel it to heal it, the more you can stay with the feeling of alarm, the more you metabolize it and the less scary it becomes.

An essential note before we move on. For many of us, the alarm holds intense pain from our younger selves and we are simply not able to stay with it for any length of time. Although I do believe this is the path to healing, we can't do this alone. True, we are adults now and have many more resources than we did in our childhood homes, but these wounds are often too much to process on our own, and a therapist familiar with alarm held in the body can be invaluable to your recovery, because our subjective perception of the pain can be just too much to bear on your own.

One last point: when I reread this chapter, it sounds like I formulated the alarm-anxiety cycle by that river in Whistler. While the inklings were there, and I saw that by focusing on the pain in my body the pain eased, it would be years until I would truly be able to explain the cycle to myself or others.

69

Changing Your Perception of Pain

I'll let you in on a big secret. Are you listening?

It is often our *interpretation* of a feeling as painful that actually creates the pain.

If we can sit with our sensation of alarm and learn to avoid adding worrisome thoughts to it (i.e., anxiety), we can stop the cycle in its tracks. We can stop feeding the feeling.

Psychiatrist Bessel van der Kolk, author of *The Body Keeps the Score*, has said that therapy is not so much about taking away the pain as it is about increasing the patient's ability to tolerate the feeling (of alarm).

For me at least, the alarm feeling is much easier to bear if I say "sensation without explanation" to myself and avoid muddying the waters by attaching scary thinking to it and just welcome the feeling even if it hurts.

I recognize that this isn't always the easiest thing to do. But you're getting better at observing what your alarm feels like and where you feel it (or at least asking the question and looking out for it), and in the same way, this is a practice that will get easier.

There is a Buddhist saying that pain is unavoidable, but suffering is optional. This is exactly how our alarm works—the pain is real but we don't need to add suffering by packing on the fearful stories and thoughts. Again, you don't have to think everything you feel!

To put this Buddhist saying into practice, bring up a worry and focus on the alarm it triggers (focusing on the heart area if you haven't located your alarm yet). Then breathe into the area. Make a conscious intention to stay in the sensation. The more you focus your energy directly into your body's sensations, the more you can "lock out" your mind's explanations.

Remember you have embodied practices to call on from this book and the Anxiety Toolkit ("I am safe in this moment," self-touch with a hand over your heart, savoring your breath, breathing in the pain in Tonglen) to help ground you. This is all about staying with your alarm and willingly taking it in.

When you connect with your alarm in a positive, loving way, you are connecting to your younger, wounded self in a positive, loving way, and that alarm will dissipate. You diffuse negative worries by removing the attention they need to survive, and you diffuse alarm by creating a safe place in your body for your younger self to live safely. You can learn that it is safe to feel again—and that's a good thing because feeling is where life is. In part 3, I'll show you another very helpful practice I've used to connect my mind and body to diminish my alarm (and the anxiety that goes with it).

70

What If You Are Pursuing Yourself?

Imagine a child in front of you, upset and holding up their arms to be held. Would you distract yourself from the child's bid for connection by using medication, addiction, distraction, or dissociation?

When you feel the pain of alarm, pushing that alarmed child away may be exactly what you are doing. Your younger self needs attention and compassion and your help in the here and now to recalibrate a system that wasn't calibrated properly when you were younger and didn't have a sea monster living in your house to cuddle with you.

This might feel like jumping into the deep end, but stay with me. There's a good chance the physical symptoms of your anxiety are really a part of your child self begging for the love, attunement, and attention it missed. The purpose of the background alarm in your system and the foreground alarm energy it creates is not to activate you to chase your tail by pushing you into fight or flight against some perceived danger or imagined worry, but rather to activate you to pursue a connection with your very own self.

Younger self? Inner child? If I had not experienced this firsthand, I would have discounted it as new-age hogwash. All this talk of the child inside of us is so foreign to what I learned as a medical doctor—but doctors were never able to fix my anxiety, or should I say: alarm. How are they doing with you? There were some MDs and psychiatrists who certainly helped me, but most relied on pharmaceuticals, and I would be shocked if any medical doctor asked me about my childhood wounds or where I felt the alarm in my body. I love the saying "When you're a hammer, everything looks like a nail." As I said in the introduction to this book, as medical doctors, we are trained to be pharmaceutical sledgehammers, and we are very quick to find a drug-based solution to any ailment or illness. I am not against using medications—in many cases they can be life-saving—but I do feel that too often they are used to simply mask the symptoms.

One of my favorite stories is about one of my fellow comedians who was a heavy smoker. I will call him Kevin because, well, that's his name, and I'm trying to get him to quit. Smoking relaxes the muscle that closes the top of the stomach, letting acid wash up into the esophagus and cause heartburn. Kevin (you hearing me, man?) wanted me to prescribe an acid-blocking medication for his discomfort. "Let me get this straight," I said to him. "You want me to prescribe you a medication so you can keep smoking?" He answered "yep" without missing a beat. Notice how anxiety could be the same—you might be taking medication to paper over the problem instead of seeing that you have the option of fixing it for good.

My best estimate is that about fifty million people worldwide take medications for anxiety. For this vast number of people—fifty million patients who you can't really say are cured but, rather, are just managing their symptoms—why not try to heal the root of the problem if we have a way to do it? Medication can be extremely helpful and even necessary in some cases, but it shouldn't be the be-all and end-all of treatment. If you go to an MD as your primary care physician, there's a good chance you *and* your inner child will receive a new prescription over a new perception. Medical doctors want to help, but outside of psychiatrists, physicians get very little training in psychotherapy. Not only are primary care doctors not trained in psychotherapy, but we wouldn't have the time to do it even if we were, so medication is seen by many physicians as the best option. This isn't a value judgment or a condemnation of doctors; it's a statement of fact. I love my fellow MDs and many more of them are embracing changes to the way they practice by incorporating mind-body medicine, but it's called "medicine" for a reason.

As humans, we are composed of mind, body, and spirit. Medical doctors are learning to embrace the mind-body part but many simply do not understand (or for the most part even want to understand) the spirit part of healing. And it is the spirit that is most in need of care in emotional disorders. Science will help us cope with emotional issues but cannot heal them, because science requires repeatable reductive processes, and the spirit simply cannot be reduced to component parts. This is one of my main issues with "science-based" or "evidence-based" therapies. Scientific therapies work for congestive heart failure but not for heartache.

The spirit, almost by definition, cannot be studied scientifically, but that doesn't mean the spirit isn't a crucial part of mental health care.

Okay, rant over. Back to that scenario of an upset child asking for your attention. Picture your own child self in front of you. Imagine Mom or Dad is drunk or raging or is about to hit you, or that you don't know when they're coming home, or that they're screaming and fighting with each other. Maybe they're incapacitated or addicted or ignoring you or being ravaged by some physical or mental disease and expecting you to look after yourself and your siblings. Or maybe your circumstances were less dramatic. No blowouts, no cataclysmic events, just an apathetic household with very little warmth or attachment. Dad was a workaholic and Mom was emotionally numb. These types of environments are overwhelming for a child and absolutely create alarm in their system.

Once you have called to mind a hurtful moment, look at your younger self as they are suffering. Imagine looking into the child's eyes as if they are your own (because they are), and in your imagination pick up the child and cuddle them, feeling their little body relax as they hold on to you. Feel their hand and arms around your neck. Place them so your adult heart is against their little child heart. Feel their alarm. It should feel very familiar—but now you've started to break the spell.

Many of my anxiety patients carry the unconscious program that providing comfort for them was their parents' job back then so why should they have to do it now? As much as we might want to believe self-care is not our job but our parents' job (and don't care for ourselves as a result), I'm here to tell you that *nobody is coming to save you.* Your parent is not coming back to fulfill their job of comforting you and looking after your needs. The child inside never got what they needed, and a part of them is still waiting. Be gentle with yourself and adopt the responsibility and make the intention that it is up to adult you to comfort and care for child you.

Once you do accept the truth that you are the secure attachment figure your inner child has been waiting for, you can provide the love and care for yourself you've been wishing you had all along. When adult you can see, hear, understand, protect, and love child you, the alarm the child still carries has a chance to heal.

Point to consider: Put a picture of yourself as a child up on your bathroom mirror or make a childhood photo of you as the screen saver on your phone as an unconscious reminder of your connection to your (younger) self.

71

Creating a Safe Place

All children need to feel safe, and usually that comes from parental attachment and connection. When children are in alarm, it is often because they are experiencing a lack of secure attachment and connection in a time of upheaval. The alarm can be acute, like losing their parents in an American grocery store, or chronic, when they perceive a constant uncertainty like having an absent, addicted, or abusive parent.

Many of us mistrust love because love shown to us by our parents was compromised, or just not there. And since at our essence we are love, in mistrusting love, we mistrust who we are. No wonder we are alarmed! When we mistrust our own selves, we split into the part that is truly, authentically us, which is love and growth, and another reactive part, which adopts the need for fear and protection. Because the brain's automatic default setting is to ensure survival, many worriers fall into protection mode by mistrusting (and then avoiding) the vulnerability that comes with loving.

If you, too, have become stuck in the alarm-anxiety cycle, it is likely that you have also disconnected from love and its vulnerability, and this rejection of love likely started as a protective mechanism when you were a child.

But the only antidote to fear (and anxiety) is love—and you need to go back there because the place has changed! Meaning, you can create a safe and loving place for yourself now that was not there when you were younger. It is now time to create a place within you where it is safe to feel safe and also safe to feel vulnerable, and also safe to feel. Period.

Healing from anxiety and alarm is not so much about feeling better as it is getting better at feeling. Creating a safe, feeling place inside of you allows your mind and body to reconnect, recalibrate, and rebalance your nervous system. Then you can allow yourself to feel *all* your feelings: the good, the bad, and the ugly, correcting the imbalance that was created by your incessant need for protection where you had to narrow all your feelings to only those based in your familiar fear. This is why it's been said that anxiety and excitement are experienced the same way (they're not, but it's close). The first step is always to connect with yourself. The alarm-anxiety cycle cannot survive inside a compassionate and functional mind-body connection.

> Try this: Right now, rub your palms together vigorously for ten to twenty seconds until you create some heat. Then close your eyes and place the heels of your hands over your eye sockets. Mentally focus on the warmth and the feeling of paying kind attention to yourself. Now focus on your breathing and notice how your breath is always there for you, and how you are surrounded by life-giving oxygen around you at all times. Repeat this as many times as you like. This is a taste of what a constructive mind-body connection looks and feels like. Know that this little practice is almost always available to you. (Except while you are driving. Or boxing. Or underwater.)

72

Alarm Blocks Connection

Simply stated, we need safety in order for our nervous system to heal, and the main problem with both foreground and background alarm is that they keep us out of safety and in a state of protection, and in that survival mode it is impossible to heal. The paradox is the SES is needed to resolve alarm but it simply cannot function properly if the system is in alarm. Another way of saying this is you cannot thrive if your system is stuck in the perceived need to survive.

Imagine you got a call that your son had been injured at school, and then in the elevator on the way to your car to be with him, a coworker started talking to you about her scheduling problems. You wouldn't be able to offer any meaningful advice, and you probably wouldn't even remember what she said afterward, right? That's because you'd be in alarm-based survival brain while worried for your son's well-being. The neurological part of you that could be socially engaged and connected with your coworker is simply offline.

We often feel this lack of connection with others when we are alarmed and anxious, but we may not be as aware of the lack of connection within ourselves. I hope it is becoming obvious to you that if you are in a state of alarm, your nervous system will be impaired and unable to connect to others (as with your coworker in the elevator above), and you will also lose the ability to connect to and soothe *yourself*.

A troubled marriage, an eating disorder, or an addiction are the effects of background alarm in the system. We have to go deeper to fix the cause. If the underlying emotional dysregulation in the body (the background alarm) is not dealt with directly, the couple will fight, the eating disorder will sneak its way back in (especially in times of acute stress), and the addiction will return.

This would be a topic for another book, but I believe addictions are just ways humans try to self-medicate their background alarm.

If the book up to this point has done its job, it has shown you what you call anxiety has more to do with a sense of alarm in the body than with the thoughts of the mind. Of course, the mind still plays a significant supporting role in holding the scoreboard up so we can see it, but ultimately the body keeps the score—it never forgets our old wounds and, courtesy of the amygdala (remember my hyperactive smoke detector?), reacts instantaneously to even the slightest whiff of familiar threat with a well-rehearsed program of alarm that got programmed into us in childhood, always at the ready to "protect" us. But paradoxically, in its childlike effort to keep us safe, that alarm constantly reminds us that we could be in danger, which causes even more alarm.

With every activation, the alarm reaction becomes potentiated—more ingrained and powerful—and even worse, by flipping us into a survival-focused state, it locks us out of our SES, so we have no way to soothe the alarm. Then we add the three Ws of worry: warnings, what-ifs, and worst-case scenarios in yet another misguided attempt to protect us that just potentiates even more alarm!

When one of my patients says, "I'm feeling anxious," I encourage them instead to say, "I'm feeling alarmed," as that is a much truer statement. If you have a friend and they are trying to understand what you are going through, I urge you to use the term "alarm" instead of "anxiety." When you say, "I feel anxious," many people have no idea what you are talking about, but if you say, "I feel alarmed," everyone can relate to that feeling.

So many of us became alarmed as children in response to a situation or event that was traumatizing and out of our control, especially if that situation or event would repeat itself. Our fight-or-flight nervous system naturally kicked in to protect us and to energize us in an effort to resolve the situation. If that alarming situation was then addressed and resolved by a loving parent or caregiver, our system could stand down and we could move into parasympathetic rest-and-digest phase. If the situation could not be resolved and a competent parent was not available, that fight-or-flight response would stay chronically active and our overwhelmed system would accumulate even more background alarm. Without a secure attachment figure to help us calm our fight-or-flight reaction and allow us to process our experiences in a healthy way, our system is like a one-way valve where more alarm can enter but none can leave.

Cells that fire together wire together in a phenomenon called potentiation. If I told you to forget how to ride a bike, could you do it? In the same way, you cannot "forget" how to ramp up your alarm. The background alarm stored from unresolved trauma and the foreground fight-or-flight activation become linked together in a well-potentiated self-reinforcing feedback loop. Again, to borrow that saying by Joe Dispenza, the body has learned to do it better than the mind.

These familiar habits can be unlearned, but it takes practice. There's an engineer who designed a bike that when you turn the handlebars left, the front wheel goes right. It's pretty funny watching people trying to ride this bike. Not many of them get farther than two feet before falling off. The engineer himself took many months to retrain his implicit program so he could ride the bike he designed. But that's how it is when we're working to retrain our alarm.

I could describe to you in words how to ride the backward bike. You could study the instructions in your mind for weeks, but that intellectual knowledge would only provide you with a fraction of the benefit of actually physically getting on the backward bike and trying to ride it.

Just as you can't talk your way out of a problem that requires action, reading about a body-based approach will only get you so far.

You won't be able to learn your new feeling-based program and reprogram your alarm until you actually get on the bike and ride it. You must say goodbye to your mother tongue, the mind's language of thinking, and become fluent in the body's language of feeling. Learning how you become fluent in how you feel is critical for the awareness of self you will need to heal from alarm and anxiety. In a way, it's like learning a language you have always known but have forgotten, kind of like learning the alphabet all over again.

So, if you're ready, let's relearn our ABCs.

But wait—in the second edition of this book I want to add a few things here before we get into the healing of part 3.

Much of what you have learned in the first two sections is how to understand your anxiety in a brand-new way, and with that new understanding of the alarm stored in your body you can feel your way out of your anxiety instead of trying to think your way out. The latter doesn't work because you can't solve a problem of rumination and overthinking with more thinking!

Here at the end of part 2 I want you to know that you can't think your way out of anxiety, you must feel your way out, and that is what part 3, Awareness of Self, is designed to help you do.

The reason cognitive therapies like CBT help you cope with your anxiety in the short term but do not heal your anxiety in the long term is that you are trying to fix a feeling-based problem (alarm) with a thinking-based solution. Further, cognitive therapies require the cognitive brain to be online to work and when we become alarmed we shut off the cognitive (thinking) brain in favor of the survival-based (feeling) brain, so cognitive therapies tend to leave you when you need them the most!

If what I have said in this book resonates with you, and you want to go deeper into your healing, I would absolutely recommend you add my video and meditation program, Your Mind-Body Prescription for Permanent Anxiety Healing, or MBRX for short. MBRX is a video and audio program that covers the material in the book in a more practical way, with deeper detail into finding your alarm along with a yoga nidra guided meditation to join your mind and body together and calm your system at the source of your alarm. My goal is to have my book and program go worldwide (it already is), and I have priced both to be accessible for everyone because I absolutely do not want you to have to suffer with anxiety and alarm as I did. I know the feeling of being promised anxiety relief from books, therapists, and online programs and the deep disappointment time after time; so I committed my life to creating something that I know works for me and my patients.

Now, let's get into the ABCs of connecting with yourself and healing your anxiety. . . .

PART III

Awareness of Self

73

Survival Versus Connection

We humans have two main drives: the drive to physically survive and the drive to emotionally connect. If you grow up in secure attachment, you and your nervous system learn to see life through the lens of growth and connection. If you do not grow up in a secure, attached environment, you and your nervous system see life through the lens of protection and survival.

This is why childhood is such a critical age to feel cared for, loved, and supported. If you experience trauma that is too much for you to bear, a metaphorical crack forms in the hull of your metaphorical boat. Then, like the groove in the snow, that crack forms a preferential pathway for further pain.

If the crack isn't repaired by your caregivers with safety, secure attachment, and love during childhood, over time it becomes a full-blown hole as the hull's integrity weakens further. That is, as more trauma spills in through the crack, the crack gets bigger, letting in even more trauma and alarm.

Once that area of weakness or damage forms, it becomes a preferential path and a reservoir for pain and the pain body—and as the pain accumulates, it blazes a deeper trail that makes it easier for more pain to follow; and as you feel more pain, you will sink even deeper into a world view of survival and protection.

Before we get deeper into part 3, I want to address a question I hear frequently: "Why do I have such anxiety when I have no childhood trauma?"

Let me say first that most people know the pain they suffered as children, but there are many who do not. The following are some common themes I see in people with significant anxiety and what they assume was a "normal" childhood.

1. **Separation from parent(s) at an early age.** Mom is sick after your birth and unable to bond with you. Parent is absent for significant period before you were five. I have seen people who were left home with a caregiver while their parents took their sibling(s) on extended vacations. I get my patients to ask their parents if they had a separation from them at an early age. Not all separations create trauma, but if the child is very sensitive, it doesn't take much separation to elicit a trauma response.

2. **Intergenerational trauma.** My friend and colleague Mark Wolynn has written a brilliant book called *It Didn't Start With You,* which I highly recommend, about how trauma gets handed down in families, especially if your parents or grandparents had very stressful lives. We can absorb trauma from our ancestors. I have seen this more times than I can count.

3. **Prenatal trauma.** When you were in utero, how stressed was your mother? There is also evidence your father's stress may play an even bigger role than your mother's stress. Perhaps a reason for this is that Mom had to deal with her own issues and her partner's issues too!

4. **Denial.** I cannot tell you how many people have told me they had great parents and great childhoods and when I question them it becomes crystal clear they had neither. Their childhoods were full of ALARMS and they couldn't (or wouldn't) see them. I think so many children had to deny that there was anything wrong in their childhood homes for so long that they actually believed it well into adulthood.

This is not an extensive list by any means, but it often helps people understand why they deal with such anxiety and alarm from "normal" childhoods.

As we embark on the last phase of our journey together, it is critical you find the alarm in your body—where it lives and what it looks and feels like. And remember, if you're not sure yet, just focus on the space around your heart. When alarm has been with you (and in you) for a long time, you can fail to see it because you 1) have acclimatized to it, or 2) simply haven't looked for it. Just as we fail to see how our parents didn't meet our needs because we were in denial, we can also fail to see or acknowledge our alarm until we choose to specifically look for it.

I've come to see there is no quick fix to resolve your alarm, and no hack that is going to suddenly make you worry-free. For a long time, I saw my worries as who I was, until I realized worries are a reflexive activity of the mind that reflects the alarm stored in the body. Even after believing my worries for many decades, I needed that "sensation without explanation" epiphany by the river to see that I had the option of not believing every worry I thought simply because I had created it. Until I separated the worries of my mind from the alarm in my body, I was convinced that I was my thoughts and my thoughts were me.

I love the quotes "The mind is a wonderful servant but a terrible master," and "There are no prison walls stronger than the ones you cannot see." For many years, I could not see I was in a prison of my own mind. I was chained to being both servant and master, never seeing that I had a choice to drop the chains by simply becoming the curious, dispassionate observer of my own paintings of scary tigers, no matter how lifelike they appeared.

Awareness showed me I was not my thoughts, that I could see my worries and therefore not to be my worries. By that river I learned that I didn't have to attach a thought to every feeling and a feeling to every thought and that was the beginning of my liberation. Once I saw my worries were only a seductive illusion, a magical "sleight of mind" (instead of sleight of hand), if you will, I saw behind the curtain to see the true source of my pain was the alarm buried in my body as a child.

Point to consider: Right now, pick a worry that bothers you and just allow the worry to stay suspended in your mind. Notice the feeling of power when you don't get sucked into resisting it or reacting to it. Alarm will likely come up and be uncomfortable, but notice where the alarm is and just stay with the alarm too. You are safe in this moment despite the discomfort.

74

ABCDE

There's a process I developed and use every day to help me heal from the alarm-anxiety cycle. It follows the first five letters of the alphabet in a cycle (although the first three are the most important).

Awareness
Body
Connection
Discipline
Ego

(You'll soon see that a couple of steps of the process encompass more than one word with the same letter, but you can use what's above as a simple and quick acronym-type way to remember the process.)

First comes awareness and acceptance. By awareness I mean conscious awareness, as discussed in the first part of the book. When you are aware of being aware, you embrace and become fully familiar with how the pain manifests in you. If you don't see how anxiety and alarm take you over, you can't change them, and when you are in the dark, digging into your worries isn't going to help you find the light. A new commitment and intention to see that you are in a state of alarm instead of the old groove to automatically and unconsciously believe your worries is the first step.

Body and breath are next. Thinking, however well-intended and "positive," is only keeping you stuck in the future-based worries of your head, and your attention needs to be grounded in your present-moment sensation in your body. When you can find a safe place in your body, your anxious thoughts lose power because you redirect the energy from thinking to feeling. The key here is to recognize when you are in anxiety and alarm and make a firm intention to move into *sensation without explanation*.

Next comes connection and compassion. Once you've opened the door to your SES to come in and soothe you, you can connect with yourself from a place of compassion. This is where you neutralize your old wounds by being the kind, connected parent for yourself now that you wish you'd had back then. In this section, you'll learn a lot more about how to relate to your (younger) self with connection and compassion.

Discipline is next on the list. It's like the old joke about a man who is lost looking for the theatre and asks a woman on the street, "How do you get to Carnegie Hall?" She replies, "Practice, practice, practice." You've lived in the groove and false belief that your thoughts and worries have been keeping you safe for a very long time. However, by overthinking, you've been digging yourself deeper into a hole under the illusion you are digging yourself out. Doing it another way—staying out of future worries and staying in the moment, in your body—is going to take practice.

Lastly (for now), ego. This is the one-trick pony (or perhaps a better metaphor is one-trick dragon—more soon) that makes you avoid vulnerability. As I'll show you, your ego dragon never forgets and will shy away from anything that has ever caused you pain. While that is functional and adaptive in avoiding a hot stove, if you avoid love out of the perception that love burns you, love is squeezed out of your box and fear jumps in to steadily fill the space left behind.

Even for those of us who don't have old pain to heal and trauma to process, there's something to be said for reconnecting with the source of our pain, the child in us whose mind was overwhelmed and protectively pushed the trauma into their body.

In the next chapters we'll draw awareness to each letter of ABCDE, one by one.

75

Awareness Gives Choice

You can't change something you can't (or your ego refuses to) see. Before you can change it, you need to see it—and feel it.

Have you found your alarm—the part of you that lights up in your body when your mind gets anxious? This is the feeling I want you to become acutely aware of. This is the ultimate source of your pain.

One of my patients, Kelly, had abandonment issues in her childhood. In the present, she was having intrusive thoughts about Paul, her devoted husband of twelve years. Kelly had convinced herself that Paul was preparing to leave her. It's important to know that Paul had never given Kelly any reason to think he would leave. When he would go off to work, she would have intrusive thoughts about him not coming back. When Kelly got really alarmed, she would search the house for a suitcase Paul might have packed to prepare for a quick exit.

My work with Kelly focused on making her aware that her anxiety had nothing to do with Paul. The real issue was old, unresolved alarm in her system from when she was ten years old. Sadly, one summer day her beloved father left for work and never came back. He was killed in an industrial accident.

Unfortunately, Kelly didn't have enough support at the time of her father's death. Her mother was too distraught to make Kelly's needs a priority. In her early adulthood, Kelly had done hours and hours of cognitive therapy trying to minimize her intrusive thoughts of being left alone, which helped for a time. But the abandonment worries always came back, often more intense (and irrational) than before.

Kelly and I went through a similar exercise to the one I laid out for you in the last section to help her find her alarm. Under my guidance, she imagined Paul leaving for work and then zeroed in on where and how she was experiencing alarm in her body. She found it in her upper abdomen, where it showed up as a sense of pressure that seemed to radiate up into her chest and throat. Over time, she was able to describe it in great detail. It was a hollow, black, empty, foggy, diffuse hourglass shape that squeezed in the middle over her heart, expanding above and below.

Leaving the story of Kelly for a moment, once upon a time, my friends and I had a regular poker night. In poker, there is something called a tell, a mannerism or habit that gives away signals about whether a player has a strong hand or is bluffing. For example, my friend Tom would always look at his cards over and over when he had a strong hand. If he was bluffing, he would barely look at them at all. These were his tells. Once I figured this out, I rarely lost big hands to him.

Like poker players learning to read each other's tells, we can look out for our own tells once we know what they are. In Kelly's case, it was when she would catch herself looking around the house for a suitcase or when she'd find herself off in her head somewhere spinning a story about why Paul was leaving her. These were the signposts telling her she was deep in alarm and had lost her rational mind.

Then she directed her attention to her body, noticing the familiar hourglass shape squeezing in her chest, and would put her hand over that sensation of alarm. Next she took a deep breath or did a few rounds of the physiological sigh, focused on the feeling of her feet on the ground in the present-moment sensation, and then reminded herself that the alarm in her body was the problem, not Paul. She made a conscious effort to move away from the worries of her mind down into the "hourglass" sensation squeezing her heart, even though that sensation was very uncomfortable.

Instead of letting the worries spiral, she now changed the direction of her attention and intention to get in touch with her alarm and get grounded in her body.

Once Kelly became familiar with her alarm and knew what to look for—or rather, *feel* for—she noticed it more and more. She became extremely skilled at localizing her alarm and learning to recognize it earlier and earlier as it came up as the hourglass-shaped sensation in her chest. She described it as a messenger telling her to get out of her head and into her body. It became a kind of early warning system for her.

Kelly didn't know this at the time, but what she was really doing when she was connecting with alarm in her chest was connecting with and reassuring the little ten-year-old inside her who had suddenly lost her daddy. Instead of bypassing into unsupported worries and self-created stories that Paul was also never coming back, she went right to the source of the pain in that little girl. Adult Kelly developed a relationship with child Kelly through the sensation of alarm in her chest, and her fear of Paul leaving disappeared. This took time, but she was able to use her anxiety and alarm as a route to a direct connection with her wounded child self, and she told me, "For the first time in my life that I can remember, I feel whole."

My hope for you is that you too will learn to see your own alarm as a direct connection to your younger, wounded self. When you are aware and connected to the younger part of you that suffered ALARMS, that part no longer needs to cry for your attention by creating and maintaining a state of alarm in your body.

When you are grounded in your body and the child in you, you're able to see your worries so you no longer need to be your worries. In short, your worries become obvious as an attempt to dissociate and disconnect from your (child) self and the pain that child still carries.

We worriers often make an automatic leap up into our heads into worry when we feel alarmed, but awareness allows us to see there is another option: to move down into our body. This will feel unnatural and uncertain at first because you've conditioned yourself to feel a perverse sense of security in the certainty of your worries, and your worries have created molecules of addiction in your brain. However, with practice, going down into the body will start to feel more natural, and create a more integrated, connected neurochemical state. Be kind to yourself and understand that you've automatically and unconsciously trained yourself to overthink, and so, when you try to do the opposite and go into your body instead, you may "lose your balance" a few times and find yourself right back in your addictive thoughts. Keep practicing, and soon moving down into your body with self-touch, breath, and self-compassion will provide a new, more holistic security. Your previously automatic, unconscious reaction to jump into unconscious worry will start to be replaced by a willful, conscious choice to redirect your energy into the present moment of the feeling body and connection with your younger self.

It's natural to question why you would want to move deeper into the painful sensation of your alarm, but if you see that your alarm is your younger self crying for your attention it will make more sense. The more you connect with your alarm, the more you connect with the child in you that needs to heal and go back to resolve the pain at its source.

Point to consider: Did you put that picture of your child self up on your bathroom mirror, or do you have a photo of younger you as the screen saver on your phone?

76

Body and Breath Break the Cycle

Remember the story from an earlier chapter where a man constantly hits himself with a hammer and when asked why, he says, "Because it feels so good when I stop"?

This is exactly how worries work. Remember the sense of relief I'd feel as a child when I got myself all worked up envisioning horror stories each time my mom was late coming home from work? The dopamine and endorphin rush felt so good each time those worries resolved with the sound of her key in the door.

But just because there's sometimes a payoff (in the form of feel-good chemicals flooding our brains) when worries turn out not to be true does not mean it's a good idea to pour our energy into worrying. I also believe we get a little shot of dopamine when we make the uncertain appear more certain and a bit of endogenous opioid in an attempt to ease discomfort of the worry, so worrying has the potential to manipulate our brain chemistry with a chemical payoff in both the short and longer term. In the longer term, the truth is that worrying adds more to the alarm we feel in the long term than its chemicals ease in both the short term. This is the definition of addiction: something that appears to help initially but makes things worse over time. Now, you consciously know that "worry is bad" already, but your unconscious holds on to worries like an addiction because the chemicals in your brain helps to make it one.

So, what's the solution?

I'm so glad you asked!

Once you become aware of your signals (or "tells") that you're heading into alarm, you can intentionally change your focus from the thoughts up in your mind to the sensation down in your body, *even if the sensation is uncomfortable or painful.* This move away from hypervigilant thinking may go against every coping strategy you learned in childhood, and your ego will likely get all fired up trying to suck you back into your worries, but I promise you can do this—and it may even save your life. I know it saved mine.

One way to begin to step away from the worries of your mind and into the stillness of your body is to intentionally focus your attention on the sensation of your breathing. We might think of the breath as neutral or "just there" without any particular quality, but you really can go into quite a bit of detail if you tune in. At any given moment, your breath has a sound, a scent, a temperature, and a speed.

> Right now, how deep is your breath? What parts of your lungs is it touching? What other parts of your body do you feel moving? Can you notice the little pause as inhale stops and exhale begins and vice versa? Try a few rounds of breath elongating that transitional space—holding it a little longer in awareness. There's so much to notice when it comes to our breath, and it's an infinitely better use of your energy than worrying. I often use a focus on my breath as a great transition point from explanation to sensation, and you should too!

If we worriers were able to focus on the nuances of our breath one tenth as much as we focused on every little %^$@#* thing that could go wrong in our lives, we'd give Wim Hof a run for his money.

Here's how this might look for me. I'll become aware that I've been taken over by some worry, like "I wonder if this book will be rejected by my medical peers?" Once I become aware that I am hitting myself with a hammer with my worries, I put my hand over my solar plexus and move to the sensation of my breath. This slows me down and reverses the direction of my energy from explanation to sensation. When the worries have taken me over, I always find the feeling of alarm is there in my solar plexus as well (because, frankly, the feeling was there first!). I will use that point of awareness and say to myself, "Hmmm, I wonder why I need to think a painful worry right now?" or "Hmmm, there's my old familiar feeling of alarm. I wonder why that's there?" Committing to a strong sense of curiosity gives me a degree of separation from my worries because curiosity is grounded in the rational mind, not the survival brain. Curiosity distances me from my worry by taking the painful urgency out of it, and that makes it so much easier to get out of my head and move into the sensation of my body and breath.

When you make a firm intention to direct your attention specifically into the sensation(s) of your body, you remove the energy and attention that were previously feeding your worries. This is the liberating moment when you separate the thoughts of the mind from the alarm in the body. With your curious intention, you re-channel the destructive energy of anxious thinking into the constructive energy of present-moment sensation.

You can't stop thinking. It's just what the mind does. But you consciously redirect your attention to your body and can starve thinking of its energy source—and this is the main goal of the letter *B*. Redirect the attention to your body and the thoughts have less ability to aggravate your alarm.

When our worries trap us in the future, we have no grounding or secure place to do anything else but more worrying. When we stop and create a space between feeling and thought that connects us to the present, we have solid ground to stand on—and with that solid ground, we can go from a fear-based belief system (governed by survival and focused on the future) to a love-based belief system (based in compassionate connection to ourselves).

Your adult self is exhausted by the chronic need to think and distract. Your habit of escaping into the worries of your mind has turned from a coping strategy in your childhood to a distinct liability in your adulthood. But by becoming grounded in your body and breath, you can begin to overwrite the childhood adaptation of worry that is now creating much more pain than it is numbing. You can stop hitting yourself with the hammer of your worries.

It's important to note that just because something sounds simple does not mean it is easy. You've had this groove in the snow for a long time and it will take time and effort to melt the old habit away. This takes practice.

But don't worry, Carnegie Hall is just around the corner.

Point to consider: Right now, take a second and direct your attention to your body and breath for five to ten seconds. Then bring your attention back up into you thinking mind and think about a worry that is troubling you at present. Then move back into your body and breath, saying to yourself, "sensation without explanation." Then back up into your worry and then back to your breath. Repeat this process a few more times. I want you to have a felt sense of what it is like to consciously change your energy from thinking to feeling and vice versa.

77

Your Thoughts Are Your Sirens

Before we move on from the letter *B,* I want to tell you a related story from Greek mythology: that of Odysseus and the Sirens. On their long journey by sea (the Odyssey), Odysseus's crew hears beautiful voices singing to them. They've been warned about these singers in advance—so powerfully beautiful is the Sirens' song that it's enticed many a ship to steer onto the rocks of their island. So as they prepare to approach this area, Odysseus orders his crew to plug their ears with beeswax so they cannot hear the singing. He is so curious to hear the song himself that he leaves his own ears open, but straps himself to the mast of the ship with strict orders to his men not to release him under any circumstances. As the ship passes close to the Sirens, Odysseus hears the song and sees maidens of indescribable beauty beckoning to him. He struggles so hard to get out of his restraints that the ropes cut and tear his skin. Meanwhile, for the crew members who cannot hear the song, the Sirens appear as grotesque monsters.

In this scenario, your compulsive thoughts are the Sirens. They seductively promise to be the answer to your fears, but they hold nothing but pain. Awareness and seeing your thoughts for what they are—and that you have a choice in what you believe—is like plugging your ears to the Sirens' song. Only once you see your worries in dispassionate curiosity can you keep rowing past their seductive call and reach into the sensation of your body, where you have the opportunity to heal both your adult self and your child self.

When you steadfastly row past the rocks and reach the sanctuary of your body, you break the Sirens' spell. You may need to "strap yourself to the mast" because you've been deeply conditioned to see your worries as protective and have allowed them to "hook" you since childhood. This compulsion to run to your worries is why setting an intention to move away from your mind and into your body (see the next chapter for how to do this) is a pivotal step—but once you learn to resist the seduction of your worries, you gain a felt sense of truly being in control of your worries instead of the opposite. I can tell you from personal experience that seeing my worries and consciously steering away from them gave me a felt sense that for the first time, I had the power to heal myself. Once you learn the critical first step of moving from awareness of your worries into your body and breath, you can undertake the next hero's journey: the letter C, developing a compassionate connection to yourself and the wounded child that still lives in you.

78

Connection and Compassion Push Out the Fear

Developing a compassionate connection with myself has been the cornerstone of my recovery from chronic alarm and its accompanying compulsive worry. Cultivating this internal connection is the part of healing from anxiety and alarm that is so often missed in traditional therapies that are focused on changing thinking instead of changing feeling.

The reason I needed to dump all that trauma into my solar plexus when

I was younger is precisely because I never had a secure attachment that could support me in neutralizing it at the time. To finally heal, I had to teach myself how to be the security for myself now that I needed back then.

When I am truly connected with myself, I do not need to conjure up a convoluted roller coaster of worrisome twists and turns to distract me from the pain of alarm from my childhood. I can bring awareness and compassion to the alarm right to its source. I can go right to the heart—or, in my case, to the solar plexus—of it.

Go ahead and try it for yourself. Place your hand on your chest or over the site of your alarm if you have found it. Form an intention to connect with yourself. As you breathe in and out, focus on the stillness and sensation of your body. Savor the air as it comes in and out of your nostrils and chest. Stay focused on the temperature, pressure, and texture of your hand against your chest, and focus deeply on the sensation of your chest rising and falling with your breath. As you stay with the sensation of your breath and body, close your eyes and stay with these sensations for five slow, deep breaths. If you can focus on seeing your child self in your mind's eye and looking into their eyes, all the better. As you breathe in, imagine the breath traveling right into the place of your alarm. Summon as much compassion and love for yourself as you possibly can, knowing that the alarm you feel in your chest (or wherever your alarm is felt) is your younger self that would have given anything to feel this connected attention from your parents. Stay keenly aware of the sensation of alarm in your body, sending it breath and love with the intention of holding your alarmed younger self in loving presence. Keep picturing that younger, scared version of you in as much detail as you can, and tell them that they hold the very best parts of you. (Because they do.) This may bring some tears up for you and that's a good thing!

What I wouldn't give to be able to collapse time and show my med-student self a glimpse of future me. He'd probably think he was hallucinating because there's no way Dr. Russell Kennedy is ever going to be talking about something as "woo-woo" as a connection to your younger self—especially not as being more effective than pharmaceuticals and talk therapy.

But if I know one thing, it's that developing a compassionate connection to myself has allowed me to heal my alarm at its source and has been infinitely more effective than any of the traditional treatments I received in mainstream Western medicine. As I'll soon show you, we worriers often have an adversarial, inner critic–type relationship with ourselves, and this is a major factor that blocks our healing.

A note of caution: if you spook the ego by trying to say "I love myself" too early and try to go straight from fear into love, you may trigger the same (over)protective resistance to love and vulnerability that created your alarm in the first place. Reintroducing a loving relationship with yourself must be done in manageable increments so you can gradually overcome your ego's resistance (more on this soon).

It's like if you've always been in abusive relationships, and finally you learn to be curious about your patterns and end your (repetition) compulsion to seek partners who hurt you. Even once you consciously choose someone who is going to treat you well, it's still going to take you a little longer to trust that they are safe, whereas someone whose relationships have always been healthy and peaceful can trust from the beginning, since their experiences haven't shown them any reason not to.

Time and patience will help as you stay committed to your intention of treating yourself with compassion. But later in this section, you'll learn about what I call the ego dragon, an omnipotent creature that you created as a child to keep you safe in times of deep fear and uncertainty. The ego dragon is powerful but not that smart, and it sees its job as stopping you from doing anything that has ever caused you pain, ever. If you have been hurt by love (like I was with my dad), it is the ego dragon that gets all fired up in an attempt to block that love. Much of your alarm is created by the ego dragon's resistance to love. Like worry hurts you in an attempt to keep you "safe," the ego dragon hurts you by blocking access to love. To heal, you need to overcome the ego's resistance to love and vulnerability, both for yourself and for others. An important point: your ego believes it has kept you safe by keeping you in a narrow range of emotion away from (the pain of) vulnerability for many years. For me, and probably you too, the ego doesn't want us to experience love if it perceives that love has hurt us in the past.

Point to consider: When, where, and who was it not safe to love when you were a child? (Note: This point can be very painful, so be compassionate to the child in you that still feels this.)

79
Discipline Versus Distraction

You've been seduced by the siren song of your worries for a long time, and this distraction provides a sense of relief—but it's very short-term. As you continue to practice your ABCs, distraction will continue to call to you and there will be a compulsion to reach back for the addiction of worry, especially at first. As much as the protective dragon of your ego is going to try to convince you that worrying and thinking keeps you vigilant and therefore safe, it's a trap. You must discipline yourself to avoid those addictive worries of your mind and instead stay firmly in your body's sensation (without explanation).

As you learn to be your own healer, it will likely feel as uncomfortable as Odysseus resisting the Sirens. The urge to rip off the ties holding you and rush to be with your worries will be intense. But as you sail past the island of the Sirens and resist the call of those worries—once, then again, then many, many more times—you will feel a liberation unlike any you have ever felt before. You will see that you are in control of your worries more than your worries are in control of you, it just takes consciously practicing the right thing instead of unconsciously defaulting into the wrong thing.

Remember that in many ways worry operates like an addiction, rewarding you with dopamine and a little shot of the brain's natural morphine each time you do it. Just as smokers know they shouldn't smoke but the urge is overwhelming, worrying is something you know you shouldn't do but you just can't help yourself—but people do stop smoking, just as you can stop worrying. You will teach yourself to stay present with yourself in compassionate connection down in your body versus abandoning yourself to chase the addiction of worry up in your mind. Self-worrying, like self-hammering, can feel so good when you stop! (Not my best sentence, but you know what I mean.) Here is the hard part. Initially, you are caught between a rock and a hard place because moving away from the worries in your head to the alarm in your body still hurts, because the alarm hurts! But even though the pain of alarm will still be present, you've stopped throwing the matches of worries on the fire of that alarm. You've stopped hitting yourself with a hammer. For me, consciously choosing my pain (alarm in my body versus anxieties of my mind) provided a liberating sense of control I never knew I had access to. So even though you still feel pain, for the first time, it is pain you have some agency over. It is *pain for a purpose* in finding your liberation instead of useless pain that keeps you locked in worry. It is the pain of your child that your adult can embrace and resolve. In other words, the adult in you can patch the hole in the hull, instead of the child in you being left endlessly bailing water.

I can't tell you how many times (especially when learning the ABCs) I've gone into awareness of my tells and triggers and moved into my body and breath, only to be jerked back into my worried mind. I cannot tell you how many times I thought I had grounded myself in my body with sensation, touch, and a focus on my breath, and maybe the smell of a calming essential oil, only to find myself right back into the anxious thoughts of my mind. The same goes after I have moved into compassionate connection with myself, only to find myself right back in anxiety and alarm. The process is not linear. I often tell people healing from alarm is two steps forward, one step back. Two steps into your grounded body and then one step back into your worried mind. Be patient, practice, practice, practice, and you'll see you are not only steering your boat past your worries, but also patching the hole in the hull!

Especially early on, your ego dragon (I'll explain this concept in more detail soon) is relentlessly going to try to pull you back into the place where it feels most familiar and in control—holding you frozen in your worries and alarm.

There is a process that neuroscientists refer to as neuroplasticity. This is the brain's ability to make new pathways. Even though there are critical periods for certain types of brain development, the brain also has a phenomenal ability to learn and develop throughout our lifespan, given the right conditions. Neuroplasticity has its work cut out for itself when there is a previous pattern (or groove) to overwrite, but I am living proof of someone with severe anxiety that started with a deep groove of protection and fear who has used the ABC process and created an even deeper groove for growth and love.

Creating this deeper groove was definitely a "two steps forward and one step back" process, and like the stonecutter story I'll tell you soon, early on I didn't feel a great deal of progress early on, but I intuitively knew I was on the right track. As I cultivated a deep commitment to awareness and perhaps an even deeper commitment to being kind and connected to all parts of myself, the process progressed and I broke through to a new way of thinking and being.

In the time I've been using the ABC process (about five years now), I've seen there are two parts that seem to be the hardest for my patients: 1) developing an awareness of their anxiety and alarm cues that allow them to initiate the ABC process in the first place, and 2) staying with the process.

When I worked with patients who were trying to quit smoking or drinking, many times they would describe finding themselves with a cigarette or a drink in their hand, not really knowing how it got there—the habit was so strong that their unconscious took over. The unconscious desire to soothe with medication, addiction, distraction, and dissociation (MADD) simply overrode what their conscious mind wanted to do. The human program to fall into MADDs is an automatic and unconscious one. Worrying is like this too—we suddenly find ourselves back in it without any idea how we got there.

Trying to avoid worry only gets harder when your mind is impaired by the alarm in your body. I still sometimes spend some time in anxiety and alarm before I notice I am back in the toboggan racing down the hill in the old familiar groove of my worries. But with practice, the time it takes me to notice and change course has decreased considerably.

As you train yourself to recognize your signature worries and state of alarm, you'll get better at bringing awareness and dodging your ego's efforts to sabotage you back into worry. And for this, you need discipline.

One way you can start practicing awareness to make it a habit is to just pause a few times a day and ask yourself with loving compassion, "Where am I right now?" Are you in your body, feeling life, being connected and open, experiencing all your feelings? Or are you in your head, thinking? If you find yourself in worry, with intention, put a hand over where your alarm usually is and check in with how you *feel*. I often get my patients to set the timer on their phone at the start of the day to go off in three and a half hours. When the timer rings, hit "repeat" to start the timer again and ask yourself, "Where am I right now?," connecting with your body. Then repeat when it goes off again in three and a half hours. Do not underestimate the power of this self check-in. You can even start it by asking "Am I safe in this moment?" and affirming you are. You can also ask yourself "What *is* working in my life right now?" and develop a new focus on thriving instead of surviving.

I go through a version of the ABCs multiple times a day, and it takes me only two to three minutes each time. I close my eyes, check into my physical connection to myself with a hand on my chest, savor a few breaths as my hand rises and falls, and focus on something I like about myself—like my sense of humor, or my generous spirit, or my intuitive gifts. Sometimes I will bring up a mental image of my wife or my daughter or one of my grandkids, or if I'm at home I'll go over to one of my dogs and give them a cuddle and a few kisses on the snout. I'll end by thanking myself for taking the time to take care of my own needs, and I'll move back into my day. Again, this is part of "What Is Working" from the Anxiety Toolkit. It is so familiar for the wounded child in us to live in chronic apprehension and worry that we must break the spell by changing the direction of our default "doom and gloom" programming of doom to a conscious and directed focus to what *is* working in our lives.

The discipline of doing the process of checking in and looking for what is working, even when I am not worrying or in alarm, is invaluable. Remember, your protective ego wants to keep you in your head and out of your body so it will often make you "forget" that you are safe in the moment and forget to check in with yourself (that is what the phone timer is for). The better you get at disciplining yourself to do the process during good times and bad, the more it will become a part of you and you'll trust growth over protection versus the opposite.

We are neurologically wired to pay attention to the most intense sensation in our body and in this way our alarm takes the lion's share of our attention, whether we are aware of it or not. The result, at least unconsciously, is we feel like the alarm is all of us, because we don't notice other parts of our body that feel neutral or good. We can train ourselves to consciously look for parts of us that feel good, and for me that is my breath as it goes in and out through my face and chest. I find my alarm in my solar plexus and my presence in my breath and spend a little time every day consciously going back and forth between these sensations. Focusing on pleasure and pain simultaneously shows my unconscious mind that there is both pleasure and pain in me and that *the alarm isn't all of my experience,* because as a child I'm sure the intense discomfort of alarm did usurp all of my experience much of the time. This moving back and forth between sensations is called *pendulation* or *oscillation,* and I'll explain more soon. If this seems like too much trouble, consider that spending five to ten minutes consciously practicing pendulation every day is infinitely better than spending hours a day unconsciously practicing and ingraining your worries!

You may have noted that nowhere in the ABCs do I say to examine your worries for accuracy. That's because it's a losing battle. From a neurological perspective, when you are in alarm and survival physiology, you turn off your rational brain. So why are you trying to use reason when the reasoning part of your brain is off-line? Sure, your worries are irrational and unlikely to happen, but when you argue with your worries when you are in alarm/survival physiology, you are using an irrational brain in a futile attempt to find a rational conclusion. You can't beat thinking with more thinking, especially if the alarm has shut off your rational brain! Trying to disprove your worries is like trying to reason with the Sirens. If the temptation is strong to examine your worries (and most likely go down a path to other worrisome scenarios), remember to put your hand on your chest, do a few rounds of the physiological sigh, and once you've grounded yourself in your body, if you still feel you must think, then ask yourself, "Am I safe in this moment?" But I would prefer you just go from worry to sensation without explanation. (If you're getting sick of hearing "sensation without explanation," then I've ingrained it deeply into you and I've done my job.)

I am not saying that examining your worries for truth is not helpful. Asking "Is this worry true?" along the lines of the work of Byron Katie is very helpful (I have completed her program), but I have found her four-question process of "the work" much more effective and resonant after I have used the ABCs to ground myself in my body beforehand.

80

Let's Practice Our ABCs

Committing to a sense of awareness is the start of taking your life back. Training yourself to be aware of your mind and body from moment to moment gives you tremendous power. And all it takes is developing a ritual of sorts, in which you ask yourself "Where am I right now?" multiple times a day as I showed you in the last chapter.

A. If you find yourself feeling grounded and your breath is slow and deep, continue on with an intention to move deeper into your body, putting your hand on your chest, closing your eyes, and focusing deeply on sensation.

B. If you find yourself in a worry or rumination, simply stop and make a conscious intention to move into your body and breath (and therefore away from your thoughts). Close your eyes, put your hand on your chest, and move fully into breath and sensation. You can still do this if you're stressed while driving, just keep your eyes open. (We don't want the ABCs to stand for awareness, breath, collision.)

C.   If you find yourself in alarm, put your hand over the alarm and breathe into it. Close your eyes and, as you focus on the sensations of your breath and your hand rising and falling, create a place where you can focus on a pleasant (or at least neutral) sensation in your body like your breath. Allow the sensation of alarm to be present, but focus your attention on savoring your breath and the pleasant and supportive feeling of your hand over your alarm.

D.   You can even breathe in the pain, Tonglen style, as I showed you in chapter 67. There is no "right" way to ground yourself. Find what works best for you. Once you've grounded yourself in your body, move into a state of compassionate connection by bringing to mind something you like about yourself (or a person or place or pet that brings you joy) and staying with the emotion of that in your body. Generally, the more anxious thoughts you have and/ or the more alarm you feel, the longer you should stay in **B** and **C.** You can often tell you need to go back and start the ABCs over again if you fall back into the original thoughts or worries. The goal is to break the destructive alarm-anxiety cycle and start reprogramming a new, constructive path that connects you to your true, innocent self in your body and out of your mind. This is when being "out of your mind" is a good thing! The more loving connection you can create to your innocent child self through present-moment sensation in your body, the less the ego dragon needs to fire up your alarm, because one of the big reasons that alarm was created in the first place was the scared child's attempt to cry for help. When you hear the child's cries and offer that connection to your child self now that they didn't have at the time of the original alarm event(s), the alarm settles.

Doing this several times a day retrains your nervous system to move into a parasympathetic, relaxed state. It also gives you something constructive to do with your mind and diverts you away from the ego's

destructive habit of compulsively worrying in a futile and counterpro-
ductive effort to keep you safe.

The more you practice the ABC process—becoming aware of awareness, breathing into your body, changing your focus from rumination to
sensation, and compassionately connecting to yourself—the more you
will start creating a positive environment where your reactive self fades
and your authentic self emerges. Over time, you'll gain more confidence
to move away from a powerless, reactive victim self and spend more and
more time embodying a powerful authentic self. I can speak from experience when I say your confidence in your own ability to consciously
choose to move away from worry and not default into MADDs anymore
may be your most prized accomplishment. I know it's mine.

An important note: the ego is slippery and it will do everything in its
power to undermine the ABCs. The best way to deal with this masterful
saboteur is to develop a ritual that you do the same way every time, so
when you do spot the ego's tricks you can go right back into the ABCs.
I know I have offered you a number of options in this book, so try them
out and pick the ones that work best for you, and do them ritualistically
as often as you can. Practice, practice, practice.

Just a word of caution: if you find that your alarm is especially strong
and you are consistently getting sucked into the endless loop of triggers and
worries, please call on a therapist who knows how to deal with trauma and
alarm stored in the body. You should not be afraid to try the ABCs—in
and of themselves, they'll be healing—but there is no harm in enlisting
additional help while you're learning to untangle your well-worn patterns, especially early on. I have had many patients take this book to their
counselor, therapist, or doctor and use it as a guide to healing their anxiety. I get messages from therapists all the time telling me how they have
incorporated my work to help their anxious patients.

Healing anxiety is a challenge but it can be done. As I said way back in
this book, if you heal your anxiety, you might look at easier challenges like
being a blind bomb diffuser or amateur astronaut. The ego has tricked
child you into (over)protection so often since childhood that adult you
doesn't even see those tricks anymore. Out of a relentless pursuit of safety
that it can never provide, your ego dragon will try to pull you away from

the ABCs and back into its lair of worry and hypervigilance (this is the one step back from the two steps forward I talked about earlier). The dragon pulls you away from loving connection because it was incarnated in an atmosphere where love couldn't be trusted, and it's just trying to protect you from the vulnerability of love for that very reason. Now you must show love to that dragon and you do that by embodying adult you and fully taking charge of and loving child you, and that will show the dragon that it can turn off the fire (alarm), stand down, and take a smoke break!

> **Point to consider:** *The very best parts of you come from the child in you,* so stop taking JABS at him or her and tell your child self how much you are grateful for the wonderful, authentic traits they have provided. You can even tell that to their picture above your bathroom mirror. (Did you do that yet???) Do an internet search for "positive traits" and see which ones you get from the little version of you, and really feel gratitude and appreciation for those parts!

81

Ego Awareness

E is for ego.

I mentioned the dragon sitting atop a treasure chest earlier. I interpret this image from Scandinavian folklore to represent the ego as the dragon, evoking a fiery sensation of protective alarm in our bodies. The treasure inside is our innocence, our authentic love for ourselves. And you have to win over the dragon to access the treasure.

By winning the dragon's favor, we can turn it into an agent of growth and love—just as fiery in love as it once was in protection.

Not to put too fine a point on it, but the ego is our love for ourselves, and it is fierce. This is why it has fought so hard to protect us. The ego is not our enemy: what it lacks in foresight, it makes up for in raw power.

The ego's job is to keep you alive no matter what. And the sad truth is

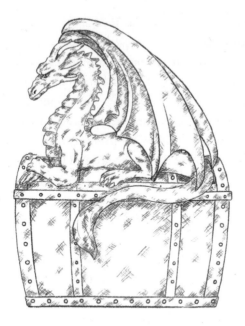

that on some level, the ego is comfortable with the alarm and anxiety in your system because you haven't died yet—and it's taking the credit for that. If the ego creates worry that hurts you but keeps you from moving into new territory that might harm you, it pats itself on the back.

Pain is a prerequisite for growth, so by shielding you from getting hurt, the ego also shields you from growth—and in blocking love (because sometimes love hurt when you were a child), the ego is causing you an enormous amount of pain under the guise of protecting you.

So, if pain in general leads to growth, why doesn't this pain inflicted by the ego lead to growth? Well, if you're reading this book, it has. I know without a doubt you've been strong enough many times in your life to "feel the fear and do it anyway" (to borrow a phrase from Susan Jeffers, PhD, who wrote a great book by that title). By the fact that you're here reading this book, I know you've experienced enough growth, and enough pain, to know you want to find a way to *heal* from your anxiety instead of just learning to *cope* with your anxiety.

Pain caused by the overzealous ego is mostly a reflection of our inner child's wounding. This is why the seemingly omnipotent dragon was in-carnated in the first place, to protect a child that felt they weren't being protected by their adults, or worse, their adults were the source of their pain. When the hypervigilant amygdala recognizes anything reminiscent of our original pain, it activates our familiar background alarm and sends a message to our brain and body to mobilize foreground alarm as well. In this activated survival state, we paralyze our rational brain and our SES, and this loss of grounding and connection causes us to age-regress back to the child we were at the time the pain occurred—a scared little being with only the resources of that frightened child at the time.

The purpose of this book is to ground you in the ABCs so you can meet your child self's pain of yesterday as the resourced adult of today, so you both climb together out of the shadows of that dark hole of chronic worry.

This may sound melodramatic, but I would like to propose that the most heroic journey you can take is gaining your innocence back by seeing that it never left; it just got trapped inside that protective chest, guarded by your powerful but single-minded, overprotective ego dragon. The dragon's chest acts as a protective structure, in some way shielding you from painful experience, but at the same time preventing you from growing and expanding beyond it. And the ego dragon is just fine with that bargain, but you, my worried friend, are seeing and feeling that overprotective structure is a hopeless place to live the rest of your life.

Goldfish secrete a substance that limits their growth to prevent them from getting too large for their pond or bowl. In the same way, your protective strategies minimized the pain you felt in childhood but at the cost of keeping you small and separate from the fullness and fulfillment of your authentic self. Your innocence and your authentic self are locked inside that chest made up of all the mechanisms that sheltered you from both the bad and the good, and they're blocking your access to the love in you.

For example, relationships thrive on trust and vulnerability—qualities you had as a child that may have been stamped out of you by traumatic experience. Perhaps now you have a strong desire for deeper friendships and romantic partnerships, but you can't seem to let anyone get close to you and really get to know you.

You're not defective. You have the same human capacity for trust and vulnerability as everyone else, it's just your nervous system got WIRED in pain: worry, inertia, resistance, ego defense. The ego dragon saw your WIRED pattern and locked your child self away in the chest because that was the only thing it could do. The dragon was created by your child self as a form of protection and therefore the dragon is itself a child. Your nervous system is not abnormal, in fact it's reacting exactly as it should to protect you and help you survive. The ego dragon helped you to survive, but now it's time to form an alliance with it, so you can thrive.

It's not your fate to have your overprotective dragon cut you off from love and social connection this way. You have the ability to develop a connected and caring relationship with your ego dragon, and indeed, all parts of you. You can stop acting like a goldfish secreting a neurological substance that keeps you constricted in fear, and, with the ego dragon's assistance, open that chest and let the child in you become the authentic, expanded, thriving version of you now, instead of the reactive, constricted, surviving child you had to be back then.

Patients often say to me, "My anxiety makes me feel like I don't know who I am anymore." They disown their wants and needs and the dreams of their authentic and innocent heart—because someone hurt them or didn't have the capacity to care for them in the way they needed. This abandonment has left them, so many years later, as a reactive self, not knowing how to get past their defense mechanisms and tune in to the love they should have received so they can access those wants and needs and dreams again.

Remember, all anxiety is separation anxiety and all alarm is separation alarm. By allowing the dragon to keep sitting on top of the chest, you've unknowingly been reinforcing its reason to guard the chest so tightly. First, your alarm came from separation from a caregiver—but what's feeding your alarm now is more of a separation from yourself.

So, come on. Let's make friends with that dragon that is keeping you separated from yourself, shall we?

82

Ego and the Abuse of Power

Your ego dragon was created by the frightened child in you, and in many ways it is like leaving a petrified child in charge of your safety. Indeed, part of you (via your amygdala and insula) still believes and feels you are back in your childhood pain, and your dragon will fight to the death to protect the child that created it. The ego dragon fires up automatically and unconsciously to protect you at any sign of threat reminiscent of that old trauma. Oftentimes, that threat is only imagined. (For you neuroscience geeks like me, a part of the brain close to the amygdala called the *bed nucleus of the stria terminalis* may be involved in responding with alarm to our self-created worries.)

Remember my story of having my alarm triggered at a concert when I heard a trumpet? When my amygdala was activated and my protective ego took over, I lost the rational ability to see I was perfectly safe. Part of me was transported back to a time where hearing a trumpet was a sign that I was trapped in a situation where I felt annoyed, uncertain, fearful, and powerless. I age-regressed and lapsed into an angry, fearful young teenager in an instant.

The reason I gave myself for wanting to leave was that the music was too loud and there were too many people. And that overreaction was evidence of the immense power of the protective ego—I convinced myself of something that just wasn't true because I was enjoying it just seconds before the trumpet solo.

Luckily, I have been able to get curious about my reaction and come to understand it after the fact. The trumpet still triggers me to this day (especially if the trumpet player is not so skilled). But now I'm fully aware of what's happening. I can see it so I don't have to be it—and not only that, but my ego dragon and I can even laugh about it . . . sometimes.

Again, it's not about defeating the ego dragon because the dragon cannot be defeated. You must learn, young Jedi, that the more you fight with the dragon, the more it feeds your alarm, which drives you deeper into an age regression. In many ways, the ego is the child in you, for the "time-deaf" amygdala has frozen you (and your body) there. But now, when you notice the pull to be dragged into the past pain or future worries, learn to immediately snap into the ABCs just like the jet pilots snap on their oxygen masks when they notice the signs of hypoxia in their bodies. In other words, when the ego tries to move you forward or back into a painful time, you immediately learn to snap on the oxygen mask of your ABCs to keep yourself in your body and breath and firmly rooted in the present.

When my ego dragon blocked my ability to let love in, I had nothing to counter the ever-increasing fear. The ABCs do not create love—they merely reveal, and allow access to, the love for yourself that was always there. *It is only your resistance to love that keeps you locked in anxiety.*

When we compassionately "come alongside" (to borrow a Gordon Neufeld term) our ego dragon, we let the dragon know that it's safe to open the chest. We can genuinely thank the ego dragon for doing what it thought was best when we were children and come to a new understanding with our dragon as adults.

In accepting and embracing all parts of ourselves (especially those parts that are anxious and alarmed), we can create a secure connection to those frightened parts and begin to correct the separation that fed the alarm in the first place. If all anxiety is separation anxiety and all alarm is separation alarm, we win over the dragon by showing it that our adult self will protect our child self. The adult in us will resolve the alarm so the dragon can cool off, stand down, and be able to finally release its hypervigilant fixation to (over)protect our child self. The dragon can be released from its vigilant protection because it sees our adult self, via the ABCs, is finally looking after our child self in a much more adaptive and loving way.

Point to consider: Do you look at your anxious parts with contempt and stigma? Can you open to the possibility of nurturing those frightened, childlike parts?

83

You're an Innocent Soul and You're Here to Remember That

We are born innocent, and that is our true nature. We are all innocent souls at our core, and if we are lucky enough to be securely attached to a parent or caregiver without significant trauma, we gain a felt sense of our innocence and our nervous system learns that life is about connection and growth, and our authentic personality emerges naturally.

But if our attachment was not secure and we experienced pain and trauma that was not resolved, our nervous system learns that life is about protection and survival and that's when we develop defensive adaptations and coping strategies that favor protection over growth. With unresolved pain, our worldview and personality are then forged more in reactivity and self-protection than authenticity, and a reactive personality is exhausting to maintain. (People pleasing, narcissism, victim mentality, anyone?)

When a child is abused, experiences great loss, or is abandoned or rejected, we often say the child has "lost their innocence." What people usually mean by this is the child lost their opportunity to be "just a kid," and had to mature too early (the *M* in ALARMS) and worry about their safety and security. But using the terms of this book, we can say the child's innocence is not lost, but instead stowed away under lock and key by an overprotective ego dragon. That innocence can be reclaimed later, but until it is, the person loses access to many of their gifts and much of their loving nature as those gifts are held back from both self and others. Your relationship with others can be no better than your relationship with yourself, and if you don't allow access to your innocent gifts out of a dominant need for protection, everyone loses, but especially you.

Nobody has gone into a nursery and said, "That baby is a narcissist," or "That baby is a people pleaser," or "You see that baby over there? It clearly sees itself as a victim." A newborn baby cannot be a narcissist or a people pleaser or see itself as a victim. These attributes aren't born—they're earned. We develop reactive personality traits and behaviors that society deems unacceptable when we see the world as a place we need to guard against.

We are not born addicted to shopping or sex or lying. We adopt those addictions because on some level we perceive them as an adaptive buffer to the pain of our background alarm. Then, because all addictions have negative consequences, we judge ourselves for having those addictions. In strongly judging ourselves for our "flaws," we become locked in them. Yet another thing I learned from Brené Brown: you cannot heal an addiction if you are still holding yourself in shame and contempt for that addiction. You can't shame someone into changing. In fact, shaming someone (including yourself) for an addiction will only increase the destructive influence of that addiction. Shame fires up alarm and we need something to soothe the alarm, so we fall into our addiction, which creates shame, which fires up alarm, and the cycle repeats itself until the ABCs and self-compassion show a new path. When you give yourself connection and compassion, you soothe the alarm at its source and the addictions (as well as the dragon) can take a smoke break since they are no longer needed to soothe the alarm because adult you has done that for child you with the ABCs.

Addictive traits or behaviors are hard to change because 1) they helped us feel better at one time (usually in childhood), so they served some adaptive purpose at a very influential time in our youth; 2) we deny their existence or impact; and 3) you can't change something you haven't accepted and embraced in yourself. If you refuse to see it you are destined to be it.

Addiction is one of those topics that deserves a book of its own. I don't have space to explore it in detail, but I did want to note that alarm and anxiety play a massive role in developing addictions. Although more intensive help is likely to be needed, the ABCs will help you get out of your shame and break the cycle that keeps pushing you back into the addictive behavior—and it starts with truly seeing your own innocence. In fact, I believe all emotional healing starts with clearly seeing your own innocence, and the ABCs absolutely relax the dragon and open up the chest to expose your true and innocent gifts. Once you fully accept your innocence, there's a flow that allows you to stay more in the safety of your parasympathetic rest-and-digest nervous system. From there, you can enter a place of engagement with yourself and others, using the SES that is wired into all of us as a factory setting at birth.

I firmly believe that nurturing and engaging this SES would help or resolve so many emotional disorders since the vast majority of them have their roots in the loss of connection in childhood, compounded by the reproach—separation—we inflict on ourselves in adulthood. Even for such severe conditions as narcissistic, antisocial, and borderline personality disorders, connection with self and others can contribute significantly to healing. The SES activation from compassionate connection in 12-step groups is a major factor in their success. I believe that the human interaction in 12-step groups actually matures the SES through neuroplasticity, helping people see their own innocence, which reduces the judgment, abandonment, blame, and shame we direct at ourselves (see the next chapter on JABS).

When you rediscover your innocence and allow it to come out to play, the overprotective ego can just stand by and watch us have fun. When you truly see your own innocence, you realize you've been creating your own alarm all along, and you can move into loving growth and away from fearful, alarm-based protection. But like anything, if you don't clearly see how you separate from yourself, you can't see how to come back together, so let's spend some time looking at the tricks the ego uses to keep you split and embrace some valuable ways to stay connected.

84

Connecting with Your Inner Child

With all this talk of reconnecting with the inner child, does the idea bring up some resistance for you?

I ask because the term "inner child" does bring up resistance with a lot of people, including me. Many view it as overly "woo-woo" and spiritual.

I do find many people object strongly and even ridicule the inner child concept, but curiously I find the people who most strongly object to the term turn out to be the ones with the most childhood wounding! For me personally, the inner child concept has been one of the most important in my healing, but it also brings up resistance in me, even to this day, because it's painful to go back and visit the child in me who was so hurt so long ago.

This is not a concept that was introduced to me in my training as a medical doctor, and in fact, I suspect that if you ever used the term "inner child" with your doctor, they would probably roll their eyes so far back in their head they'd fall off their stool. But although conventional physicians may not be on board with using that term just yet, there is an increasing awareness of the importance of childhood experiences, and physicians are starting to ask routinely about traumatic events in childhood.

The adverse childhood experiences (ACEs) study, published in the late 1990s, made a crucial contribution to our understanding of how trauma in childhood leads to physical and mental illness in adulthood, and some doctors receiving their education today do learn about it. Examining a sample of more than seventeen thousand people in the US, the study found that ACEs like neglect, physical, sexual or emotional abuse, parental addiction or alcoholism, or any significant loss greatly increased the risk of mental and physical illness and disease in adulthood.

Another sobering finding was just how common ACEs were. Participants in the study were not from typical at-risk populations. They had solid incomes and steady employment with access to high-quality healthcare since the prerequisite to enroll as a subject was to be a member of the health system that conducted the study. Yet, in this relatively well-off population, more than one-quarter reported being physically abused as children, and more than one-fifth reported being sexually abused. About two-thirds of the sample reported having at least one ACE (a list that includes neglect, abuse, parental addiction, divorce, death, incarceration, or mental illness). Just search "ACE questions" if you are interested in seeing the actual questions used to assess childhood trauma.

In my terminology, ACEs are ALARMS that aren't resolved by a caregiver and both ACEs and ALARMS lead to background alarm stored in our body, and as adults we then separate from our body (and move into our worried minds) because it holds our childhood pain. But when we cut ourselves off from our bodies for fear of running into that old pain, we also deny ourselves access to the child in us that holds that pain. The ego dragon is incarnated to keep the child protected, but it's more like solitary confinement as we learn to cope alone, cut off from the connections that would allow us to heal and thrive.

Your inner child is waiting for you to stop judging, abandoning, blaming, and shaming them. That child wants to be seen, heard, accepted, and loved.

And you can do that with the ABCs.

Become aware that your hurt little self is inside you, and make an effort to see them. Move into your body, which is their body too, and both of you can learn to feel together. Show them that it is safe by providing them with the compassionate connection they needed when they experienced those ACEs and ALARMS. Be the comforting, competent parent to them now they SHOULD have had back then. (Another acronym! I'll explain later in chapter 100.)

People often tell me they've been trying to reconnect with their inner child but they just can't seem to reach them—and I just tell them to keep trying. Imagine that you have numbed, medicated, judged, abandoned, blamed, and shamed that child for so long they've lost the ability to trust you or have faith in you. Isn't that mistrust and distance an understandable response? Consistently show that child you're not going anywhere and you will be there for them whenever they're ready, and they will show up. You can trust me and the therapy I recommend in this book—after all, I *am* a doctor, but not like the doctor Jackhammer Johnson played in the move *Funny Bone Therapy*.

Here's the story about a stonecutter I mentioned earlier. There is a skilled stonecutter who is faced with the task of breaking a very large stone in half. His tools are so heavy that he can only manage a few strikes before resting. He examines the rock and sees the line he must strike in order to split the stone evenly. When he begins his work, each blow is precise and delivered with intention.

After exactly one hundred well-placed strikes over many days, the stone is still intact. As the sun sets on another day, the stonecutter sets down his hammer and chisel and walks home with a heavy heart, wondering if he's taken on an impossible task.

But he wakes up the next day with renewed determination. When he examines the stone that morning, he sees a crack he's never noticed before. When he places his chisel in this crack, the ensuing strike breaks the stone clean in half. A passerby witnesses this strike and exclaims in wonder, "You broke that stone apart with a single blow!"

That's how it is with connecting to your child. It may seem like nothing is happening, and then, suddenly, you break through.

Each time you practice the ABCs is another strike to open to the heart of the matter.

In doing the ABCs some people may feel an immediate connection to self, like they've found the missing piece of the puzzle. For others, it may take a while for the ABCs to break down the ACEs that created the massive stone of anxiety and alarm.

Point to consider: A for awareness, B for body and breath, and C for compassionate connection to yourself. The ABCs are available to you in every second of every minute of every day.

85

Ego Tricks That Keep You Separate (JABS)

When I first met my patient Anne, she described herself as "high-strung." That was an understatement. In her early forties, with short blond hair and intense blue eyes, she was one of those people who always seemed like she had just drunk three cups of coffee. She spoke quickly, and when she talked her hands flew everywhere. This dynamo was a tiny, wiry person—just a little over five feet tall—but she carried a big personality and a lot of alarm from the trauma she experienced in childhood. Her anxious thoughts mostly involved her three daughters, who at the time ranged in age from thirteen to nineteen.

Anne was a classic people pleaser. Her husband and kids always had fresh lunches and fresh laundry. She was very good at keeping her family fed and taken care of, but she rarely looked after herself, especially when it came to food.

She had grown up the oldest of three sisters. Her mother was narcissistic and demanding, and Anne performed the vast majority of the work around the house from a young age, along with looking after her two younger sisters and having dinner on the table when her mother got home. Her mother was tall and striking and garnered a lot of attention for her looks. She would often comment to Anne, "Don't ever let yourself get fat," even though Anne was naturally slim (even tending toward skinny). Every few months, her mother would go into a fit of rage that was almost always directed at Anne.

Anne learned that she was not important for who she was but for how she looked and what she could provide for others. Her only measure of control was the rare praise she got from her mother for being responsible enough to look after her sisters. Her father was affectionate when he would come home after a few drinks, but without alcohol, he was unemotional and seemed to "go through the motions" of being a father, attending school plays and community events out of obligation more than interest.

Remember, when a parent abuses, abandons, or rejects a child, the child doesn't stop loving the parent—the child stops loving themselves. And when you block love, the only thing left is fear. Anne started to attribute the dysfunction in her family to something that she was or wasn't doing, and the fear in that created and fueled Anne's inner critic. And what fuels the inner critic?

Judgment, abandonment, blame, and shame, or JABS.

Anne became the poster (inner) child for the acronym JABS. She judged herself as being unworthy, or only worthy when she abandoned herself and her own needs to look after others. She blamed herself for her mother's rage (or any of her family members' anger) and shamed herself for eating because she feared the dreaded weight gain her mother harped on about.

JABS show up in many forms I'll elaborate on soon—resistance, victim mentality, inability to receive love (or even compliments), defensive detachment—and they all block access to your ability to heal. You just keep on hurting and alarming your inner child, not realizing that the enemy you're trying to protect the child from may not even be present anymore.

As Anne rejected herself, she created a deeper split between her authentic self (her innocence) and her ego-created reactive self—and as this split grew wider, her alarm increased. She was caught in the alarm-anxiety cycle with her old alarm feeding the JABS she took at herself and the JABS reciprocally feeding the alarm. There was no way out as the external critical voice of her mother was replaced by the internal critical voice of her ego dragon. Ironically, the ego had adopted Anne's mother's criticisms under the unconscious impression those criticisms were constructive and protective, when in reality those JABS her ego took at herself were destructive and damaging.

When I explained all this to Anne, just hearing it gave her some immediate relief. She told me for the first time she could see that what happened was not her fault. And over time, as we worked on accepting and loving the lost parts of herself, she was able to regain control of her life.

Anne was a sensitive person by nature, too, and she had cut off that sensitive side of her to protect it. Once she became aware that her ego had adopted her mother's critical voice of judging, abandoning, blaming, and shaming her under the illusion of protection, she started to see she was worthy of protecting that little girl inside of her. And that little girl was worthy of her own compassion, attention, and self-care.

Once again, there is no healing from anxiety and alarm until you gain access to your innocence. You can do that by becoming aware of the JABS you take at yourself and the messages that you internalized from what your parents said to you directly or the unspoken messages they gave you in their treatment of you.

For example, when Anne would feel shame as she was about to eat something, once she became aware of it, she could label it and then set the intention to shift her attention to sensation. Once she placed a hand on her chest and connected with her breath, she could move into a compassionate connection with herself, using phrases such as "I like that I've made a safe and comfortable home for my family" and "I accept and embrace all parts of me." This conscious action releases shame and promotes self acceptance in both thinking *and* feeling.

Anne felt better quickly when she practiced the ABC process multiple times a day. It worked well for her in part because she was so intensely disciplined about it. She started to have an easier time looking after herself, telling me, "The more connected I felt with my body, the more I wanted to take care of it." She told me the ABCs process helped her feel more empowered and less like a helpless victim just waiting for her anxiety and alarm to pass.

Like so many of us worriers, instead of Anne assuming she was generally safe with fleeting moments of danger, she assumed she was in danger with only fleeting moments of safety.

> So, right here, right now, let's break the alarm's spell on us where we sense that danger is all around, shall we? Take a moment to look around, take a breath, put your hand on your chest, and assure yourself that in this moment, right here and right now, you are safe. It's that quick and easy, so I encourage you to do this multiple times each day. Adding sensation creates a *feeling* of safety, as opposed to just verbally telling yourself you are safe. Notice that when you focus on your breath it naturally becomes deeper and slower. Your breath *wants* to help you!

Good! Now, before we leave this chapter on JABS, if you feel up to it, ask yourself these questions. You don't need in-depth answers—I am just priming your brain for the next sections.

Where do I judge myself? Where do I abandon myself? Where do I blame myself? Where do I shame myself?

Where do I judge the child in me? Where do I abandon the child in me? Where do I blame the child in me? Where do I shame the child in me?

Again, you don't need to go into these questions in depth right now. If any answers came up that really struck a nerve with you, please write them down as the intensity they bring up can help you find some nuances in your alarm. Also, these can be emotionally evocative questions so be sure to ground yourself first before you move on with the book.

86

Ego Trick: Self-Judgment

In the coming chapters, we'll look at some of the ego dragon's common tricks because (all together now!) when you can *see* them, you no longer have to *be* them. Along with JABS, the ego uses victim mentality, resistance, compulsive thinking, inability to receive, and defensive detachment among others (I told you the ego was crafty!) to trap you in alarm. With all these tricks, the ego unwittingly creates pain in its efforts to shield you from pain.

Along with each trick, you'll learn ways to move past them. Know that these are not a replacement for the ABCs; they are meant to help you gain awareness of the ego in real time and move into the ABCs when you notice one of your tells revealing your ego dragon in action.

Let's look first at self-judgment.

We may have been born sensitive, but we weren't born specifically judging and disliking parts of ourselves. Two-year-olds don't tell themselves they are getting too fat or they should stop crying because it makes them look weak.

Tibetan monks live in an environment of compassion and acceptance and find it hard to believe it's possible for a human being *not* to love themselves. But if we grow up in an atmosphere of trauma and compromised attachment, which is becoming more common, being compassionate to ourselves is unfamiliar. With no direct experience of compassionate attachment, it's difficult to conjure it up on our own.

As noted before, when there's trouble at home, children often blame themselves. On that foundation, it's not hard to see how you probably wouldn't have a positive self-image if you judged yourself to be the cause of problems in your family. Because we depend on our parents for our survival, it's too painful to believe they are the cause of the problems in the family—so the cause must be us.

It makes perfect sense where self-judgment came from. But over time, it's learned and ingrained with repetition until it has nothing to do with our parents anymore—we just do it because it's what we've always done. Self-judgment, like all the ego tricks I'll show you, is self-reinforcing, just like the groove in the snow we make deeper and deeper and faster and faster the more we follow its track.

The first part of the solution is to make the specific intention to be fully aware of the judgments you make toward yourself.

This most often shows up with statements that sound like "I'm too _____" (anxious, fat, selfish) or "I'm not _____ enough" (nice, smart, productive). View it as detective work—you are a private investigator gathering intelligence on the habits of your ego dragon, following it around in the shadows.

If you have a supportive friend or partner you can share this journey with, I'd recommend asking them to tell you when they notice you judging yourself. Sometimes it takes a while for it to sink in how pervasive and harsh our self-judgment really is, not to mention invisible! When you *notice* that you're being critical of yourself, you've taken the first step of bringing your unconscious habit of self-judgment into the light of conscious awareness. By labeling it as an intrusive thought and not something you automatically need to believe, you bring it into the light and take away much of its power to control you from the shadows. Now, recall that we're not trying to slay the ego dragon; we're trying to make friends with it. So, the solution is not to "think positive" and tell yourself the opposite of the negative thought ("I'm so unselfish! I'm very svelte! I'm sooooo productive!"). This is where the self-help movement gets a bad name. We are not Stuart Smalley (the Al Franken character on *Saturday Night Live*) looking in the mirror saying to ourselves, "I'm good enough. I'm smart enough. And doggone it, people like me!"

Instead, we need to bring compassion to the qualities in ourselves we thought were not acceptable—but first, as always, we need to get grounded in our body.

Personally, my ego dragon often judges me for being too sensitive. Once I notice it (using my awareness to label the thought as intrusive and self-judgmental), I'll pause and move into my body and stay there in sensation until I feel grounded. Then I place my hand over my alarm, savor my breath—by now you can pick your favorite way to ground yourself in awareness of your body.

Once you've mastered the basics of getting grounded in your body, there's a way to look a little deeper into awareness that can be especially useful in bringing all of the ego tricks out of the shadows, but let's start with self-judgment. Awareness is not so much a thinking; it is an openness to observing your thinking. Thinking is expressive; awareness is receptive. We are not trying to replace or contradict our expressive thoughts as positive psychology would tell us to do. Awareness is not a convergence to a specific goal but a divergence into a curiosity. In awareness, we first pay close attention to cultivating a receptive feeling state before we move toward expressive thinking. Awareness is embracing a sense of not knowing, suspending our preconceived notions and judgments of ourselves and an openness to the wounded child as if it was a scared child you didn't know that you encountered on your street. Grounding ourselves in feeling and compassion for the innocent child in us is the platform from which we can change our habitual, judgmental perceptions of ourselves. Simply stating an affirmation by rote will do little unless there is a connected, compassionate feeling that is energizing it.

I mentioned the somatic experiencing practice called *pendulation* earlier. In pendulation we consciously oscillate our attention back and forth between two sensations—typically one comfortable or neutral and the other uncomfortable.

When I notice my self-judgmental thought, for example that I'm too sensitive, I stop and acknowledge that I'm being critical of myself and then, as I said earlier, I go back and forth between the pleasant sensation of my breath through my sinuses and the feeling in my body as I have the thought "I am too sensitive." For me, my JABS toward myself all seem to energize the well-known alarm in my solar plexus, but you may find different body sensations of alarm are associated with different worries or self-criticisms. You can absolutely have more than one alarm stored in your body.

As I shift my focus back and forth between the two sensations, the rhythmic back and forth of my breath through my nostrils, and the purple, sharp pressure sensation in my solar plexus, it breaks the illusion that the alarm is infinite and inextricably coupled with my self-judgment. As I ground into my body, I am no longer in a sea of danger with a few islands of safety. I focus on the sea of safety in my breath with the island of alarm in my solar plexus.

It's like adding a bit of ice-cold water to a cup of too-hot tea so it's no longer hot enough to burn my mouth. I can now take a sip of the alarm and see it no longer has to burn me. I always have a safe place in my body to return to—the place I've created with my own caring and compassionate touch and the reassuring sensation of my breath.

Now moving on from *B* to *C,* I will take the original thought and, with compassionate connection to myself, question the thought in curiosity. I'll ask "Am I really too sensitive?" and I might even go through Byron Katie's four questions and a turnaround, *but only once I have grounded myself in my body and breath.*

Is it true I am too sensitive? Do I absolutely know it's true? How do I feel and react when I believe I am too sensitive? Who would I be without the thought "I am too sensitive"? And the turnaround: "How is it more true that I am *not* too sensitive?" And then I will respond, "My sensitivity is a gift," or "My sensitivity is what's allowed me to help so many people in my career." Or it could be a broader statement like "I used to see my sensitivity as a weakness that I now embrace as a gift and a strength."

If these four questions and a turnaround appeal to you, check out Byron Katie's book *Loving What Is.*

Another approach is saying, "I am too sensitive and I can love that about myself!" The key is cultivating a felt sense of love and compassion for yourself and then dealing with the self-judgmental thought. Do not try to process self-judgment without first going through the ABCs to put yourself in a curious, open, and grounded place.

Do you see how this is all different from Stuart Smalley's approach? Poor Stuart is trying to counteract his self-judgments, but he's probably just digging himself deeper into a hole because he doesn't believe what he's saying to himself in the mirror. There's no feeling to what he says to himself, only words. Feeling is what changes our thinking—not so much the other way around. Statements grounded in the feeling of compassion let us know that we are joining within ourselves, and that is the best antidote to the internal split that created and maintains our ego trick of self-judgment (and all the ego's tricks) in the first place.

When we are able to reframe our perceived "flaws" and view them with compassion and curiosity in grounded physiology, we truly see them so we no longer have to be them. When we pendulate traumatic thoughts with grounded feeling, we neutralize alarm. And the best part is we're not trying to fool ourselves by quoting some rote phrase like Stuart Smalley—our statements of compassion are heartfelt! I now fully embrace my sensitivity, as I know that without it this book would never have been written. As a teen I hated my sensitivity because I just felt . . . too . . . much, especially the alarm. As an adult, I embrace my sensitivity as the trait that has the most to do with my success. I also acknowledge the child in me for my sensitivity, because it comes from him.

The emotional component of the ABCs is why the process has been so healing for people. If we could simply think our way out of emotional issues, talk therapy would work wonders and only take about seventeen minutes—but you need more than a cognitive solution to fix an emotional issue.

When I started with the ABCs, every time I got to the compassionate connection part, I would find a way of discounting myself. I became adept at awareness, and then moving directly into my body, but developing a compassionate connection to myself was by far the most challenging aspect of the ABCs for me. You may find this as well, but as you persevere you build more faith in your connection to yourself, and the JABS and ego dragon tricks naturally fade. I found it fascinating that I became aware that doing this pendulation work made me much more gentle and kind to myself, as well as lowered my alarm considerably. Perhaps the most obvious benefit was a distinct lowering of my irritability. Alarm in the system is a profound source of irritability in myself and so many of my patients. As I integrated the disparate parts I judged, abandoned, blamed, and shamed in myself and brought them into a functional whole, my alarm ceased to control my emotions and my behaviors. I can't explain the relief I feel after being in therapy for thirty-plus years with no real benefit and then finding this relief for myself!

When you do the ABCs and focus deeply on the positive parts of yourself, you begin to break down the ego dragon's strategy of self-judgment. You'll notice that I say "the positive parts of yourself" and not "the parts you love about yourself." If you do have parts you love about yourself, then by all means use those in your ABCs—but many of us have a hard time with loving parts of ourselves because of a strong inner critic. By the way, the inner critic is just the ego dragon hiding in a different-colored ninja suit.

For many, especially early on in the process, finding and focusing on something you love about yourself can be a tough proposition, because your inner critic has been after you (in their crap-colored ninja suit) for a long time. Don't feel that you have to love yourself before you are ready. When you've spent many years unwittingly focusing on the negative parts of yourself, it may take a while to create a new groove. But once you commit to developing a compassionate connection within, you might be surprised how much you start to see what you truly do like about yourself. What you focus on, you'll get more of—so if you focus on what you like about yourself, you'll see more of it, and it starts to form a new groove in the snow.

Your statements are so powerful because you're taking the time to get grounded in your body and connect with emotion before saying them—unlike poor old Stuart, who's just repeating words into a mirror without any feeling behind them. The more intention and feeling you invest into your words, the more power they have to create change in your system.

Again, whatever you focus on your brain will give you more of.

Focus on self-judgment and you'll see more self-judgment. Focus on self-connection and you'll renew your perception to see more self-connection.

87

Ego Trick: Self-Abandonment

There is perhaps no greater propagator of chronic alarm than self-abandonment, because the feeling of being abandoned replicates the original separation in your childhood that created the alarm in the first place. Any hint of abandonment will fire up the amygdala like a faulty toaster can light a house on fire.

Self-abandonment typically begins 1) automatically when there are family ALARMS; 2) early in childhood; and 3) under the guise it is keeping us safe. Over time, leaving ourselves becomes a pattern (like people pleasing), and this is why we find ourselves still doing it as adults. The antidote to self-abandonment is to 1) see it consciously; 2) act as your own connected "parent" now as an adult; and 3) keep yourself feeling safe by consciously and compassionately connecting with your very own authentic, innocent self.

One of the most devastating ways self-abandonment shows up is putting others' needs ahead of your own. In medical school, we were trained to do exactly this. It didn't matter if you had been awake for the previous thirty-six hours; you still had to be there for your patient. The doctor's code is that the patient always comes first. Every med student accepts it, and nobody is allowed to complain about it. Nobody spoke up to say this is unrealistic and unsafe, but after an epidemic of physician suicides, medical programs have started to take notice that doctors need to be taught how to look after themselves. Sadly, this culture of self-abandonment in medicine is why I believe doctors continue to have such a high burnout and suicide rate.

Self-abandonment arises when we get into the habit of putting our own needs last, or we stop speaking up for ourselves because we have learned it doesn't do any good—and may even hurt us. Children raised in dysfunctional families often come to believe their only value lies in what we can do for others, and sometimes we give up our own authentic dreams and passions because we've been told they are unrealistic or impractical—or simply because they take time or attention away from another person.

Before I leave this chapter, I want you to see where you leave yourself for others, but in general it's more important to see when you leave yourself, period. Since all anxiety is separation anxiety and all alarm is separation alarm, it stands to reason you need to separate from yourself for you to experience anxiety and alarm—and when you engage in any of the ego tricks, you abandon your innocent self. Much of the power of the ABC process is to make the conscious intention to expand the connection to yourself because it was the lack of attention to that child in you that created all this alarm in the first place. When you connect to yourself with the ABC process, the alarm begins to heal and resolve because you are showing the child in you that they are seen, heard, understood, loved, and protected now in a way they just weren't back then.

I know I've suggested this before, and I repeat it because there is likely to be resistance to the vulnerability this creates, but consider putting a picture of your child self up on your bathroom mirror. Or make that picture the screen saver on your phone as I do. Stop judging that child and start connecting with them! But, if you think this is going to trigger you and you're not ready to go back there just yet, don't do it! (Yet.) I don't want you to put up a picture of your younger self if you don't feel you can connect with them (that in itself would be a type of self-abandonment).

88

Ego Trick: Self-Blame and Self-Shame

"There are no prison walls stronger than the ones we cannot see."
We blame to discharge energy. Physiologically, when we blame someone else there is a temporary decrease in stress chemicals like cortisol. It feels

good to us to see someone held accountable for their negative actions. When someone is sent to prison for a crime, we feel justice has been served and some of the negative energy experienced has an outlet for discharge. Humans have an innate sense of justice, and the urge to blame serves that desire for justice—the desire to see wrongdoing named and atoned for. We use blame as a way of making sense and discharging pain. So self-blame is related to self-judgment but is not quite the same.

As children we learn that blaming others discharges pain, but as we often blame ourselves for the dysfunction in our families, this holds the self blame in suspended animation within. Children can't judge or blame their parents because they depend on them for survival, so the blame gets boomeranged back to the child. This self-blame loop is unresolvable and overwhelms the child's conscious mind, and then their nervous system freezes in response to the futility (as an animal would that is hopelessly cornered by a predator) and this dumps alarm energy directly into their little body.

I view self-blame as a child's way of holding themselves in alarm's prison for a crime their parents committed. A child that consciously or unconsciously blames themselves becomes an adult who cannot (or will not) see their own innocence, and therefore cannot heal.

Blame and shame are similar but manifest very differently. Self-blame is summed up with the statements "I made a mistake" or "This is all my fault." The blame keeps what I have done in my awareness, and although it hurts, in awareness I can use that self-blame as a way of preventing myself from making the same mistake. When we use the ABCs to bring self-blame into conscious awareness and see and embrace our innocence, the guilt has much less negative charge and it is infinitely easier to work through because we don't take it so much as a personal failing. With the ABCs we can see our self-blame in nonjudgmental curiosity, which goes a very long way to helping us resolve it without abandoning ourselves in self-judgment. Like the alarm-anxiety cycle, the JABS have a way of energizing each other too!

Compared to guilt, shame is more paralyzing. When we blame ourselves we can use awareness to point to an action. Shame, on the other hand, is like kryptonite for awareness. We can't look at it because it just reignites too much alarm. Even if we want to look at shame, our ego dragon buries it deep in the shadows of our unconscious. What shames us is who we believe we are at our core. We don't want others to see it and we especially don't want to see it ourselves.

For many of my anxious patients, they were bullied at home or (especially) at school. School is a petri dish for shame. When my patients bravely access their experiences with being bullied, the shame is palpable. They often felt it wasn't something they did that was wrong; it was their essence that was being attacked. Even though the bulling or rejection came from the outside, the shame is felt at our core. Shame is an inside job.

Entire books have been written on shame, but I am going to go back once again to Brené Brown. She says shame is toxic because, from an evolutionary perspective, we feel it threatens our very survival. To be shamed in our history as humans could mean ostracization from our tribe, and that would literally be a death sentence.

Shame is an extremely potent potentiator of self-separation and alarm because it lives in the shadows and feeds our dragon big chunks of our self-esteem (or whatever dragons eat). I cannot tell you the number of people I've known or treated who saw their mental struggles as shameful and held off on getting the help they needed because of it. The dragon has a field day with shame over having a mental illness or even having a family member with a mental illness. I remember being deeply ashamed of my dad, even though I knew his illness wasn't his fault.

One of the biggest sources of shame I see in people is the shame over taking a psychiatric medication. I've written many thousands of prescriptions for different kinds of psych medications, and I've noticed that people never shame themselves for needing to take antibiotics to treat an infection, or eye drops for glaucoma, but they sure do when the prescription is for a psychiatric medication.

When we see our self-blaming and shaming in the light of awareness, often we can use what we blamed and shamed ourselves for as an avenue to connect with ourselves. Using addiction as an example, there is tremendous power in embracing a part of you that you previously kept in the shadows. When you see it (and accept and embrace it), you don't have to be it. When you have an addiction and say, "And I can love that about myself," you have broken the dragon's shame spell and taken major steps toward healing it. (Yes, of course dragons have magic, haven't you seen *Game of Thrones*?) So what are *you* blaming and shaming yourself for? Chances are your dragon has been using blame and shame for a long time to keep you separated from your authentic self and, therefore, exacerbate your alarm and anxiety which keeps you frozen where you are, and the dragon avoids change because it deeply fears uncertainty. You may hold shame from many decades ago, and it's still keeping you stuck in alarm. If you feel a lot of self-blame and shame (or if you are suppressing them), that will both supercharge your foreground and background alarms and lock you in them.

Telling another person about what shames you is a powerful practice in itself. Just by doing so, you are giving yourself the message that you don't need to be ashamed and there's nothing to be deathly embarrassed about. The shame is less of a negative force because now it's been brought into the light and somebody else knows! Whatever you were or are ashamed of, even if it's still not something you're immensely proud of, getting it out into the light removes that "I must keep this hidden at all costs" energy. Not only that, but telling a trusted friend or therapist engages your SES, forming a connection with someone who can help you hold compassion for yourself and help you metabolize that shame. I am amazed at how many people believe they are the only one with their particular brand of embarrassment and shame, and how surprised they are to find out that countless other people harbor exactly the same shame they do.

There is nothing negative you have said, thought, or done that is unique to you. There is nothing you could shame yourself for that has not been done by countless people before you and will be done by countless people after you. There are no new shames, only recycled ones.

Shame cannot live in the light of conscious awareness. Bring it into the light. You don't have a secret; a secret has you. You don't have shame; shame has you. Your dragon is blackmailing you and holding you hostage. Are you going to keep paying the ransom in alarm, or are you ready to escape?

In the ALARMS acronym shame is the last component but arguably the most influential as shame is one of the most powerful originators of alarm, and neutralizing shame is one of the most powerful ways you can neutralize alarm.

The antidote to shame is to choose to see your innocence. You cannot change something you keep in the shadows and continue to reject in yourself.

Unless you bring your shame into the light, see it, fully embrace it and accept it, and see your innocence in it, you are at the mercy of the alarm it creates. The curiosity "trick" works very well with shame. Bring in some shame from your childhood, perhaps a time of embarrassment or bullying. Sex is a big source of shame, especially at a young age. When you see the option to embrace shame with curiosity and self-compassion you move away from ego protection and toward your innocent, authentic being. Seeing your innocence is the most powerful antidote to shame.

Point to consider: Shame comes from a place of lack, fear, and separation. If you were getting your human needs met, there would be no reason for you to do anything shameful. You … are … innocent. Anything else is a lie.

89

Ego Trick: Victim Mentality

I haven't met anyone with chronic anxiety who didn't see themselves as a victim (including me). They might not be aware that they are in a chronic victim state but they sure feel it!

Creating a victim mentality in us is arguably the most devastating trick the ego dragon uses to keep us locked in alarm. In short, the ego dragon maintains our sense of alarm so we are too afraid to challenge ourselves to do anything that might hurt us. The dragon figures if it can keep us immobilized in fear and alarm we will just stay frozen in place and not risk doing anything that might hurt us. This is also why it keeps us locked in the chest, to prevent us from being hurt.

Victim mentality is one of the hardest tricks to overcome because it insidiously forms part of our identity when we are young. Having a pervasive sense of alarm makes us feel like a victim to the world and that everything is dangerous. This "fear without eyes" gives us the impression that we could face a significant threat at any moment. As a result, we are constantly trying to protect ourselves from an invisible enemy. The background alarm in our system keeps our sympathetic fight-or-flight nervous system active and that foreground alarm activates the background alarm, so we feel alarmed without an obvious precipitant.

So to resolve the uncertainty (that we worriers hate more than almost anything), we make up a threat in our mind to make sense of the fear and alarm we feel in our body. This is worry.

A victim mentality becomes a self-fulfilling prophecy because the weaker it makes us, the less able we are to stand up to it and the more we confirm that we can't handle it.

There is no bigger factor that keeps us locked in alarm and anxiety than our victim mentality. This might sound harsh, but until you see your proclivity to see the world as a victim, you will always be a victim, and you'll always be alarmed and anxious.

A victim mentality makes us lose faith in the world to help us, and making matters much worse is a sense that everything is up to us. We believe the world is stacked against us, and our anxiety and alarm make us weak so we just get crushed, especially as children. Victim mentality becomes part of our identity and that is a life sentence, keeping us imprisoned in anxiety and alarm.

This is going to be triggering for many, but the most pervasive form of victim mentality is blaming one's parents. There are some horrendous parents out there, and many are at fault for creating anxiety and a victim mentality in their children.

But the vast majority of terrible parents had terrible childhoods. This is not an excuse by any means. It is just a way to stop making yourself a victim of your parents, for as long as you see yourself as a victim (to anything, really), you will not be able to heal from anxiety and alarm.

Our ego wants to blame, for it perceives blaming and judgment to be forms of justified retribution and therefore resolution, but it just keeps us locked in victim mentality. Again, I have heard some horrendous stories of parental dysfunction, but please believe me when I tell you the only people I've known who've been able to move out of alarm are the ones who were able to break the victim mentality of blaming their parents. This is not to say they did not have good reason to blame their parents— only that those who were trapped in a victim story about their parents were never able to resolve their alarm.

Just reading this may feel alarming. Blaming your parents can be a way of making sense of your life, and know that you have my complete sympathy if you had a horrendous parent (or two). So many people with anxiety disorders had caregivers that were absolute nightmares. I get why they deserve to be blamed—I really, really, really do. I just don't know of anyone who still blames a parent who's been able to resolve their alarm.

I am not saying to immediately gloss over pain by simply realizing the innocence of your parent(s) and the world at large. There are losses that absolutely need to be grieved.

The inability to grieve our losses contributes greatly to unresolved trauma that leads straight into background alarm. There are millions of people who had a dysfunctional or abusive parent who still carry that pain, and I've said before that a massive amount of anxiety and alarm is due to unresolved grief. But I reiterate: horrendous parents almost always had horrendous childhoods themselves. I have seen many a wounded child inside of one of my adult patients soften when they accept and embrace that their parent was steeped in alarm when that parent was themselves a child.

Know it is well worth putting in the work to let go of blame and stop viewing yourself as a victim. Independent work, like what is described here, can be combined with talk therapy and body-based therapies so you have a robust support system to help you change the belief that you are a victim.

I did this exercise in the mirror and if you are brave enough you should try it too. Look yourself in the face and say, "I am a helpless victim," then add, "and I can love that about myself." When I did this I started to laugh! It seemed silly but it really showed me how much I believed something JABS-like about myself and then turned it on its ear. Doing this in the mirror and adding that I love something about me that I clearly hold myself in judgment for allowed me to really see it, accept it, and ultimately take responsibility to heal it. Strangely, and I don't know how this happened, but when I said right to my face, "I am a helpless victim... and I love that about myself," the ridiculousness of it showed me how deep this victim mindset went, and how it impacted all aspects of my life—and it astounded me how pervasive it had become in my system.

We move out of victim mentality by realizing it is our ego trying to trick us out of taking responsibility for our own healing. Your ego does not want you to take any risks; it wants to keep you frozen in alarm and anxiety, right where you are. Once I became aware of the tendency to fall into victimhood, that awareness allowed me to see that nobody is coming to save me and take responsibility for my own life. By simply seeing it and saying to myself, "I am blaming others," or "I am shaming myself," or "I victimize myself when I stay in worry and don't do my ABCs," or "My anxiety is not my fault, but it is my responsibility to fix." This taking control was a *massive* awakening for me.

There is a little trick I learned from transformational comedian Kyle Cease. Kyle and I were speaking at the same event in Phoenix, Arizona, in September 2023 and I thanked him personally for this tip. I'm paraphrasing a bit, but Kyle takes anything that is negative or shameful or judgmental and adds, "And I love that about myself." So someone might say, "I worry all the time," and he would turn it into "I worry all the time and I love that about myself." Anything negative people said about themselves, Kyle would add, "And I love that about myself." It sounds silly in a way but it makes sense from a neurological point of view because it takes a cold, judgmental statement that is frozen in fear and removes the shame from it enough that we can open the door to perceiving the statement in the exact opposite direction. We are taking a victimizing statement that was closed and assumed to be true and entertaining that the opposite may be equally (or more) true.

I am willing to bet that, even while in the grip of your ego dragon, there have been many times you were afraid to do something but you felt the fear and did it anyway. It might be a relatively big thing, like speaking in front of others, or a relatively small thing, like taking your dog to the park. Perhaps it was going to a social gathering where you didn't know anyone. In those moments, you made a choice not to be a victim. Now, when I see myself adopting a victim stance, I use my compassionate connection to myself to mobilize me in a much more caring and empowered stance. And sometimes I will use anger and faith to help with that mobilization.

ANGER AS AN ANTIDOTE TO VICTIM MENTALITY

Once you find yourself in victim mentality, get mad if you have to. Anger is a great antidote to victim mentality because it removes the freeze aspect of it that is so paralyzing. Victim mentality needs immobility and freeze to do its dirty work, so dance, move around, do anything that mobilizes you to overcome the paralysis of victim mentality. Then, you have the building blocks to adopt the opposite mentality, which substitutes victimhood with faith in the world—and in yourself.

FAITH AS AN ANTIDOTE TO VICTIM MENTALITY

The more faith you create inside yourself, the less danger you will feel. The more faith you can create that the world is indeed a safe place (as hard as that may be), the more you escape from victim mentality. Faith assumes that whatever is happening is happening *for* you and not *to* you. Because faith is a belief from the inside, it's not something that can be manufactured or outsourced. Faith is an inside job and it's a brilliant antidote to victim mentality.

Your faith in yourself will grow from the inside, and your victim mentality will have no choice but to be pushed out by your increasing faith.

In yourself.

And instead of unconsciously feeding into the problem, you are now consciously part of the solution.

Soon, I will revisit anger and faith and other ways to see victim mentality so you don't have to be it. Victim mentality is a huge player in anxiety and alarm. Know that there is more coming on how to escape this devastating mindset.

90

Ego Trick: Inability to Receive

When we don't receive the care and support we needed as children, we will often adopt a coping strategy of telling ourselves we just don't need it. It is more often an unconscious protective reaction than an authentic and conscious decision to deny care and support from others. If we don't allow it in the first place, we see the lack of support as less painful than experiencing the repeated disappointment of anticipating care and having it not be available or withdrawn.

In adulthood, this shows up as a dynamic where the ego resists external positive attention from others and, more important, resists positive internal feedback from ourselves. You can see how this inability to receive might be an especially sneaky trick, since the ABCs rely on us being supportive and compassionate to ourselves, and the ego dragon tricks us into blocking self-support!

Many worriers develop a coping strategy of putting our needs below the needs of others on the priority list. We literally stop being able to see what we need in favor of looking after someone else, and it usually starts with a parent. As I talked about earlier, when our parent is not safe we know we are also not safe, so many times we will step in to meet the parent's needs. Children are exceptionally intuitive and learn how to read their parent very well, but the cost to the child is they lose the ability to read themselves and get their own needs met. This is the beginning of codependency and people pleasing. With time and practice those patterns are potentiated and rewarded by those who benefit, deepening those family-liar patterns that poison all the child's relationships for the rest of their life.

My patient Anne (whose mother told her "don't get fat," remember?) blocked her own ability to receive, and it showed up most in her relationship with food. She was extremely good at looking after the needs of her family but very poor at looking after herself. Anne would feed her family elaborate meals while she would allow herself to eat very little. I believe this is because she held so much alarm in her body that she lived in the worries of her head and wasn't able to detect when her body was hungry. I'm sure her mother's comments to instill fear of gaining weight played a big role in this behavior as well, blocking Anne from receiving.

Once Anne became aware of her pattern of self-neglect, when she would notice that she was denying herself food, she would say to herself, "This is my inability to receive." Then she would get grounded in her body with the ABCs and usually observe a sensation of desire for the food she had just made. She would put her hand over the area in her upper belly and chest where she felt hunger and really connect with the sensation, while at the same time allowing the pleasant sensation of her own touch and the flow of her breath. She told me how she always got a feeling of reassurance from sensing the rhythmic rise and fall of her hand with her breath. Then she would give herself a taste of the food and savor that sensation in present-moment awareness. Finally, she would cap it off with a compassionate connection, saying how proud she was of her own creative cooking and appreciating herself for how good she was to her family. And, she didn't just say it, she *felt* it.

This took time and practice, but when Anne was able to consciously connect with her body and become aware of her hunger, she was able to observe and respond to her own needs. She went from being blocked from receiving the pleasure and nourishment of a healthy, delicious meal to the opposite—gratefully receiving. I like to think she was both allowing herself to receive the food and receiving her younger self at the same time. Anne's ability to embrace food became the gateway to embrace all of her needs, because the inability to receive food was just the tip of the iceberg for so many other things she habitually denied herself (massages, hikes, fun, etc.) as well. The inability to receive infiltrates all aspects of our lives and impairs our ability to release old alarm, as well as making life suck. I have seen many patients with anhedonia (inability to enjoy) and most of them had a significant element of inability to receive as a longstanding pattern.

When we cannot (or will not) feel ourselves and our bodies, we may start to fill our needs in maladaptive ways. This is often how addictions start. Any addiction (alcohol, drugs, porn, social media, shopping, gambling, food) is often a way that we allow ourselves to overcome our own resistance to receive. Our ego dragon often blocks healthy, loving emotion because that loving emotion was untrustworthy or inconsistent when we were children. As an example, people will take opiate medications because the drug "forces" them to feel warm and connected, essentially overwhelming the ego dragon's overprotective resistance to love. Heroin addicts have described the initial hit as an all-over warm, loving embrace. For many who did not feel loved as children, and learned to reject love and connection as adults, drugs and alcohol may be the only way to bypass their ego dragon's resistance to receiving love and feeling good in their body. A perhaps trivial but poignant example is when men say "I love you, man" to each other—but only after a significant amount of alcohol.

Speaking of resistance to feeling love. Do you feel uncomfortable receiving a hug? We all feel uncomfortable getting a hug from someone that we don't feel comfortable with, that's just normal humanness, but what about a hug from someone you like or even love?

For fun, I get my patients to create some awareness of who releases the hug first. Many of us worriers are the first to "tap out" (ha ha) because of that pesky inability to receive. It may sound trivial, but just be aware if you are always the one to release the embrace first, and try to hold it a little longer, just to show your conscious and unconscious you can and will receive!

How we respond to a compliment can be another tell that we are blocked from receiving. If you tell your friend you love her new haircut and she says, "Really? I thought it might make my nose look too big," this may be a sign she's not comfortable receiving or entertaining kind thoughts about herself.

Sometimes I would give my anxious patients a compliment as a simple way to assess their ability or inability to receive. (I always gave a true, genuine compliment that I meant, not just one made up to test them.) If someone responded by simply saying "Thank you" or "I appreciate that," they passed my little test and were able to receive, and I used that as an indicator they may not have a lot of negative self-talk. But if they tempered the compliment, deflected it, or made a joke, I wondered if receiving was hard for them.

The inability to receive is devastating. But like all the other tricks of the ego, it can be unlearned with the help of the ABCs.

Literally and figuratively, after you feed yourself, you can feed others if you choose to.

A critical part of the ABCs is to give to yourself—to create a compassionate connection where you are both giver and receiver. As you learn to give to yourself, you reactivate the part of you that shut down when you began to deny yourself. Helping yourself puts you in a sustainable position to help others because you are filling yourself up before giving to others, in contrast to compulsive people pleasing.

When you consistently give to yourself, you take responsibility for your own needs. Then you can *choose* to help others from a place of growth instead of feeling obligated to do so from a place of protection.

91

Ego Trick: Defensive Detachment

Defensive detachment (DD) is another term Gordon Neufeld uses to address the dissociation and withdrawal that occur to protect us when we feel too emotionally vulnerable or threatened. It is exactly what I did when dealing with my father as I got older. Loving him and seeing him suffer became too much for me, so my dragon stepped in to block my vulnerability and I went into withdrawal and dissociation. Because my ego perceived that connecting emotionally was too risky, I closed off to real connection as a way to protect myself.

Defensive detachment is simply withdrawing from connection out of the fear it will be taken away. The classic example is leaving someone before they leave you.

Using defensive detachment as a form of protection does block out some of the acute feelings of pain, but it comes at a significant cost. Going into defensive detachment creates more alarm in the long term, because when you detach from connection, you are separating from your emotional body and denying your own human need to be seen, heard, and loved, both by your own self and by others.

This is why it's so hard to connect with people when we are anxious. I often tell the partners of my patients with anxiety about defensive detachment and why their partner seems to "leave them" in an emotional sense. I explain to the partner that their mate is not detaching from them but, rather, from their own self. This helps clear up confusion and helps the partner not to blame themselves for the separation that they clearly feel. As I talked about earlier, you can't connect when your body is deep in alarm and shuts off your SES, even if that "danger" is purely imaginary worry.

The ego trick of defensive detachment is very hard on relationships because, whenever we get close to the other person, our dragon gets scared and pulls us away. (In attachment theory, defensive detachment is a causative mechanism in the avoidant attachment style.) DD is often the first stage of distraction and dissociation, two other entities that damage relationships and maintain alarm. When I am alarmed, I will feel the urge to distract into my phone or completely zone out in dissociation. When Cynthia sees me detaching, she warmly touches me (making a physical connection) and asks, "Is there something uncomfortable you feel you need to withdraw from right now?" And there almost always is. Sometimes I feel like talking about it and sometimes I don't, but just creating awareness of what triggers me into DD helps breaks the pattern for the future, keeps me more connected to myself and others, and helps me to stay much more present and out of alarm.

It is so important that when you see you are heading into a defensive, closed state, you use the ABCs to bring you back into a compassionate connection with yourself. When you provide that connection with yourself, you can better provide that sense of attachment to your partner, parent, friends, kids, dog, dragon, pink elephant, and even a metaphorical monkey in you that won't let go of a banana.

The tricky thing is, DD is often hard to spot within yourself because there is a real sense that you need to protect and withdraw. But just like when someone has a panic attack in a grocery store and then will avoid grocery stores, they are misunderstanding and mislabeling the problem. The goal in reducing alarm is to minimize the separation from yourself and others. Once you see you are withdrawing, you can use that as tell to engage the ABCs so you can reconnect to yourself.

Once you've connected to yourself, your SES comes back online and you no longer feel the need to go into defensive detachment from others, and this compassionate self-connection resolves the problem at its source.

I still hit the odd "anxiety patch" (like black ice, you don't see it until you're on it and start sliding) and still feel like I want to withdraw into defensive detachment. But it no longer surprises me—I recognize my dragon firing up this old pattern. I can notice my solar plexus alarm going into high gear, and this is my tell that it's time to follow my ABCs back to a connection to myself. Once I have reconnected to myself, I'm back in a place where I can reconnect to the other person.

Just as Anne would say to herself, "This is my inability to receive," when I see my urge to defensively detach, I call it out: "I'm going into defensive detachment." I can then breathe into my alarm and find something I really like about myself and about the person or people I am detaching from. This helps me get back into social engagement with myself and others, which gets me out of defensive detachment, which soothes my alarm. This one realization has changed my life. It allows me to connect to myself and others before I am so deep into detachment that I become frozen in it.

Can you make the intention to become aware when you start to detach, distract, or dissociate? It is the child in you going back to a time they were in so much pain they had to withdraw and detach. Learn to recognize when you move into this daydreaming default state of separation from yourself and others. The antidote to these is to bring yourself into the present moment with the ABCs and make a conscious, compassionate connection to that scared child inside. This is a challenge because DD, dissociation and distraction, are ways we default into unconsciousness and are hard to recognize as they begin to take you over. But the more you are aware of what they feel like, the more you can flip your oxygen mask immediately into conscious self-connection instead of unconscious self-abandonment.

Before I leave this chapter, I wanted to say the distraction and dissociation I mentioned are forms of defensive detachment but could also be considered as (over)protective tricks of the ego dragon.

92

Ego Trick: Resistance and Regression

Just like I have never met a person with anxiety and alarm who did not have a victim mentality, I've never met a worrier who wasn't full of resistance. Often that resistance is to change and uncertainty, but the most devastating kind is resistance to love and connection.

The ego dragon wants to keep you exactly where you are, frozen in anxiety and alarm—again, not because it wants to hurt you but because it wants to keep you "safe," and it perceives that if you move into more connection with yourself or others, that vulnerability will put you in even greater danger. As you know by now, because connection to my father was so painful, my overprotective ego made me resist it. To allow love for him was to put myself in danger of losing it (again and again). In blocking my connection to my dad, I blocked connection to everyone else, including the connection to myself!

The ego acts like you are behind a tree, hiding from a predator or some ill-defined danger. There is real safety a relatively short distance away, but you resist allowing yourself to break cover long enough to get there. You are paralyzed with fear, but the ego resists any chance to escape, as it tells you things may get worse if you try to move. Of course, in this state of freeze and alarm, you lose access to your rational brain and fully believe your anxious thoughts. Specifically the thought that your immobility is protective and you'll be worse off if you attempt a dash to safety.

The amygdala has no sense of time and it never forgets, so if there's a situation remotely similar to the original trauma, you're emotionally transported back to that time—with the same emotional resources you had at that time. Let's say you experienced being verbally abused by your mother when you were six. Now today, if you hear a woman yelling (even if it's not at you personally), your amygdala will light up, and in some sense a part of you is experiencing life as that frightened six-year-old. I believe that future research will show that a part of our brain called the insular cortex, working in concert with the amygdala, is involved in creating an *emotional signature* of sensation in your body when you are traumatized. This emotional signature is held for life, generating the same sensation now that you felt when the original trauma happened. So when you hear the woman yelling, your amygdala and your insula act in concert to activate your body so it feels the same way now that it did back then. In other words, much of anxiety and alarm is a regression to a time we felt powerless and afraid.

So, if you know hearing someone yell is one of your triggers, when it occurs you can use your awareness of that trigger as a switch to move immediately into your ABCs in your body, using present-moment sensation to keep you in the now before you get whooshed back into the past. But sometimes the trigger is just too powerful and the groove of the old trauma too deep, and the old alarm will overwhelm you. This is exactly what happened to me when I heard that old musical phrase my father used to play on the trumpet. I got triggered and age-regressed into anger and frustration before I could realize what was happening.

But that reaction has faded considerably. Since then I've heard people playing the trumpet and, although I felt I did not like the sound, I didn't get angry or dissociate. I recognize that the sound of the trumpet is still a trigger for me and I use it as an entry point into the ABCs. With awareness, I move into my body and breath and connect with that boy who endured the opening phrase from "Dream a Little Dream of Me" thirty times in a row. I now move into compassionate connection with that boy and support him.

Anytime you feel pain, if you set an intention to stop resisting, the pain may not go away completely but it will be reduced. (This is the basis of "Objecting Without Contracting" in the Anxiety Toolkit.) The psychiatrist and spiritual teacher Dr. David Hawkins in his book *Letting Go* tells the story of deeply cutting his thumb and not being able to tolerate anesthetics or painkillers, so he just had to accept the pain. He said that when he resisted the pain, the discomfort became intense, but if he stayed in full acceptance and flow, the pain eased considerably.

By definition, resistance blocks flow. When you flow from awareness to body to compassion, you are creating a state of acceptance and nonresistance that eases pain.

The message around worries is very easy to fight and resist because you don't want those worries to be true. When you resist something, you close around it. But your goal is to let the worry pass through, not grasp it tighter. What we resist persists, but what we can yield to, we can heal through.

Here is a massively important point: your ego will resist you doing the ABCs. Your dragon will try to keep you in your familiar state of anxiety and alarm and dissuade you from doing anything that moves you out of that freeze state because it's familiar, aka secure with that pain. The biggest obstacle you will encounter as you begin to heal your anxiety and alarm is that your ego dragon will not feel safe with your newfound calm in the ABCs, because you likely grew up with the unconscious program that it's not safe to feel safe, and feeling like the other shoe is going to drop at any moment. As an unfortunate result, as you start feeling more grounded, the dragon will pull out all its tricks in an attempt to pull you back into that familiar, alarmed freeze state and its accompanying worries. To counteract the dragon, you must tune your awareness to look for its tricks and be vigilant in consciously creating a connection with yourself with the ABCs. The hardest phase in healing for many is when they finally begin to feel it's safe to feel safe and the ego dragon freaks out because it can't "protect" you anymore by keeping you trapped in a familiar freeze state that feeds your worries. How about we take a second and I bring you into your body? Would you resist that?

> Feel your body right now. What is your jaw doing? Is your breath easy and slow, or is it shallow and tense? What are your shoulders doing? Are they relaxed, or are they up around your ears?
>
> Consciously make a point of slowing your breath and relaxing your jaw and shoulders, with an energy of allowing, not commanding. You can even close your eyes for a moment and put your hand on your chest. When you do this, you are consciously easing your resistance (again see "Objecting Without Contracting" in the Anxiety Toolkit) and your alarm. This awareness of your body and the grounding it creates is available to you in every moment of every day. And it's what enables you to flow out of alarm-based freeze and live your life, not resisting your alarm but using the sensation as a somatic reminder to use the ABCs to connect with all parts of yourself.

Point to consider: Think of something you do not want to do right now, and then see if you can get a felt sense of your resistance in your body. Just notice how resistance feels in you.

93

Ego Trick: Compulsive Thinking

Compulsive thinking is nothing more than resistance to a quiet mind. As you learn to use the ABCs consistently to create and move into a safe place in your body, your resistance to calm is reduced. Initially though, the dragon may rise up to block the feeling of calm and this is why you need to practice, practice, practice the ABCs to break through the dragon's resistance.

As you shine the light of awareness on your compulsive need to think and worry, that can be a beacon telling you to get out of your head and into your body. You redirect the chaotic energy that was previously devoted to distracted and disorganized thinking and funnel it into the feeling presence of being. The chaotic energy that was keeping you frozen in alarm is consciously directed into flow and ordered movement.

Strange that movement is more orderly than being frozen, right? But that's how it works. Think of a computer with so many programs open that it just freezes and you get the spinning wheel of death. Your cursor will move a lot faster and you'll be able to work more effectively once you close down some programs—your anxious thoughts, alarm, and ego tricks—and free up some space to get things moving again and focus on the task at hand.

When our minds are worrying at gold-medal levels, it makes us feel like we are doing something. But although it may seem like we are moving, we are essentially digging ourselves a hole in place. The more we think, the more we dig. Frenetic worrying was something we did as kids to distract us into our head from pain in our body as it accumulated energy from ALARMS. Worry and rumination helped us feel like we were doing something when in reality we were powerless children, but now as adults it's just keeping us stuck in our heads and that isn't where life is.

If you get nothing else from this book, know that when you are in alarm, thinking will only make it worse. You have a choice to turn down into your body and feel, instead of turn up into your mind and think. In a way, we worriers lose our minds while we are in our minds, believing that this time, by some miracle, the worry will show us the answer.

To be in alarm and choose to feel instead of think is the most powerful advice I can give you. I cannot tell you how liberating it is to be in alarm and make the conscious choice to redirect energy away from the thinking of your mind and into the feeling and sensation of your body, even if it hurts. And finding the alarm in the body and committing to feel it will likely hurt initially, but you have to feel it to heal it. You can't metabolize thoughts by thinking them; worries just make more worries. But you can metabolize feelings by feeling them. In many ways, anxiety and alarm are the result of unfinished emotional business! Stay in sensation without explanation and as Dr. Bessel van der Kolk says, you will learn to acclimatize to the discomfort.

I have found that once you can consistently feel the alarm without resistance and stay present with it, the alarm loses much of its power to push you into compulsive worry.

When you can stay in the presence of the sensation of your body safely in the now, you no longer need to regress back to the time of your original wounding or leap into the future with worry. *I am not teaching you how to get rid of your anxiety. I am teaching you how to acclimatize to your alarm and neutralize it so that you have a safe alternative down in your body so you don't have to reflexively and compulsively retreat into the worries of your mind.* Simply put, as you soothe the root of your pain (the alarm), you'll no longer need to escape into your worries to distract from it. And the more you practice the ABCs, the more this safe place in your body expands. You feel more and you worry less.

You need to take your power back from the dragon and show adult you that you are no longer stuck in child you whose only option was trying to escape into your head to avoid the alarm in your body. You are now an adult and you have much more power to stay present with your alarm. When you get scared, the child in you still will want to default into worry and try to think their way out of the pain, but adult you knows the only way out of the pain is to go into it with a compassionate connection to all parts of you.

You are no longer that child who had to get tiny bits of relief from distracting into worry, trying to relentlessly think your way out of a feeling.

You can now take that child by the hand and heart and show them how to feel their way out.

94

Moving a Body That Is Frozen in the Past

For many of us with alarm, our bodies are frozen in the past. As children, it was progressively less safe to be in a body that was filled with alarm. Perhaps the most detrimental by-product of having alarm in our body is being stuck living life in a "neck-up" cognitive space and not a body-based feeling one—and feeling is where life is truly lived.

I used to give a tremendous amount of credibility to my thoughts, and as a result, paid much more attention and credibility to my worries than those worries deserved. The more I ruminated on my pink elephants and painted tigers, the more real they appeared—becoming not only plausible but probable as my rational mind became paralyzed by the alarm in my body. In the process of absorbing myself in the world of my thoughts, I lost feeling. I lost much of life, and I regret that more than almost anything else. It gives me comfort to know that my pain helps you find feeling again, because living in your head is a waste of your life.

I know now that I was divorced twice because I was unable to feel connected to *myself.* My story was that I was disconnected from my partners because of something in them, but in truth my own body and mind were separate, and I was disconnected from my own ability to feel. Since my relationship with others could be no better than the relationship with myself, the disconnect I felt from myself was the real cause of my failed relationships—but just as we might expect from an overprotective dragon, it's much easier to blame failure on someone else. I was pinning my hopes on outside relationships to save me, but saving myself was an inside job.

There is no question that other people can help you along the way, but you can't simply offload all the responsibility to some magical other who is going to show *you* how to love *you.* In addition to my work with practitioners of somatic experiencing therapy and other body-based practices, I have found my own yoga practice to be one of my most powerful tools in getting myself out of a frozen state into flow. When your mind is in resistance, your body is your most powerful ally to release that resistance. Besides overcoming the resistance and stiffness in the body, qigong, tai chi, and yoga also create a flexible, aware mind.

I became a yoga instructor because I had a felt sense when I did yoga that I was connecting to a place of comfort. I also had the distinct sense this place had been untouched for a long time.

The body language and somatic signature that go along with dissociation are slouching and shallow breathing. Movement practices like yoga, qigong, and tai chi help you break that pattern in a way that is gentle and safe. When you are in movement and flow with your breath, you are showing yourself a direct way out of harm. The deeper your breath, the deeper your ability to feel.

The practices described above (yoga, tai chi, qigong) also increase flexibility. While any type of exercise gets us into our bodies, certain types of movement are more effective at bringing us into the present. Personally, I find it very hard to motivate myself to move when I am in alarm. There is a frozenness to it that is reminiscent of my childhood pain. In a meditation years ago, I was shown an image of myself with my body frozen in ice and was given the message that my anxiety (I had no concept of alarm at the time) was the ice, freezing my joints. As I imagined moving those joints, I felt and heard the cracking of the ice as I saw and viscerally felt it fall away.

That was an image I received years ago and to this day, whenever I do yoga I have the image of moving and freeing my joints, breaking the stagnation of alarm in my body. There is a point, usually about ten minutes into my yoga session, where I enter a flow state. I feel the distinct change when my breathing shifts markedly from shallow to deep, and I feel like my shoulders drop and a weight has been lifted from me.

I do believe anxiety and alarm keep me frozen in both body and mind. I also believe that anxiety results when our adult self is separated from our child self and our mind is separated from our body. One of the reasons I believe yoga is so helpful is that when body and mind are joined together, more flexibility and flow are naturally created in both than either could attain on their own. When both body and mind are flexible and flowing together, this creates a flow state that dissolves the emotional and physical rigidity that maintains alarm. This is one of the reasons yoga (and tai chi, qigong, etc.) eases anxiety and alarm.

Countless patients have told me how hard it is to exercise when they feel alarmed. It makes sense that if you are feeling like you are frozen behind a tree with a tiger on the other side, it's going to be hard to move! Returning to Mel Robbins's book *The 5 Second Rule,* if you are hesitant about moving, to the shower, to the gym, to ask someone out, just count down 5, 4, 3, 2, 1, and just do it! Neurologically we have programmed ourselves to follow ordered sequences since we were children, and inertia keeps us going once we start. Saying "5, 4, 3, 2, 1" creates a sense of momentum and inertia that makes it much easier to initiate movement than if we just come from a standstill. Again, it's hard to move if you are frozen in alarm! So use this little trick and count 5, 4, 3, 2, 1, and stand up for a few stretches. Just break the ice. For me, more often than not, this flows into doing a few more, and then my breath settles and my body opens into a flow state. You don't have to run a marathon; simply stretching and moving your joints will begin to unlock the rigidity you hold in your body, and that quickly moves into your mind as well. The trick is 5, 4, 3, 2, 1, start. Just do it, just start.

When our bodies are rigid and inflexible, that state is transferred to the mind and when the mind is rigidly following your warnings, what-ifs, and worst-case scenarios, your body will want to mirror that rigidity. The mind may be going a million miles a minute, but it's not flexible—it's frozen in the compulsion of ruminating on the same damn worries. Anyone who lies in their bed frozen in worry knows exactly what I mean. When we improve flexibility in the body, the mind follows. Body and breath are connected in reciprocal flow. But if you've had anxiety and alarm for a while, the body and mind have separated, and it takes effort to get them to dance together again. Speaking of dancing, never underestimate the power of music to ease the transition into movement.

In the late seventies I was nineteen and "Disco Inferno" by the Trammps never failed to get me moving. Still does.

For many years, I resisted breath and touch, yoga and meditation, tai chi and qigong, and thought they were new-age brain droppings. I hated my early yoga classes. At the time I told myself it was because everyone was better than I was, and my ego hated that—I felt like an elephant in a ballet class. But in retrospect, I think my resistance came up because yoga brought me directly into the alarm stuffed in my body, and my ego hated that more. Still, I kept going back. Some part of me knew it was good for me.

I would repeat the same pattern: resist going to yoga like the plague, then get there and feel uncomfortable as I entered my body, go through class and finish it out feeling a sense of peace. That peace was a very rare occurrence during a very troubled time in my life. I am sure that I coerced myself to sign up for yoga teacher training as a way of forcing myself not to quit yoga. If I became a yoga teacher, I thought I would be forced to practice, and if I felt competent by actually learning how to teach yoga, I would be much more likely to continue the practice. I knew my ego would resist, so I needed to cut off my escape route. As Tony Robbins would say, I got to the island and burned the boats by signing up for teacher training.

And I absolutely loved it. For twenty-eight straight days in the summer of 2007, I took the intensive yoga teacher training under Shakti Mhi at Prana Yoga in Vancouver. It gave me a brand-new relationship with my body.

Now you can start developing a new relationship with your body. You can regain access to its truth and wisdom.

One of the saddest things to me is when people who are out of touch with their feeling bodies assume it's too late in life for it to be any other way. It is such an ingrained and unconscious habit to remain up in their thinking minds that they don't even see they could go back to their feeling bodies. It reminds me of a sad story about how they keep elephants from running away. They keep a shackle around their leg tied to a thirty-foot chain that is tied to a stake in the ground. For the first few months of the elephant's life, it is bound by the chain, so it can only move within the thirty-foot radius. But then they remove the chain and the elephant won't go outside his familiar radius. Human children are the same in a way—if they grew up with trauma and worry, they don't see the option not to worry. No matter how old you are, no matter how silly you might feel trying a yoga class when you've never heard the names of any of the poses and don't even have any idea what to expect, I promise you, it gets easier. And it is such an incredible gift to get out of thinking and into feeling.

In the disconnection where the mind moves too quickly and the body hardly moves at all, there is no reciprocal flow. We need a flow of energy to be in optimal physical and mental health. Your body holds the treasure—your innocent self. Embracing movement and flow can greatly enhance your ability to feel safe in your body. And remember, living in your mind is what got you where you are now. Isn't it worth at least trying a different way?

95

A New Default Setting

After my LSD trip, I was curious (there's that word again) as to why psychedelics allowed me to see the alarm in my body that had been invisible to me when my mind was not impaired. A frequent observation of people on psychedelics is they seem to lose the boundaries between self and not self and between conscious and unconscious—essentially, there is no separation. They feel "one with everything."

This is the polar opposite of what the ego does. The ego reinforces the separate idea of self. You definitely aren't one with everything, you're not even one with your own self! The ego also keeps our conscious, accessible-on-demand mind separate from the deeper, unconscious, "hidden" mind. The ego is a separating, not a joining, force. The ego is born of reaction, protection, and survival and it splits your mind from your body out of a sense of protection.

Now let me introduce to you a network in the brain called the *default mode network* (DMN). The DMN is a relatively recent discovery in neuroscience. In short, it is a pattern of brain activity that occurs in identifiable brain structures that link together in a firing pattern when we are not focused on a particular task. Think of it like the daydreaming mode of the brain. It's what the brain falls into when we are not focused on a particular task. The DMN may be a type of self-protective state when we are not actively involved in conscious processes like reading a book or solving a math problem.

The ego protective state may be linked to the DMN. This would make sense, since for us worriers, rumination and worry seem to be our default state. That is, we fall into unconscious, compulsive worry automatically, seemingly by default. There is evidence that a particular part of the DMN called the *posterior cingulate cortex* may be linked to self-referential thinking (what we think about ourselves), for example, self-judgment, worry, rumination, and shame. It has been postulated that the PCC may play a role in the voice of our inner critic. So, in effect, we can be worrying automatically, unconsciously, and passively when we fall into the brain's default mode. In other words, when we worriers are not focused, our brain defaults into overprotective worry and critical self-talk.

This is why awareness is so critical. Advanced brain imaging studies show that when we focus our attention on something specific, we switch out of the DMN. Those imaging studies also show that psychedelics shut down the DMN. In other words, activity in the DMN is diminished by both conscious attention to a task and psychedelic substances. The DMN acting in concert with the ego creates a type of anxiety and alarm daydream so, as you fall out of awareness, you fall into the nightmare of anxiety and alarm. When you are present, aware, and connected to yourself, the DMN and ego do not have the power to keep you in their daydream of anxiety and alarm. That is, awareness snaps you out of the grasp of the DMN and ego. This is one of the reasons I spent so much time showing you exactly what anxiety of the mind and alarm in the body look like in the first two sections. On a physical level, the DMN may be responsible for JABS we direct on ourselves because that is self-referential thinking. The ego, acting with the DMN, may be using the default state of worry in the mind to keep us away from our old alarm in the body. The DMN and the ego form a formidable pair in making us feel badly about ourselves and adding worry on top of that self-reproach to make certain we are sidetracked away from our alarm. What a combination! A commitment to mindfulness and present-moment awareness brings us out of both the DMN and the ego and gives us the best chance to connect with our best, authentic selves. This is why awareness is always the first part of the ABCs.

96

Change Your Focus

The dragon wants to keep you in your head, but if you stay there you'll be stuck in worry forever.

The paradox is you must use your head in awareness to see how to get out of your head—but the dragon doesn't want you to see you have a choice to move to awareness at all. The ego dragon gets paralyzed in present-moment awareness because it only sees life in the painful past or the predicted future. In other words the ego cannot exert its tricks unless it transports you out of the present moment. When your overprotective ego scares and distracts you with worry and JABS, all your energy goes into survival concerns and there is no energy left for rational awareness in the present. Unless you learn to live in the present moment with the ABCs, you are always going to be tricked by your ego into staying in chronic worry.

It is critical you bring yourself into the present moment so you see you have a choice. Again, the ego dragon and the DMN are like vampires—they cannot live in the light of present-moment awareness. So let's make an intention to move them into that sunlight, shall we?

The ABCs at their core are all about creating the intention to stay in present-moment awareness so you create fertile ground to change the habitual alarm-anxiety cycle. Instead of unconsciously making the problem worse by allowing it to continue, you can consciously start to make it better by creating an awareness and choice to do something different, starting with getting out of your head and into your body.

Much of this book has been about learning to see exactly where you have unwittingly and automatically turned up into thinking and become trapped there. By learning the ego's tricks—judgment, alienation, blame, shame, resistance, defensive detachment, inability to receive, and compulsive thinking—you can recognize them in the light of awareness and consciously choose a new path.

But even if you don't know which trick the dragon is firing up right now, it doesn't matter. When you feel alarmed or catch yourself in worry, the path is always the same. Use awareness to see that you are in your head and then turn down into your body and breathe. Do not try to fight your anxiety or alarm with reasoning because you can't beat thoughts on their own turf, and alarm has turned off your rational brain anyway. Changing your focus to grounding yourself in your body is always the critical first step to change.

As you become more aware of your own personal dragon's tricks, you will spot them earlier. And you will see the trap and move away, into your body, faster and faster. You will see how your body can never lie to you, but your mind constantly does.

97

Moving into the Present-Moment Body

Here is a quick way to tell if you are in your body or in your anxious mind: *focus on your breath.*

When you are predominantly in your anxious mind, your breath will be high in your chest, with frequent, shallow, and relatively fast cycles of inhalations and exhalations. This is not to say you are breathing quickly; it's more like you are not breathing slowly.

When you are in your body and with your non-alarmed, authentic, innocent self, your breath will be slow and deep.

When you are in your head, your dragon is controlling your breathing. It's keeping you frozen behind that tree. Your dragon believes you need to stay with short, shallow breathing so you won't get spotted by a predator. In other, deeper words, the peaceful innocence that is your underlying and perpetual presence is not breathing you into expansive growth and movement. Rather, your protective ego dragon is breathing you with the mandate to keep you protected and frozen in place. Anyone who has been too afraid to get out of the house or even move from the bed to the shower knows exactly what I mean.

Our minds and bodies take their cues from our breath to assess safety or danger. If our breath is shallow and rapid, the message sent to the brain is that we are in need of protection, and the shallow, quick breath of protection continues to reinforce itself. This is why it is so important to move into body and breath with the ABCs. When we consciously move into our bodies, our breath naturally slows, switching the control away from the unconscious, mind-based ego dragon of protection.

Your breath is the best conscious link to your parasympathetic nervous system—but when your dragon is in control, it keeps the seesaw up in fight or flight in the belief that it is protecting you. I would sometimes go for hours before I checked in with my breath and realized I'd been in shallow, rapid breathing for who knows how long. This is why it's so important to make a habit of checking in with your breath and putting a reassuring hand on your chest. But you have to choose to consciously connect with yourself or otherwise the DMN will keep you locked in the inertia of protection, alarm, and anxiety.

Right now, pause for a second and check the depth and quality of your breath. Put your hand on your chest and connect with your touch as you feel your chest rise and fall. See how your breath naturally becomes slower and deeper as your focus drops out of your head and into your body. If you have an essential oil like lavender or chamomile that calms you, breathe that in.

Go ahead, I'll wait. It's worth it to get you into your senses.

Welcome back. Now think of something you appreciate or are grateful for about yourself, like appreciating yourself for reading this book. Don't resist! You can receive this. Put one or both hands on your chest and compliment yourself and say thank you in appreciation and gratitude for your own self-care. If you really want to supercharge the effect, thank yourself face-to-face in the mirror. When you look into your own eyes, I believe you are speaking right into the emotional part of your brain, so it can be pretty intense, but that is also what makes it so effective!

This self-gratitude exercise is a mini version of the ABCs, and you can do this multiple times a day. In addition, there are other ways to tell if you're in the *feeling* of your body. Here are a few:

YOUR JAW

When I talk about breath as a barometer of being in your body or your anxious mind, my wife always reminds me to remember to talk about relaxing the jaw. She likes to tell me that you can't breathe fully when your jaw isn't relaxed, and while I remind her she is not a doctor, she reminds me to try breathing with a tight jaw and then with a relaxed jaw, and there is a marked difference. (I guess doctors aren't the only people who know anything.)

So, what is your jaw doing right now? Is it relaxed and loose or are you holding it tight? Make a conscious effort to focus in on the muscles on both sides of your jaw and allow them to loosen and relax. You can even use your fingers to give your jaw muscles a little massage.

SMELL

I discovered essential oils a few years ago in my search to help people relieve anxiety and alarm and found they are often very helpful in getting people into sensation. I look at essential oils as a kind of switch to make it clear to the system that the focus is to be on sensation and not on thought. I also think a strong scent (pleasant or even unpleasant) breaks the daydreaming DMN and helps bring us into deeper conscious awareness.

Out of all our senses, the sense of smell is the only one that goes directly to the limbic, or emotional, brain. Touch, hearing, sight, and taste are all "preprocessed" in the brain center called the thalamus before their information reaches the other parts of the brain for processing. Smell is not filtered by the thalamus; rather, smell sends the raw data to the limbic brain, and it has an immediate and powerful effect.

This is a throwback to thousands of years ago when we relied on smell to warn us of danger and give us pleasure (which had the biological function of drawing us closer to food or an attractive mate). This was information we needed quick access to for survival purposes.

Although we don't have the same keen sense of smell we had thousands of years ago, this sense is still strongly linked to emotion and memory, and it is still something we can use to calm our limbic brain and bring us out of thinking and into sensation.

I have found that telling my patients to have a little vial of an essential oil they find grounding and stimulating is a great shortcut for moving into sensation. If you imagine a boxer being brought back to his senses with smelling salts, an analogous thing happens to us when we smell something pungent like an essential oil. In the ABCs, after the awareness phase, I often suggest people use an oil they like as a way of making a distinct signal to move into sensation, and the essential oils do that quite well. Aromatherapists have made entire careers on finding essential oils that help people soothe pain, anxiety, and myriad other conditions.

TOUCH

Your awareness will automatically go to the place of sensation, and touch is a key part of sensation in your body. In my wife's work as a somatic experiencing practitioner, she uses touch to bring her clients into the sensation of safety of the present moment. But even touch on your own self is grounding. Touching the area around your heart or putting your hand on your belly to feel the rise and fall of your breath is soothing and relaxing. If you feel your alarm in your belly, you can touch there. If your alarm is in your throat, touch there. Keep it slow and focused—the opposite of the superficial quick pace of the regular world. The slower the better.

I find touching my chest over my alarm and really savoring the sensation of my breath helpful. Once I commit to awareness and see that I am being seduced by my worries, I call out those thoughts as intrusive and set an intention to move into sensation. I use my hand on my chest and savor my breath (often with smelling an essential oil) as ways of reinforcing that intention, telling my entire system we are moving into present-moment sensation.

You don't have to rely on putting your hand on your chest and focusing on your breath. That is what I find works best for me, but there are other options you can use. The point is to get out of your head into your body—so whatever you find works best, use that.

Patting your shoulders and upper arms with opposite hands, rubbing your hands or fingertips together, or rubbing your face like you are pretending to wash it are great touch exercises to redirect attention from thinking to feeling. Because so much of your brain is devoted to the sensation of your hands and face, touching these areas at the same time really gets your brain's attention. Many people use EFT tapping and that is often helpful to get you out of explanation and into sensation.

Doing a rhythmic beat with your hands on your chest (or over the place you feel alarm) is a wonderful way into savoring sensation in the present moment and out of ruminative thoughts of the future. When you withdraw energy from rumination and worry and bring yourself into the present moment, you lessen the power of those ruminations because the mind energy that had defaulted into rumination and worry is now consciously directed into the body energy of sensation.

Worry has a self-reinforcing quality to it, likely due to activating the dopaminergic addiction circuits in the brain. Many of my patients find it hard to jump right out of worry and into sensation, and self-touch is a great bridge to help with that transition from mind to body.

Here's another exercise you can do. This one is like giving yourself a hug. Take your right hand just under your left armpit and your left hand over your right shoulder (or vice versa if that feels better). Hug yourself with the pressure you feel most connected and comfortable with (you may have to experiment with different levels of squeeze to find what feels best for you). And remember, don't tap out, stay with it!

Some of my patients really love support on their head and neck. Although most people experience their alarm in the torso and abdomen,

I've seen more than a few who feel their alarm in the back of their neck and even their forehead or face.

Go ahead and try it now. Put one hand behind your neck and the other across your forehead. Many of my patients have told me the hand on the neck reminds them of supporting the head of a young infant. Who knows—it may even bring back a distant sensation of physical support when you were an infant. For me, my mother would use her fingertips to make circles on my forehead or rub my back when I was child, and I still ask my wife to do the same thing. I find it very relaxing. Replicating a touch or smell that calmed you and brought you into sensation when you were young is a very potent way to induce that relaxation response in the body.

Know that your tools for getting into your body don't have to be anything fancy or even a specific "practice." They can truly be whatever works for you—even if it's something silly. My friend Angela bought me one of those soft rubber stress balls. It feels really squishy and changes color when you squeeze it. She bought it for me as a kind of a joke, teasing me about being a stress doctor (she's a lawyer)—but I love that thing and I use it all the time. It sits on my bedside table and I squeeze it every night. I really devote my attention to all the sensations with it. It feels soft and pliable. It's yellow but it turns to orange when I stretch or squeeze it. I'll hold it up to my ear and listen to it as I squash it against my face. I'll even smell the rubber. I know I am more than a bit obsessed with it—but that's okay because it really is good at bringing me into sensation in my body, which is such a welcome change to being trapped up in my head.

One thing to keep in mind when moving into your body: go slow—and then slow that down by half. Your mind goes very quickly, and that becomes a habit. The mind is whirring away and you probably don't notice how fast it's going until you decide to move into sensation. One of the reasons our mind and body get out of sync is because the mind moves so damn fast in comparison to the body. When we slow down, in general, the mind and body have a chance to sync up.

The word "yoga" comes from "yoke," which means to join, so the ancient yogis were on to something. Here's another bit of priming or foreshadowing: Anxiety and alarm result from two separations, a separation of your mind from your body and separation of your adult self from your child self, so anything that joins those things together will relieve your alarm and anxiety.

98

The Social (Dis)Engagement System

Did you know the face is the only place in the human body where the muscles are attached directly to the skin? That is why so much connection and warmth can be transmitted through our facial expressions. We are social animals, and social connections start as early as birth. I delivered many babies in my medical career, and over the course of my years as a doctor, getting the baby to the mother as soon as possible after birth became more and more of a priority.

Early in my career, when a baby was born, the nurses would dry the baby off and we'd do an examination. And that took time. The medical community has since realized how important it is to start the mother-child connection as early as possible. Provided the baby is not in distress, it gets skin-to-skin time with its mom before anything else happens, such as cutting the cord and washing and weighing. This first moment of connection is often referred to as bonding and is a way of engaging the child's SES from the start, with lots of oxytocin in mom and baby.

I've talked about the SES earlier, but I want to go a little deeper because it is so important in soothing and healing. The SES is a two-way system that has both expressive and receptive qualities that guide interactions between people. Put very simply, the SES modulates the expression and reception of love and compassion from ourselves to others and the flow of love to ourselves. Starting from infancy, the more secure connections you have with your mother and other important people in childhood, the more the SES matures. And the more the SES matures, the more resilience and capacity is created in the nervous system, so we can better give and receive love with others and ourselves.

The opposite is also true. If you do not get enough engagement, love, and compassion from your caregivers from birth onward (or worse, your caregivers are the source of your alarm), the SES fails to fully mature, and your ability to self-soothe and give and receive compassion and love (both to others and yourself) is also impaired.

We learned a lot about how this system develops from heartbreaking research on Romanian orphans in the 1980s. While living in orphanages, these infants received no emotional nurturing—no touch, no play, no books read to them or "baby talk" to help them get used to their caregiver's patterns of speech and expression—even though their physical needs (food, clothing, toilet, bathing) were met. This wasn't your typical randomized, controlled trial (to treat children this way would actually be completely unethical), but given the conditions in the orphanages because of Romania's economic and political situation at the time, researchers followed the children through life to see the lasting impact of their early years. When the country opened up after dictator Nicolae Ceaușescu was overthrown, child development researchers who visited the orphanages reported the eerie silence inside; sadly, the children had simply stopped crying because they had learned that nobody would respond. Compared to children who had not been raised in institutions, the orphans had different patterns of electrical activity in their brains, and their brains were observably physically smaller, with lower volume of both gray matter and white matter.

Foster and adoptive families that took in these formerly institutionalized children noticed a pattern as the children got older: the children would hold their arms up to be picked up and held, and when they were, they pushed to get away and be put back down. This process would repeat itself over and over. It was like they craved love and attention, but once it was available, they were unable to tolerate the connection. I find this both fascinating and curious, as it is reminiscent of many people with anxiety: they desperately want to trust the nurturing and connection, but the increase in vulnerability that goes along with that connection sets off their extra-sensitive smoke alarm.

When the SES fails to mature, we develop strategies such as resistance, inability to receive, and defensive detachment in a pattern similar to the exaggerated version seen in the Romanian orphans. The good news is the brain is incredibly plastic and you can mature and enhance the brain's ability to connect with self and others at any age. (There is hopeful news about the orphans too: their language, IQ, and social-emotional functioning improved as they spent time in loving families, especially if they were adopted out of the orphanage before the age of two.)

If we are going to embark on this project, it might help to know a little more about how the system works. In the interest of keeping the technical aspects of this book to a minimum I have left the talk of polyvagal theory until now. First named and studied extensively by Dr. Stephen Porges and adapted specifically to therapy by Deb Dana, LCSW, this theory has provided valuable and practical insights to understand how anxiety and alarm affect the human nervous system.

One of the main nerves involved in the SES is the vagus nerve, which is the tenth cranial nerve and the longest nerve of the parasympathetic rest-and-digest nervous system.

The vagus plays a major role in the SES/HRC, inducing relaxation and relaying the presence of safety and connection. The vagus is also thought by many to be intimately involved in the more emotional "heart-to-heart" connection that is so important in the feeling of comfort and safety.

In the polyvagal theory, the vagus nerve has two main branches—the dorsal vagus and the ventral vagus. Dorsal and ventral refer to the differing positions of the nerve; the dorsal is toward the back of the body (think of the dorsal fin on a whale) and the ventral is toward the front. The ventral side of the vagus nerve is thought to attune to cues of safety and emotional connection. It supports a sense of physical safeness and a calming and reassuring emotional connection to others, similar to what I have explained about the SES. In contrast, the dorsal part of the vagus nerve responds to cues of potential danger and the freeze response.

If you grew up with trauma, the dorsal vagus learns to be on a hair trigger, ready to spring into protection and freeze at the slightest provocation. In those of us with stored alarm, we see threat in things that are not dangerous and we actually create threat by our own worry, so the dorsal vagus in worriers gets lots of activity. When we experience a cue of danger (and this can even be just worry), the dorsal vagus will shut off social engagement and we can even feel frozen. This makes sense from an evolutionary standpoint since you do not need to be socially engaged and connected when you are in physical danger—your energy is needed elsewhere, and there's no need to be "open" to social connection when you are face-to-face with a poisonous snake, especially if it's your ex.

The dorsal vagus, in concert with the amygdala and the ego dragon, pulls us away from connection, out of awareness, and into a state of social disengagement. I have called this protective mobilization with loss of emotional connection the social disengagement system (SDS), in contrast to the SES you know about already.

For our purposes, it's useful to know about the chemicals in the body that play a role in the SDS and the SES: cortisol to move us into protection and away from perceived danger (the SDS), and oxytocin, serotonin, and vasopressin to move us toward growth and love (the SES). Cortisol is often referred to as the stress hormone because it acts in concert with adrenaline (aka epinephrine) to mobilize the body for protection and survival, and oxytocin is known as the love hormone because it creates a sense of emotional bonding and thriving. (This "love hormone" view of oxytocin is far too simple but the general idea is logical.) When you start a new relationship and you are smitten with each other, oxytocin is secreted in great quantities, and you just want to be around your new mate all the time. Oxytocin is also responsible for bonding between mother and child during that skin-to-skin time after birth. In general, cortisol is thought to play a role in *protection* through the dorsal vagus, and oxytocin, vasopressin, and serotonin help mediate *connection* through the ventral vagus.

The ventral vagus is the main pathway used in the SES. The ventral vagal system relies heavily on input from the head and neck, especially tone and prosody of voice, facial expressions, and eye contact. When we feel safe, calm, and connected, we are in a ventral vagal state. We feel relaxed and receptive to connecting with others. When the ventral vagus is active, we make eye contact, our voice has a pleasant and even lilting quality, our facial muscles are relaxed, and we readily smile and laugh.

If you struggle with significant anxiety and alarm, your "set point" may be leaning in the dorsal vagal direction. This encourages your system to resist connection because your body simply isn't open to warm human connection if it senses background alarm. This resistance keeps you separate from others, which activates your sympathetic nervous system, aka foreground alarm. In resisting connection, your body secretes cortisol and epinephrine, giving you that flushed feeling so many of my patients complain of. The foreground alarm increasingly activates your background alarm, and your system moves into freezing behind the tree, aka dorsal vagal shutdown, even further blocking the loving connection you need to push the fear out of your box. A feeling of disconnection potentiates the foreground and background alarm resulting in even more disconnection and freeze, which not only blocks us from resolving our alarm, but creates even more of it! Dorsal vagal shutdown is also the likely precursor to dissociation as well, and while we are at it, defensive detachment too!

One of the most frustrating aspects of alarm and anxiety is that we become alarmed at the prospect of human connection because of the vulnerability and pain that connection meant in our childhood. The catch-22 here is that warm connection with others is exactly what we need to mature our SES and be able to soothe ourselves and break the cycle of alarm and anxiety. In essence, anxiety and alarm are so hard to resolve because the alarm state makes it very difficult to accept and absorb the warm social connection we need to heal the alarm state! The protective, freeze-inducing dorsal vagus, once it gets grooved into protection (childhood trauma, anyone?), creates one hell of a groove in the snow.

The dorsal vagus state plays a lead role in social anxiety disorder. Imagine you want to go to a party but you struggle with anxiety and alarm. As you get closer to the party, you move into dorsal vagal immobilization and maybe become frozen in outright dissociation. As you move deeper into foreground alarm (with a little background alarm thrown in as a ping-pong partner), you lose access to ventral vagal SES skills. You can't make or hold eye contact, your voice is flat and monotone, and you misread other peoples' social cues or perceive body language as intimidating when it is not. Someone politely excusing themselves to go and talk to someone else is seen as a personal affront when it was merely that they hadn't seen that friend in a long time. The perceived affront intensifies your dorsal vagus freeze response, encouraging your system to disengage even further. Of course you hate parties!

If your response to social interactions is repeatedly one of freeze and alarm, your system learns to fire up your protection faster and faster (potentiation), and of course you are going to shy away from those social interactions. Without access to your ventral vagus and SES, you can't "speak" the social language, so you go into a protective freeze state, which locks you out of any possibility of being social. I believe social anxiety disorder should be called social alarm disorder or maybe even social freeze disorder because that is exactly what it is. You simply cannot be social and connected when the physiology of your mind and body is telling you (unconsciously) that you are in danger, even if you (consciously) know you are perfectly safe!

(And, yes, I see the paradox of a fire-breathing ego dragon creating a freeze state.)

99

A System to Engage Your Social Engagement System

You may have noticed above I mentioned something called a vagal "set point." You've probably heard this phrase used when it comes to our weight and the fact that for some people it settles within a small range and it's very difficult for them to gain or lose weight outside of that range, regardless of diet or activity levels. What if I postulated a set point for intrapersonal and interpersonal engagement that is mediated by the vagus nerve based on the quality of social engagement, love, and connection we had in our childhood? We still go into and out of dorsal and ventral activation at different times, but the set point we return to varies from person to person and is influenced by our experiences. In addition to governing how much time we spend in alarm, your vagal set point would determine how open and how often you would be able to be emotionally connected to yourself and others.

Albert Einstein is reported to have said, "The most important decision we make is whether we believe we live in a friendly or hostile universe." While I don't disagree, I don't believe it is a decision until we are aware of the question. I believe we see the world the way our nervous system learned to perceive it, and this happens mostly outside of our conscious awareness and subsequent decision-making. In other words, we see our current adult world in a way that is determined by the way our nervous system experienced our child world.

Have you ever thought of yourself as someone who directs your empathy and attention toward others and not enough into yourself? I have seen many people like my patient Anne who looked after her family well but abandoned herself. I would propose to you that you can shift that self-abandonment by bringing your level of love and compassion for yourself into your awareness.

Just making yourself aware of the JABS you take at yourself and seeing your ability to love and be empathic toward yourself can begin a path to being more fulfilled and connected to yourself. This conscious, intentional shift in self-connection makes us less vulnerable to painful alarm and dorsal vagal shutdown and more able to access and stay with pleasant ventral vagal activation and peaceful connection. The more you commit to ventral vagal connection, the more you deepen that groove of caring for yourself. The groove in the snow can work for us too! The SES and the ventral vagus combine to help us be more deeply connected to ourselves and others, which begins to creates the felt sense of safety we need to release our alarm.

It's wired in us to be connected to each other. In recent years, the medical profession is seeing just how devastating it is to our physical and mental health to be lonely and disconnected. You have a neurohormonal system innate in you that is designed to connect mother to baby and person to person. The system is optimized when it has a healthy dose of connection and compromised when it doesn't. When we make a firm intention to let the SES do its job of creating an empathic connection to our own selves and others that it's been designed to do over thousands and thousands of years of practice, we truly begin to heal our alarm and anxiety.

The fact that you are here reading this book makes me very confident that you truly want to live a better life. I want you to connect the scared child to the competent adult using your own SES to boost your vagal set point toward the ventral side (love) and away from dorsal side (fear) and heal your alarm. I did this for myself and it literally saved me from suicide. My life's work is to show you how to heal yourself because, frankly, nobody is coming to save you. It is up to you to save you. And that is much of the point. When you realize that your connection to yourself is in your hands, you also see your healing is in your hands. So much of anxiety and alarm began because nobody was truly connecting with you, and as you got older you didn't allow anyone else to truly connect with you, and then you didn't allow a true connection with yourself.

So, what can you do to consciously work on allowing this connection that can finally heal you? Repeatedly use the ABCs process like your life depends on it, because it just might. We always come back to the ABCs as our foundation, and here are some additional tips to help inspire a true connection within yourself.

EYE CONTACT

One of the things that helped me greatly was very simple. Before I even knew much about the ventral vagus and polyvagal theory, I had read an article in a psychology magazine about increasing eye contact with someone you feel connected to as a way of increasing oxytocin and soothing anxiety. I tried it in fifteen-second increments with my wife and the results were immediate. It wasn't to the point of a staring contest; it was just to make a commitment to do it more often and hold it for longer than usual. If you are lucky enough to have a person in your life you trust, this is a great way to deepen your connection. (PS, this even works with your dog—a 2015 article in *Science* showed a 300 percent increase in oxytocin levels in humans and a 130 percent rise in dogs with mutual eye gazing.) So, if the love from humans is too vulnerable, you can start with your pup! Eye contact is a big part of your SES, and your ventral vagus helps process the sensory input from eye contact. If you are *really* brave, you can even make eye contact with yourself in the mirror and express what you like about yourself and the child in you. You can even make eye contact with that picture of you above your bathroom mirror that is undoubtedly there by now. A little tip about eye contact with another person: you can't meet both eyes in yourself or your partner at the same time, so pick one eye and direct your focus there, and you can certainly alternate which eye you focus on with humans (or dogs).

At first, I noticed I had some resistance to eye contact, and that didn't surprise me since my ego dragon's job was to protect me from connection and vulnerability. The resistance was there, but I also felt a distinct benefit, so I stuck with it. And, initially, I didn't tell Cynthia what I was doing (I was just holding eye contact with her for a little longer than usual), so there was no pressure from anyone but myself to maintain my little eye contact experiment. I'll also let you know that doing this eye contact exercise in the mirror can be very intense, but also intensely helpful. It's like taking your SES to the gym! And if your real gym has mirrors, you can even make eye contact there, but not for too long or you might alarm people. The idea is to be more connected to yourself in ventral, not to scare other people into dorsal!

SINGING, CHANTING, VOCALIZING, LAUGHING, CRYING, FACE YOGA

The recurrent laryngeal branch of the vagus nerve connects to our voice box, with vibration and stimulation of the voice calming our whole system. When you sing, chant a mantra, or use any form of rhythmic vocalization, you create more stimulation or "tone" in your ventral vagus, releasing oxytocin and building capacity in your SES. This is why singing and chanting make us feel good.

Laughter, by the way, has oxytocin-releasing power all by itself. In addition, laughing creates a form of breathing that is soothing and also stimulates your vagus nerve. Thousands of years ago, laughing was a sign of safety and connection as we would laugh in a safe group of our tribe, and laughter in a group setting especially releases oxytocin. I saw this for myself—there were few feelings as good as having a great set in a packed comedy club!

Crying also has oxytocin-releasing power all on its own and involves vocalization and vagal stimulation. Tears are a powerful mechanism for self-soothing and connecting with ourselves after a painful event such as a death or a breakup (or a divorce or two). After a good cry, the external reality of the loss has not changed, but tears soften our internal perception of the event. Tears have a soothing activity on our nervous system. As a sobering observation, I think this is why men have a much higher suicide rate and higher rates of addiction than women because crying has dried up in boys and men due to shame and social stigma. This isn't popular for a man to express, but I can feel when alarm energy is building in me and I know that tears will help me release it. Accepting and allowing my tears, although it strongly goes against my conditioning as a male, is a small price to pay to get myself to discharge that energy, because I know that if I don't, I'll experience a significant rise in my alarm.

A little tip for those stoic males (and females) who have a lot of pain built up and can't release it or find their tears: car screaming. Get into your car and drive to an area where you can just let go. Don't be surprised if after the screaming the tears come, and don't stop them. Physical motion moves emotion that is stuck, but be careful about doing a round of car screaming outside of your gym and then going inside to stare at yourself in the mirrors.

Lastly, there is something called face yoga. Yes. It's a thing. I won't get into it too much here, but there is evidence that the tone of your facial muscles plays a role in your mood by sending signals back to the brain. It's been shown that if your facial muscles are formed to create a smile, you feel happier, and if your facial muscles are formed in a frown, you'll feel down. We often think that we smile because we are happy but new research suggests we may be happy because we smile! Your posture also affects your mood and vice versa. Studies at Harvard and Columbia Universities have shown that the "Superman pose" (puffing out the chest with hands on hips) increased testosterone and lowered the stress hormone cortisol and had people feel more powerful before a speech. The main premise of this book is that your physiology (alarm) affects your psychology (anxiety), so these studies make perfect sense to me.

COMPASSION

You probably knew this would be on the list as self-compassion is the *C* in the ABCs.

Giving of yourself releases oxytocin. Giving to yourself releases more. Oxytocin helps you befriend your dragon and opens the treasure chest that holds your innocence and your true, authentic self.

Like I couldn't feel alarm when I was full of love on MDMA, you can't feel loving compassion and alarm in the same moment. (Go ahead, try it, I'll wait.) So all you need to do is expand the time you feel compassionate and loving and you automatically decrease the time you spend in anxiety and alarm. (Self) love indeed pushes fear out of your box. Because we worriers tend to be hard on ourselves and use sticks more than carrots (story coming soon), this book is designed to show you exactly what you need to do to increase compassionate connection to yourself, which boosts your ventral vagal connection, makes you more compassionate to others, and boosts your oxytocin. Win-win-win!

Alarm (dorsal vagus) and compassion (ventral vagus) have an adversarial relationship. One suppresses the other. Building compassion into your life as a daily practice is hard when your alarm constantly blocks it. The dorsal vagal effect of unconscious alarm is precisely why you need to make the unconscious conscious and commit to making self-compassion a frequent conscious intention. Simply, when you are kind to yourself you send an emotional signal to the universe that you view it as friendly rather than hostile, and what we focus on, we will perceive more of, and we will *think* better when our body *feels* better!

RHYTHMIC BREATHING

Your vagus nerve innervates the throat and lungs, and breath is a highly effective way of moving into a ventral vagal state that is more socially engaged and connected. When you are alarmed, your shallow, rapid breathing is an indication the dorsal vagus is more active, but note that this is both cause and effect. Just as (unconscious) vagal nerve activity can negatively influence the quality of your breath, consciously taking control of your breath can positively influence your vagal nerve tone. The physiological sigh from the Anxiety Toolkit has a profound effect on moving vagal tone from dorsal to ventral, and does it quickly.

In yoga, we have breathing practices called pranayama that are tremendously effective in increasing vagal tone and creating a more grounded state in our minds and bodies by consciously breathing and bringing a keen sense of awareness to the breath.

You don't necessarily need to do much. When you stop and focus on your breath, it naturally slows and deepens. Any process (even holding your breath) that puts you in control will break the ego dragon's pattern of alarm unconsciously pressuring your breathing cycle. Again, three to five rounds of quick inhales and long exhales of the physiological sigh has never failed me.

I encourage you to look up Ujjayi breathing as it is a very potent way of stimulating the vagus nerve. To give you a brief sense of it, put your hand up to your mouth and pretend you are fogging up a mirror or the lenses in your glasses before you clean them. Now see if you can hold your throat in that position as you breathe in and out. Darth Vader was an exceptional example of how to do Ujjayi breathing. (He did seem to hold a lot of alarm, though.)

You might also look into Holotropic Breathwork®, which you learned about in part 2. (Remember, it's the technique invented by the doctor who was trying to help people reproduce the effects of LSD without actually taking LSD.) Personally, it's been very beneficial for me, and another benefit is that you don't have to take LSD to do it.

MOVEMENT

There's a whole chapter on the power of movement (chapter 94), but I wanted to say a little more here because when we're talking about ways of connecting with ourselves, you really can't leave this off the list. Yoga, qigong, and tai chi are my favorites for connecting the body and mind. When we are relaxed and comfortable—which is the effect movement has on us—that's a sign of ventral vagal activation. Lastly, who knows what kind of ventral vagal connections you'll make at yoga class?

One of the causative and perpetuating factors in anxiety and alarm is a separation of mind and body, and movement helps yoke those two back together. There is an exceptional book called *Body Aware* by Erica Hornthal, LCPC, that I have found very helpful in connecting mind to body and body to mind. Erica has also created *The Movement Therapy Deck*: fifty-two cards with easy exercises that increase vagal tone and soothe the nervous system.

The separation of body from mind is a big reason alarm and anxiety are crushing us. The other causative and perpetuating factor in anxiety and alarm is something I mentioned briefly at the end of Chapter 97: the separation of your adult self from your child self. To heal we need to connect mind and body and outer adult with inner child, and much more of that is coming up.

MEDITATION

If you suffer from anxiety and you find trying to meditate difficult, you're not alone. I can offer you an explanation of this difficulty that is true for me. Meditation brings me into direct contact with the alarm in my body because I am unable to distract into my thinking. You likely know all too well how your ego dragon will swoop in with distracting thoughts to keep your mind from stillness.

But I promise that after you practice meditation for a while, you'll get more skilled at separating from your thoughts.

For a reason I can't explain—and I usually try to have an explanation for *everything*, so maybe I am finally getting out of my own head?—once I started following the ABC process regularly, I found it so much easier to stick to a regular meditation practice. Before that, I was very inconsistent with meditation. I believe that the more I practiced the ABCs, the more I created a place of comfort in my body, so I didn't resist wandering in there and hanging out during meditation.

When you're starting out, don't set a goal of sitting and meditating for half an hour. This will be the longest half hour of your life and, probably, the only half hour you ever spend meditating because you'll develop such an aversion you won't ever want to go back!

I often tell people to use the two-to-three rule: two to three minutes of focusing on your breath two to three times a day for two to three weeks. "Start low and go slow" is a line we use as MDs to describe starting someone on a medication; the same can be said for meditation!

Meditation in many ways is an embodiment of *sensation without explanation*, and the more practiced we are at detaching from our thoughts, the less worry can activate the alarm-anxiety cycle.

And there is neuroscience behind meditation's positive effects on anxiety. The anterior cingulate cortex (ACC) in the front of the brain has been shown to have a calming effect on the amygdala, and meditation has been shown to increase the size of the ACC. Ommmmmmmm . . .

CREATE RITUALS

Rituals are conscious activities in a repeatable sequence. I believe one of the reasons our culture is in chaos and alarm is that there is so much inconsistency in the world. As the world gets busier, we've lost touch with our rites of passage and our rituals—and without rituals, our days have no bookends, no boundaries, and no grounding.

Rituals create consistency and structure because they are performed the same way every time, which is why they are so reassuring to children. If your childhood lacked rituals and structure, it's time to create some for yourself and bring that sense of grounding and predictability to your relationship with yourself.

Remember way back in part 1 where I talked about Freud's concept of repetition compulsion, the urge to equate familiarity with security by unconsciously replicating the chaotic events of your childhood in your adulthood? A common theme I've observed in people with alarm and anxiety is they often tend to unconsciously create chaos in their lives. I know that I gravitated to chaos in my young adult life because chaos was so familiar (family and liar) in my childhood. I believe a big reason why anxiety and ADD go together so often is that dissociating into the chaos of our mind distracts us from the alarm in our body. A dissociated mind looks very much like ADD.

You may know at a conscious level that chaos in your life creates alarm, but at the deeper level where your unconscious behaviors and shadowy motivations lie, there is a pull to repeat the turmoil because it's a familiar distraction from the pain of alarm. Its familiarity gives it a sense of safety, but the chaos is the exact opposite of safety and we can't see the label from inside the bottle.

But now that awareness has let you out of the bottle and you see it has the label "Creates Chaos as a Replication of Childhood," you know better, so you can do better. You can create your own rituals as a powerful antidote to chaos.

There are morning rituals, prayer rituals, meditation rituals, and lots of internet posts and articles on creating rituals in your life. It is really about finding what resonates with you. A ritual is often about creating a repeatable, safe place for yourself in your body and mind, and I find easy, short, repeatable morning rituals are the best ways to start the day in a grounded place.

The ABCs are one of my rituals, although there is a great deal of flexibility in the way I practice them. The Anxiety Toolkit has lots of great options you can create rituals from. One of my other favorites is drinking a full glass of water when I first wake up while I look at my picture above my bathroom mirror. Trust yourself to find what works best for you and the child in you.

As soon you wake up, get out of bed and go to a comfortable chair. (Use 5, 4, 3, 2, 1, go!) When you first awaken your brain waves are still in quiet and receptive theta waves and this is a great time for a breathing practice. Wrap yourself in a cozy blanket or sweater and sit with a straight spine if you can (meditation chairs that sit on the floor are relatively cheap and great for this). Then count your breaths in and out: inhale on one, exhale on two, inhale on three, exhale on four. The numbers give your mind something to focus on to block the worries from coming in. As you become more practiced, see if you can slightly expand that little transition gap as the breath changes direction from inhale to exhale. You can start by just going to ten. That's five breaths. (I count to one hundred each morning, fifty breaths.) It's not the number of breaths you do, it's the ritualistic aspect of doing it every day. I have added holding a small glass of water with me while I count and breathe with the intention of mentally pouring compassion for my alarmed child self into the water as I breathe. When I finish counting and breathing, I intentionally drink the glass of self-compassion and imagine it reaching every cell in my body. It's a wonderful and easy start to the day and you can begin with just five cycles of breath. Again, it's not the time you spend doing it, it's the ritual of doing it *every* morning (and don't hit yourself with a stick—story coming soon—if you miss a day!).

AVOIDING SOCIAL MEDIA AND MEDIA IN GENERAL

"Comparison is the thief of joy."

−THEODORE ROOSEVELT

"Don't compare someone else's outside life to your inside life."

−ANNE LAMOTT (MY PARAPHRASE)

"Only an ego compares."

−GILA GOLUB

I do think we get a hit of dopamine from social media that makes us temporarily feel good—"temporarily" being the operative word. Even though that hit is instantaneous and doesn't last, we worriers crave any positive hits we can get (this is also why we are sitting ducks for addiction). If you struggle with alarm, the risks of social media outweigh the benefits because we artificially distract from pain by clicking for the next hit of dopamine. I see so many people with smartphone-induced anhedonia: lack of interest, pleasure, or enjoyment of life. As Dr. Andrew Huberman describes, we have exhausted our mesolimbic and mesocortical dopamine systems by incessantly scrolling on our phones—and we worriers need less manipulation of our neurotransmitters, not more.

In addition to being addictive, social media is a fantastic way to distract yourself from making real changes in your actual life. There's nothing wrong with spending a little time on social media, but if you've escaped into zombie scrolling and using up energy you could be putting into the ABCs or mindful connection with yourself or others who are important to you, it's actually keeping you away from your SES and ventral vagal state and promoting more dorsal vagal freeze. Pretend connections (or at least connections that are less satisfying than time spent together in person) are stealing your attention away from improving your connection with yourself. Again, a little social media is engaging, a lot strongly activates your social *disengagement* system.

Take it from the hammer guy—sometimes you can make something much better just by stopping what was making it worse. Having your system awash in cortisol from the twenty-four-hour news cycle and comparing yourself on social media is not helping you. Put on some music ("Disco Inferno"!), dance, do some physiological sighs, do some face yoga, or go car screaming.

PLAY AND CREATIVITY

In ayurvedic medicine, they say that creativity is the cure for anxiety. Play and creativity have been shown to mobilize the ventral vagus and sympathetic nervous system, so they can be powerful tools as you work to develop social engagement with self and others. In the coming years, I believe we will see play (defined simply as finding what you like and doing it) incorporated more and more into therapy for anxiety and depression. Engagement in play is one of the most healing and most underrated modalities. I cannot emphasize enough the role of finding what you enjoy—and doing that.

Many of my patients say they don't know what play is for them anymore. A good place to start is asking yourself what you liked to do for fun when you were young. Was it riding your bike or singing or dancing or drawing? Playing a sport or playing an instrument? Pick up one of your favorite childhood activities and see if you still like it. It might take a little while to relax and enjoy it since we are so used to telling ourselves that play is a waste of time, but that's just your ego dragon talking.

LOVING THE LOVE

There is something I've observed in myself and in most of my anxious patients. We actually love and crave connection from others, especially our family and friends. One of the crimes of the protective ego dragon is that it shuts us off from love and connection under the assumption that love can't be trusted. One of the reasons we are so alarmed is that we are pulled in two opposite directions: to crave the love and resist the love at the same time.

Wanting the love and simultaneously being resistant to it becomes this deep inner conflict that freezes you in dorsal vagal immobilization and alarm. It reminds me of the saying "You can't have your cake and eat it too."

What the hell good is cake if you can't eat it?

So, how do you "love the love" if your system has been programmed to fear it?

Let me answer you with a story of one of my patients, Anna, who was recovering from anorexia nervosa. I met Anna when she was thirty years old. She was upbeat and quirky with youthful, childlike energy. She was tall, about five feet nine, and looked to be very fit and muscular. Anna had for the most part recovered from her eating disorder, although she would not get on a scale or allow herself to go to a restaurant to eat (which made dating difficult). She told me her medical records stated that at sixteen years old she weighed eighty-six pounds and was sixty-eight inches tall.

Anna and I had an easy rapport right from the start. When I asked her how she had recovered, she told me that she woke up attached to tubes and wires and there was a nurse sitting with her, not doing active nursing duties, just being with her. When she looked at the IV in her arm, she saw it as a symbol that someone cared. Somebody had placed that needle in her arm to help her, so why couldn't she help herself? Her doctors had been telling her that she was on the verge of death. In that moment, she realized she wanted to live, and if she was going to survive, she would have to accept food.

To heal, Anna had to accept the nourishment she had trained herself to resist. I believe it is a similar situation for those of us with anxiety: we need to accept love and connection that we have trained ourselves to resist. If you want to survive you're going to have to stop resisting nourishment too, and as I said above, you're going to have to feed yourself.

After Anna had restricted her food so severely for so long, she had to begin with small meals—a bite at a time—and fill in additional calories intravenously while she gradually built up the amount of food she could chew and swallow. It took her almost two years to physically and emotionally accept enough food to begin to steadily gain weight.

That program of self-starvation is still in her, but in slowly learning how to accept food, she was able to live a full life. Despite being told she'd never be able to have children, she was able to fully nourish herself through two pregnancies and is now a wonderful mother to a boy and a girl. Anna is a testament to rewriting old programs by learning to give herself the love and attention she needed to not only survive but thrive. It is incredible what connection to yourself and others can heal.

A word of caution. Like someone with anorexia who starts to eat normally again, we need to open up to love bit by bit. If we flood our system with love all at once, it will overwhelm us. Our old ego tricks will cause resistance and likely cause us to go into protection and defensive detachment—the exact opposite of what we need to do to heal.

If you have unconsciously resisted love and connection for a long time, becoming connected again—and being someone who loves to feel love—is not going to happen overnight. Nor should it, and nor should you feel bad if it doesn't. Start with small things like holding a hug a little bit longer, maintaining eye contact for a little bit longer, consciously smiling a little bit more. Anything that creates a feeling of connection will bolster your SES, but especially things that promote more face-to-face and physical contact will reengage your ventral vagus and sense of love and connection. And before you know it, more love squeezes in and more fear gets squeezed out. I believe that as we develop our SES, we are able to metabolize, resolve, and integrate our own traumas so much more. "Increasing tone in your ventral vagus" is a more scientific explanation of the saying "Be your own connected inner parent." The more you focus on creating a compassionate connection to yourself, the more you can bring the SES back into a greater level of functionality, move your vagal set point toward connection with yourself, and have a greater connection to others, too!

If you would have asked me about my father five years ago, I probably would have told you he was severely mentally ill and I wasn't able to trust the love I got from him. If you would ask me about him today, I would tell you my father showed that he loved me in many ways and that it was his illness that created such pain in him and our family. I would add that I am grateful to him in many ways; if it weren't for him, I wouldn't be able to put this book into the world in the hope that his pain would lead to healing for so many others. I would add that I was very proud of him for coping with a devastating disease and for being able to take the pleasure in life that he did.

So, what used to be a tale of victimhood became a tale of victory through the process of integration. I have become more connected to myself (and others) than I had ever dreamed possible.

Practicing compassionate connection for yourself releases chemicals in your body and brain that foster more attachment. The more your innocent, loving, compassionate self comes out to feel safe, seen, heard, and loved, the more your SES matures. The safer you feel, the safer you will feel. Whatever you focus on you will see more of. It's a virtuous cycle, as opposed to the vicious cycle of alarm and anxiety. Self-connection becomes the new groove, and the more you focus on it through the ABCs, the more of it you will see and the more you will get!

There are so many ways to be compassionate to yourself. One of the most powerful compassionate connections you can use when you get to the letter *C* is acknowledging what a source of connection you are being for yourself. That child in you is so used to being shunned that it has given up hope and faith that a rescuer will ever come. Be the parent (to yourself) you would like to see in the world. YOU are coming to save you.

When you A) become aware of your triggering worries and alarm, (B) move into your body and breath, and then get to C) compassionate connection with yourself, it is critical that you really *feel* your compassion. Just saying the words that you will take care of your inner child without the feeling behind them can trigger your child's resistance, inability to receive, and defensive detachment. But if you set the intention to feel that compassion for your entire being, both adult and child, you will create a feeling of safety that is believable to your child self, especially if you make your self-connection a ritual. Again, it takes time to overcome the resistance of your ego, but creating compassion for yourself in small ways begins to reinforce itself. Also, a key component is being consistent with your self-connection. It is just as important to connect with yourself when you are feeling good as it is when you are feeling alarmed. When you are having a good day, share that with the younger version of yourself. Bring that child along with you and show them they are seen, heard, and loved on both good days and challenging days. More on this soon.

Ideally, and this is a bit of an advanced move, the awareness you came into the ABCs with should be reflected in the compassion part of the ABCs. For example, if you became aware you were in defensive detachment from your partner and had withdrawn, when moving into compassionate connection (after taking time to ground in your body), you could bring to mind a time you were very close and connected with your partner (maybe your wedding day or a holiday you took together) and sit in the feeling of that connection. The point is to draw on an emotional, compassionate connection that runs counter to the awareness that started you into the ABCs in the first place.

It is in your authentic nature to be compassionate to yourself, but your reactive/adaptive child self rejected the vulnerability in positive emotion a long time ago. It takes discipline and practice to commit to that compassion because, chances are, that inner child has felt judged, abandoned, blamed, and shamed for a long time and is wary of showing their authentic, innocent self. You need to show them—and believe yourself—that there are no reasons not to be loving and compassionate to yourself. Even when you find yourself caught up in worrying you can say "I am trapped in worry and I can love that about myself" as you move into your body and breath.

The cornerstone of being able to be loving and compassionate to yourself is seeing that no matter what you have thought, said, or done, you are an innocent being at your core.

(And so is everyone else, including your parents.)

> **Point to consider:** If you had a horrendous parent (or two), you can see them as a spirit energy that got tainted by alarm and that you can change your perception of them as spirit energy. I know this sounds "woo-woo" but this simple intention has helped many of my patients stay spiritually connected to a "toxic" parent they cannot be around physically.

100

Hello? Is It Me You're Looking For?

The thirteenth-century Sufi poet Rumi wrote, "What you seek is seeking you."

You have worked so diligently to learn about your alarm, to understand that you are not your worries and that they are not serving you. You've practiced your ABCs to help you choose to stay present down in your body instead of spiraling up into worry. You have learned all about your ego dragon and its tricks and how you can make friends with it so you can open the treasure chest to find your authentic self. You've learned how to activate your ventral vagus and connect with others and, perhaps most important, with your very own child self.

It's critical to your healing to open up a line of communication with your younger self to let them know you are there for them. Because your child self has been there all this time, just waiting for you to bring them into connection.

And I mean this literally: I have actual conversations with my inner child. Not out loud in public—that would be crazy—but rather when I feel calm and resourced. (When I see a troubled person on the street who looks mentally ill having a heated conversation out loud but with themselves, I sometimes wonder if they are arguing with their mid-tantrum inner child, but then I look closer and see the earbuds.)

If you had attached and attuned parents, the child you flows into a natural connection with the developing adult in you, flowing together and staying whole as you grow up. But if you had unresolved trauma early in life, this adult self / child self connection is often compromised and instead of staying whole, there is defensive detachment that splits the child and adult apart as you get older. The adult doesn't trust going back to visit the child because the child holds so much of their pain, and the child doesn't trust the adult because they've felt abandoned and on their own for so long. I certainly think that was true for adult me and young Rusty. As I reassure him that I am him and he is me and I will never leave him again, we've developed a relationship, and it's begun to feel more like we are one.

Yet another Neufeld quote: "We grow older but we don't grow up." I think that was true for me. As I developed this accomplishment-driven, "lone-wolf" adult, I left Rusty behind to hold his trauma alone. Of course he's going to be alarmed!

The ABCs have closed that gap between adult Russ and child Rusty and I have become much more whole as each part of me becomes more connected to the other.

As Rusty began to trust that I wasn't going to abandon him by distracting into my adult thoughts and worries, and as he felt my compassion for him, he became a more visceral part of me. We could have conversations, and I learned much more about his life from how he perceived it, rather than my memory of it. We could converse about where he felt judged, abandoned, blamed, or shamed, and I could reassure him that I would see, hear, understand, love, and protect him forever. I told him that we could never be apart again. I made sure he knew I loved him and cared for him no matter what he ever said, thought, or did.

When you try connecting with yourself, remember that it's not a "one and done." Just as it takes time to develop trust and increasing levels of intimacy in a romantic relationship, it will take time to develop trust and intimacy in this one too. I have had countless interactions and conversations with Rusty. If you had a childhood nickname, I suggest you try using that too, as a way of connecting to your younger self.

If you can overcome your own self-consciousness, talk to that picture of you on your bathroom mirror. Believe me, this gets easier and helps creates a real connection inside of you. Put your hand on your chest or over your sensation of alarm as that encourages an actual physical connection through the somatosensory and sensorimotor parts of your brain. Simply say to that child, "I see you and I am here for you." Do not underestimate how difficult this can be. Don't be surprised if this becomes very emotional, and also be aware if there's little emotion or numbing. You can repeat "I see you and I am here for you" as often as your emotions will allow. This can be a life-changing exercise.

Your inner child must not only be encouraged by your words but must also feel safe with you. The importance of staying present and grounded in a state of connected compassion is what brings you into wholeness and resolves alarm.

Give it time. You need to keep throwing your child a life preserver with your adult self assuredly holding the rope at the other end. That child needs to know beyond a shadow of a doubt that if they grab the life preserver, you are going to consistently pull them to safety and not just drop the rope and leave them stranded in a leaky boat once again.

It is your job to give yourself now what you didn't have then—to take your child self by the hand and See them, Hear them, Open to them, Understand them, Love them, and Defend them. That is what we all wanted as children and what we all SHOULD have received.

If you feel up to this, consider trying a little exercise I call commiserating. (It sounds more negative than it actually is.) Ground yourself in your breath, maybe do a few physiological sighs, feel the grounded weight of your body in the chair or the bed, relax your shoulders, relax your jaw, lovingly put your hand over your alarm or your chest, and make the intention to create a warm connection with your child self, knowing that you can't do this wrong. Once you've settled, create an image of your younger self in your mind's eye and say to the younger part of you, "It must have been really hard for you when _____ (you were bullied, your mom was drunk, your dad would hit you, etc.)." Pick a troubling childhood experience and see if you get a response from them. This exercise brings many people to tears. Stay with the tears. It's okay. The tears break down barriers to the child in you who has been waiting for this connection for a very long time.

Healing your anxiety and alarm is connecting your mind to your body and connecting your adult self to your child self.

101
Use It or Lose It: Self-Compassion

For many of us worriers, compassion and empathy are inherent in our (over)sensitive nature and we are often very good at showing that warmth to others. But ironically, it is exactly our heightened sensitivity that has made our inner critic and ego dragon so powerful in blocking that same vulnerability and compassion for ourselves.

The self-compassion muscle is still there. It just hasn't been exercised in a while.

Our sensitivity is fertile ground for our self-compassion. When we re-engage our sensitivity and our willingness to be vulnerable and connected to ourselves, we can create more compassion and care within. Bit by bit, self-connection comes more naturally as our sensitive inner child realizes they are safe and they won't be punished or chastised for their inherent sensitivity.

Make your inner child this promise: "I will love, guide, and care for you, no matter what you have ever thought, said, or done in the past or think, say, or do in the future. I will see, hear, understand, love, and protect you always." I suggest to my patients they put this up on their bathroom mirror beside a childhood picture of themselves. I don't know if I have mentioned putting up a picture of your childhood self above your bathroom mirror, but it's a good idea.

Then, be persistent and patient. As you reconnect to your authentic, innocent self, more of that self can emerge. As you become more authentic, you become less reactive.

When you soothe your alarm with connection, compassion, and love, the alarm can stop flaring to get your attention. Your alarm has no need to activate if it gets the love and compassion it has been asking for.

Inability to receive, defensive detachment, and resistance have blocked our kindness to ourselves for a long time. Now, with consistent self-compassion, the innocent child innate in you will begin to integrate with your adult self and begin to resolve the separation that fired up your alarm.

Compassion and care for yourself mature the SES for connection in your mind and body, enabling you to increase the connection both inwardly to yourself and outwardly to others.

102
The Biggest Obstacle to the ABCs

Perhaps the most poignant thing a patient has ever said to me is, "Dr. Kennedy, to be blunt, I get worried when I'm not worrying."

Nothing captures the ego dragon's essence better than that statement. I knew exactly what she was saying. The moment she said it, I felt it.

Before I learned the ABCs, I could stay in this worried state indefinitely. I had no idea what to do. It was like worry was an old, familiar friend whom I didn't like very much but still found a perverse comfort in their presence—a strange security in the familiarity of rumination and worry. I had been frozen in reactive worry for decades.

This feeling that there is no escape from anxiety is devastating, and it came close to killing me. I've had people tell me my anxiety couldn't have been that bad because I worked as a doctor and could do stand-up comedy. I would say that many of us worriers are infinitely stronger than we give ourselves credit for. We grossly overestimate threat and grossly underestimate our ability to cope.

To win over your ego dragon, you will need discipline. It will be a fight, but it's one worth winning—because you are fighting for your life, or, at the very least, the quality of it.

Discipline yourself to show compassion to yourself and others. Discipline yourself to limit social media or news.

Discipline yourself to stop taking JABS at yourself.

Discipline yourself to receive so you can drop your resistance to giving and receiving love.

Discipline yourself to recognize compulsive thinking and move, instead, into sensation and feeling.

Discipline yourself to recognize when you are making yourself a victim, and discipline yourself to see that you can absolutely do things your dragon tells you that you can't.

Discipline yourself to see when you are going into defensive detachment and separating from the people close to you, and discipline yourself to lean into connection with yourself.

Acknowledge your sensitivity, and discipline yourself to limit stressors that are avoidable.

Discipline yourself as a wise and guiding parent, knowing that discipline is always carried out in a compassionate way.

If this sounds overwhelming, know that it can be done—and it gets much easier with practice.

One of the most powerful strategies that helps me every day is the discipline to not add worries in my mind to the alarm in my body—just to feel the alarm, put my hand over it, breathe into it, and stop compulsively adding explanations to the sensation. Having faith (more on this soon) that I can trust the inherent safety of the world and stay with feeling without compulsively adding thinking.

Stop being afraid of living. For the vast majority of us, life is safe. You're still here, right? How many times have you assumed the worst—and yet, here you are. I can't tell you how many times I have diagnosed myself with some terminal illness and then convinced myself that I was not going to survive, yet I made it to my sixties and I'm still here. Not only that, but I'm thriving.

Just like me, you've probably used your habit of worrying to avoid going into your body, but there is a way back to your inner child, and that is through your body.

> **Point to consider:** This book will absolutely help you heal, but you need to change your programming and that takes a disciplined practice of what I suggest here. To be blunt, your overprotective ego will unconsciously try to sabotage you back into your old family and liar program of worry and this will be the reason you will stay anxious and alarmed.

103

And I Love That! Or Embrace Your Dragon

It's hard not to think of the ego dragon as an enemy or villain. It's not that your dragon is bad—it's just fixated on the impossible task of making sure you never get hurt again. But in its compulsion to keep you safe, it ensures you don't get better. Another way of saying this to the dragon is "By keeping me in your protective chest, there is no room for me to grow."

When my alarm flares up, it is usually my ego dragon breathing fire into that alarm. Much of my healing has come from being able to see the dragon's overprotective tricks so I don't have to be them.

Although the ego is often regarded as some kind of omnipotent deity, it is a child's manifestation. It may appear magically powerful, but it had to appear that way in order to protect you. We must always remember that as a child's incarnation, your ego dragon acts in protection, not growth, and it is like Schwarzenegger's character in *Terminator 2* in its relentless single-minded focus to protect.

To overcome anxiety and alarm, we must see through our ego. By that I mean we must see its attempts to "help" us and compassionately tell our dragon, "Thank you for trying to protect me but I am not a child anymore. Can you help me find another way?"

Just as arguing with worries makes them appear more real, trying to fight with the ego's primitive, heavy-handed attempts to keep you safe just puffs the dragon up so it doubles down on keeping you behind that tree, or locked in that chest. As the dragon's tricks and the thoughts enlarge, they obstruct our field of view so they appear as our only option. This may have been true when we were young, but we are no longer powerless children despite what our ego trick of victim mentality and our amygdala's age regressions would have us believe.

When we vilify and separate from our ego dragon, we are failing to see its innocence. We are also vilifying and separating from the child who created it and failing to see that child's innocence as well. It's like creating an imaginary friend to help you and then treating that friend as an enemy.

The idea is to see the dragon and consciously embrace it as only a part of ourselves that is trying to keep us safe from our old monsters. In this process of embracing the dragon it becomes smaller—perhaps so small it can perch on our shoulder. We don't want to lose it; we just want to put it into perspective so it doesn't overwhelm our adult self. Many alarmed people live their entire lives in the "protection" of their ego dragon. Giving everything over to the dragon seemed like the only deal when we were young, and the dragon helped us survive, but as adults, its tricks keep us trapped in survival and block our growth.

I want to make this book as practical as I can. Your dragon will likely have its favorite tricks it uses on you, and I want you to see how to neutralize those tricks so adult you becomes the main protector of child you, and the dragon can be more of a guide than a tyrant.

Let's look at some of the dragon's common strategies to keep you frozen in alarm and then learn how to neutralize its tricks, so our adult self can look after our child self directly without the need for the dragon to fire up and set off our sensitive smoke alarm.

SELF-JUDGMENT

Our society and our economy run on self-judgment. If none of us judged ourselves, we wouldn't have to constantly buy stuff to make us feel better. I used to judge myself a lot, especially for having anxiety. Now I go car screaming or embrace my tears when I feel that alarm build. I thank my ego dragon for firing up my alarm so I can do something to actually move that energy to resolution instead of defaulting into freeze (and adding more alarm).

So where do you judge yourself? Your self-judgment (and all the JABS) keeps you separate from yourself and adds to your alarm, so call it into the light and label it. Are you too weak, fat, skinny, dumb, sensitive, or fearful, according to your dragon? Say to yourself, "My dragon thinks I'm too _____ and I can love that about myself." While this sounds trite, I guarantee that when you say you can love something about yourself, it renews your perception of that judgment, and it also shows you how much you really do it!

SELF-ABANDONMENT

I can knock off two ego dragon tricks in one paragraph. Compulsive thinking and worrying is a form of self-abandonment. When you find yourself in ruminative, worrisome thoughts, call them out: "I am in compulsive worry, and I can love that about myself." The dragon relies on your resistance to keep you locked in or addicted to that dysfunctional pattern (like taking JABS at yourself). The ego dragon and the inner critic come from the same place, trying to protect you from pain but creating pain in the process. It's a bad deal. If you embrace the critic and the dragon's tricks by saying, "And I can love that about myself," you release the resistance and can stop holding on to what you don't want.

When you distract into social media, food, shopping, sex, drugs, or alcohol, you are also abandoning yourself. Not always, of course, but be aware of your motives. Are you using these things primarily to give yourself some pleasure, or are you doing it because you are attempting to avoid pain? Call it out: "I am distracting right now to avoid pain, and

I can love that about myself!" It doesn't even mean you have to stop distracting, but if you are conscious about it, you can see it and then have the choice to be it (or not).

Let's say someone cuts you off in traffic, and at that moment you have a choice to yell at them and ratchet up your own stress and blood pressure or just take a breath and let it go. I always say that as long as you give yourself the conscious *choice*—as in, "I could yell at this guy, or I could just breathe into this experience"—I have no problem if you yell. I really don't. The point is, rather than unconsciously and automatically beginning to scream at the other driver, you gave yourself a choice. And then decided to yell.

And I can love that about you.

(Maybe it's a sign you need a good ol' session of car screaming?)

SELF-BLAME

There is a surefire sign to see if you are blaming yourself for something: guilt.

You don't have to look too deep into guilt to see what you are blaming yourself for. The blame may be justified, but remember that the things we do that we are not proud of we likely do because of our past wounding. Again, embracing your innocence is the best antidote to self-blame.

Guilt is often a useful emotion in that it shows us where we can do better. But you can't change anything until you accept and embrace it in yourself.

Acknowledging "I feel guilty about _____, and I can love that about myself!" changes your relationship to guilt. After connecting with your body and breath, seek compassionate ways to see your guilt as a messenger for change rather than a stick to beat yourself with. (The stick story is coming up soon, I promise.)

SELF-SHAME

We can look guilt in the eye. It's uncomfortable but it's doable. Shame is different. Shame hides in the shadows. We are much more open to looking at what we feel guilty about than what we are ashamed of. But we can add "And I can love that about myself" to both guilt and shame. This is where you can start to see, embrace, and process your shadow side. Our shadow, especially when it comes to shame, is a massive driver of alarm, so as you cast the light of awareness on your shadow, you are metabolizing your alarm.

It seems almost wrong to address a topic as big as shame in just a few paragraphs, but it's important to include here. Seeing your shame, labeling it compassionately, and saying "And I can love that about myself" is a great way to start bringing it into the light so you can change your (likely fixed and alarming) perception of it. When it comes to shame, the ego dragon inflates to a monstrous size in an attempt to protect you. Your dragon will bury your shame very deeply. And, like guilt, shame becomes a more powerful source of alarm if you do not address it.

Shame is the place where self-compassion from your ABCs may have the most benefit. Shame grows in your shadow, because it tends to make you do other things you are ashamed of. An addict feels shame for their addiction and the pain of that shame drives them back to their addiction in an endless cycle. Bringing your shame into the light of full acceptance and embracing it is the only way to get free from it.

You do not have shame, shame has you. You are not your shame, but unless you acknowledge it and love it, it will always hold you hostage.

Try saying, "I feel ashamed about _____ and I can love that about myself." Saying the words alone is a start but with shame especially *you really need to feel it to heal it*. Feel the shame, put your hand over your chest, breathe in, and pendulate it back and forth by really feeling the love, too. Doing this into a mirror will change your life.

INABILITY TO RECEIVE

The next time you get a compliment and watch yourself deflect it, say to yourself, "I don't allow myself to accept compliments, and I can love that about myself." For a long time, I had a hard time receiving gifts, even small things like when a friend wanted to pick up the check for dinner. If you find yourself rejecting a gift or show of affection, call yourself out.

I am much better at receiving now than I ever have been, and I've found that when I give to myself without reservation, other people give me more! My theory (and you know by now I have theories on everything) is that I was blocking love from others as a way of protecting myself from the vulnerability of receiving, and they felt that, so they just stopped trying.

So many of my patients (especially females) feel uncomfortable with the vulnerability associated with receiving. How are you with it?

DEFENSIVE DETACHMENT

Sometimes you feel like you need to end a relationship because that's the healthy choice, but often we worriers withdraw because attachment feels too vulnerable and alarming. As I mentioned earlier, in psychological parlance, this is often referred to as an avoidant pattern of attachment. The person wants intimacy but becomes uncomfortable when things get too close. Defensive detachment has demolished countless relationships.

When I engage my awareness and find myself pulling back (especially from Cynthia), I call it out, saying (sometimes out loud), "I am going into defensive detachment, and I can love that about myself!" I put my hand on my chest, take a breath, and step back into awareness of my protective reflex to resist loving connection.

Every time I go through a successful cycle of calling out my defensive detachment in awareness, I find a little more love for myself—a little better ability to engage my SES and globally connect. Each time I neutralize one of my overprotective ego's tricks, my dragon gets a little bit smaller and softer and allows me a little more access to the treasure chest containing my innocent, sensitive, and truly loving self.

VICTIM MENTALITY

Victim mentality thrives on a principle called secondary gain, which means that as victims we get some sort of payoff or reward. We all appreciate being helped out and taken care of at times, but for someone with unresolved trauma and wounding, this feeling can be downright addictive. Victims have such a strong sense of lack, often left over from childhood when they weren't taken care of, that they keep on trying to manipulate others to fill the void instead of recognizing that they are mature adults who can, and should, take care of themselves.

One of the most interesting aspects of the human brain is it will create chemicals and peptides to support your perceptions. Once you see the ego dragon's tricks, you can choose not to automatically accept what it tells you. To some extent you can choose a different perception, and therefore choose your brain chemistry. If you see someone across the room that you would like to talk to and you command yourself to go over and courageously strike up a conversation (use 5, 4, 3, 2, 1 if you have to), the periaqueductal gray matter in your brainstem will secrete endogenous opioids (the brain's natural morphine) and the mesolimbic and mesocortical systems in the brain will secrete dopamine, and these chemicals will support your quest to make a new acquaintance. However, if you tell yourself the person is going to reject you and list all the reasons in your mind you shouldn't talk to this person, your brain develops a victim stance, and will create victim neurophysiology. The locus coeruleus in your brain will pump out norepinephrine (noradrenaline) that will put you in a defensive stance, increasing your worries and heightening your perception of potential rejection, as well as sending the signal to your adrenal glands on top of your kidneys to generate epinephrine and cortisol, all of which will make you feel more afraid and confirm that, indeed, this person will reject you and you shouldn't even try to approach them as they might try to hurt you. (I'm only partially joking here.)

Neurochemically, when we refuse to be a victim and take responsibility to solve the situation ourselves with courageous action, our brains will support us in the challenge. Also, if we withdraw from a challenge, our brains will also support our self-defeating retreat. The dragon is especially heavy-handed at creating cortisol and norepinephrine to make us retreat (or not move in the first place), and block our potential growth. In awareness, you can choose to be a victor or a victim, and your brain chemistry will match whatever course of action you decide.

Whatever you focus on you'll get more of, so focus on more courage and "feel the fear and do it anyway," and your brain will take the path of courage. Choose to withdraw from your challenges as a victim and your brain learns to preferentially take that path. Your choices determine your physiology, and your physiology will support those choices.

When we victimize ourselves with JABS today, we create victim physiology and often age-regress back to childhood where we indeed felt like victims. This withdrawal into victim mentality leads us to mistrust ourselves more and separate from ourselves more, leading to more alarm. As we feel the consequences of withdrawing into victim mentality, we use that impotence as proof that we are incapable of lovingly caring for ourselves—and the self-judgment strengthens as our self-esteem weakens, confirming our victim status in a vicious cycle. As we become weaker, we feel more like a victim (and become more alarmed), and victim mentality feeds on itself.

It's so critical to call out your victim mentality because it grows in you like a cancer and freezes you in ever-increasing alarm. Victim mentality is self-perpetuating. Although there is a "payoff," in that we appear to get sympathy or the ability to withdraw from potential pain in the short term (avoidance), we will continue to act and feel like a victim in the long term. The more you disempower yourself, the more you'll be paralyzed by alarm, and you won't (and actually can't) do what scares you. This is what's known in psychology as negative reinforcement—reinforcing a behavior by removing a painful stimulus. If you had a panic attack on the bus and then avoid buses, you avoid the (perceived) pain of getting on the bus today, but you feel yourself getting weaker as your life becomes more restricted tomorrow (and on top of that you will have to walk everywhere).

It's easy to feel like a victim when you are in alarm. I know. Been there, done that—more times that I can count. But the first step is always awareness. "Oh, I see that by avoiding this event, I am making myself a victim, and I can love that about myself!" Loving your victim mentality changes your physiology and allows you to accept it and, as I have said before, we cannot change anything we don't accept in ourselves first.

When you label your victim mentality and lovingly call it out in awareness, you can make what was invisible visible, which makes it so much easier to choose another way.

By now you may be thinking how trite this "And I can love that about myself" can sound, but do not underestimate its power as a tool of self-awareness and change, especially in front of a mirror! By grounding in your ABCs, doing a few rounds of the physiological sigh, placing your hand on your chest while you say "And I can love (my resistance, my stubbornness, my anger) in myself," you can call it out, bring it into awareness, and dissolve the unconscious power it has over you.

RESISTANCE

Alarm cannot be released if we resist it. If you're feeling pain, chances are you're resisting, so put your hand on your chest or alarm and say to yourself, "I am in resistance right now, and I can love that about myself!" When I did this, I was amazed at how aware I became about how much I resisted, how intense that resistance was, and how unconscious and automatic it was. Then, I would move into the ABCs and have deep compassion for that place in me that was so resistant! Hint: it's usually the child in you.

When you call out the ego's tricks, you can love your dragon for trying to protect you. When you "win over" the dragon, it sees that you are an adult who can make their own choices and no longer a victimized child that needs to be (over)protected from any and every source of potential pain. In other words, when you love and appreciate your ego for simply trying to protect you, it can stand beside you instead of in front of you (or maybe just perch on your shoulder).

Embrace the dragon (sounds like a kung fu movie). Embrace its tricks and its fighting spirit because that is your fighting spirit too. Remember the child in you made it your protector, and the dragon is only trying to keep you safe. It just went into beast mode as it perceived you got weaker and more alarmed. In your newfound awareness you can say, "I am in judgment, alienation, blame, shame, resistance, defensive detachment, inability to receive, and compulsive thinking, and I can love that about myself." And most of all, embrace your innocent, true child self—because as you give yourself the love and compassion you need, the dragon can ease out of protection and allow you to access growth. In growth (more on this soon), you can see and feel more of your real, authentic, and innocent self, and the more you see it, the more you will be it.

104

Carrot and Stick

Even though I often say you can't think your way out of a feeling issue, I am by no means against thinking. But I am against thinking when you are in alarm. If you struggle with alarm, you've probably been living in your thoughts for a long time—so long that you've forgotten what it is like to live in the only safe place there is, your body.

We need to be able to think, but there is a big difference between conscious, aware thinking in your prefrontal cortex and the unconscious, automatic daydreaming ruminations and JABS of the default mode network. In the former, you are in charge, and in the latter, your ego dragon has locked you in an unconscious, automatic worried state of the DMN, fueled by both background and foreground alarm.

Conscious thinking has an end point or goal that is constructive. Rumination is unconscious, endless, and destructive, creating a vicious cycle that feeds on itself, driving you deeper into even more rumination and alarm. And you can only distract and dissociate for so long. Eventually, being in your head all the time catches up with you. The alarm gets stronger, and worrying loses its power to distract you from the alarm in your body.

When you were a child, your body wasn't safe. To avoid the discomfort, you defaulted into rumination and retreated up into your head. But with the ABCs you are growing a safe place of presence and wisdom in your body. Now, you have the blueprint to connect with your body in a sustainable and self-reinforcing way. The more safety you create in your body, the less you will be driven to distract and dissociate into compulsive, worrisome thinking.

With the help of the ABCs, you can smash the one-way valve where alarm gets in but doesn't get out. In compassionate connection with yourself, your SES becomes engaged and your ventral vagus activated. You are able to see your ego's manipulations in a new light and choose to do the opposite by loving those tricks as you recognize they were an attempt to keep you safe as a child. As you move out of victim mentality, you feel more and more empowered as your successes increase your ability to feel good about your life. You no longer feel you need to heal yourself; instead, you *want* to heal yourself—and this is a crucial distinction.

I've known I needed to heal for decades, but it wasn't until recently that I wanted to heal. And this move away from victimhood has changed my entire life.

In doing the ABCs, I have seen, especially in part C where I focus on my positive qualities and compassion for myself, what a truly sensitive, caring, and giving person I am. For much of my life, my personality made me strive for accomplishments and to help others as a physician. But that came at a price because I wasn't giving enough to myself. It's no wonder I felt like I was giving and not getting anything back because I saw myself as a victim. My attempts to give were compulsive, exhausting, and often not appreciated, and I so badly needed to feel loved and appreciated in my work as a doctor. But here's my victim mentality in action: I was unable to allow myself to receive love because of the conflicted relationship I had with love as a child. I had locked love out of my life in victim-based protection and it was filling up with so much fear that suicide became my only perceived option.

That is why I am actually grateful for my Achilles rupture in February 2013 because, when that happened, I had nothing left to give—to others or to myself.

At that moment, my tank was empty. I had burned out. I loved helping people, but pushing myself harder was creating more pain than pleasure. When being a doctor wasn't enough, I tried harder, becoming a yoga teacher and stand-up comic. It was just another attempt to get the love and attention from others that I was, as it turned out, unwilling to receive or give to myself. If I had carried on that way, I'm quite sure I would have died.

On that tense note, I am finally going to get to the carrot and the stick I have been alluding to in the last bunch of chapters! If you have a mule and you want him to move, you can hit him with a stick or entice him with a carrot. My ego dragon spent much of my life hitting me with a stick, and now I am enticing my inner child self with carrots. It's a much kinder and more productive way for me to be.

Point to consider: What are your sticks? What do you use to drive yourself? What are your carrots? What do you like? What makes you feel good, and can you receive it?

105

Your Thinking Hurts More than It Helps

On your journey to healing, your ego will try to convince you that there is a thinking solution.

There isn't.

Of course, you need your thinking mind to be aware of the ego's tricks and to label them and embrace them. But after that awareness stage, most of the healing comes from feeling.

You can't heal what you refuse to feel. But when you are on your own side, using carrots instead of sticks, feeling becomes the better option and your emotional range increases. You begin to get better at feeling.

On the other hand, when we are stuck with the sticks and stones of compulsive thought and scary ruminations, afraid to go into the body and feel, we become victims to our own painted tigers and our emotional range progressively narrows. It's almost like our ego dragon signs an unconscious agreement as children to keep us in a narrowed range of emotion if that prevents us from feeling deep pain. Anytime we venture out to feel and go into our bodies, we use the sticks of thoughts and worries to beat ourselves back up into our heads.

You are much more than your thoughts. Your thoughts and worries are only a small part of your life experience but they seem so overwhelming and scary because the alarm has shut off your rational mind. You have a complete and beautiful range of emotions you can live in, now that you've given your ego dragon a carrot (or whatever dragons like to eat) to let you begin to experience all of your emotions, not just the painful ones.

As you practice the ABCs, you'll feel the awareness in yourself that love can be trusted, especially from yourself.

You may perceive that a *person* may not be trustable, but love is love. I know my father loved me very much, but as he got older, his illness got in the way. You can be sensitive and thin-skinned in a safe environment or you can be thick-skinned in a challenging environment, but both my dad and I suffered the worst combination—being highly sensitive in a challenging environment. And the odds are strong that you had that latter combination as well or, at the very least, the sensitive part.

I've learned a new feeling story with my father. He loved me very much, and I remember all the things he would do for me as a young child, taking me fishing, showing me how to ride a bike, catching and hitting a ball, and playing chess with me. You know, dad stuff. The more I focus on the good memories with my father, the more good memories I recall. I don't know if you've heard me say this but what you focus on, you will perceive more of (ha ha). I am lucky in many ways because I knew my father loved me, and I can focus on the feeling of that.

So I focus on the good parts of him. It's much more compassionate than the alternative—to myself and to him. He did the best he could, and his real self would shine through sometimes, even in the late stages of his illness. As I focus on his playfulness, sense of humor, and his natural teaching and coaching ability, I remember more of that, and I am more willing to see myself in him.

It is so easy to blame our parents, but I always ask my patients, "How was your parents' childhood?" Then I remind and assure people that for the most part, you can't give what you didn't get. We are all innocent souls, but trauma, especially childhood trauma, moves us away from our authentic selves and toward our reactive selves, and reactive selves can to damage. You've probably heard the phrase "hurt people, hurt people." My father hurt me, no question, but he also put me on a path to help others and write this book. Even just before he died, my dad would share music or a book with me, or an interest in me becoming a physician. I even believe his suicide was a compassionate way of releasing the family from more pain, as in lucid moments he could see how hard it was on all of us—but especially on him, of course.

Simply put, the more you focus on practicing the ABCs and embracing feeling over thinking, the more you'll heal. And the more you heal, the easier it becomes to feel (and be) truly connected to yourself in all the feelings you hold. As your connection within yourself grows, your relationships with others grow too because your SES expands to feel the joy and the pain without the ego's protective need to narrow a feeling sensation with a thinking explanation. Again, healing from anxiety is not so much about feeling better (although that happens) but getting better at feeling.

106

Belief

I said earlier that I would return to beliefs. Did you believe me? Even if you didn't, I can love that about you.

Just because you believe something does not make it objectively true. Beliefs can be an accurate representation of reality, or not. Of note, for us worriers, if we are in survival mode created by alarm, the chances that our belief is valid and true decrease significantly when compared to the exact same belief when we are in a calm, peaceful state in the mind and body.

Beliefs begin as thoughts which, with repetition, are then elevated to perceptions. Those perceptions turn into hypotheses. If those hypotheses are confirmed by repetition, they become beliefs. Much of this goes on outside of awareness, usually in childhood. Here is a critical point: those perceptions and subsequent hypotheses are *subjective*. The child-generated hypothesis can be (and often is) completely false. (Remember how children wrongly blame themselves for the pain in their households?)

Our experiences shaped our perceptions of ourselves and the world. The ego gathers information throughout our existence and, along with our amygdala (and other brain structures), guides our subsequent perceptions and behaviors based on those earlier perceptions. If those perceptions are repeated, we create a belief system that we rely on to inform us if the world is safe or not. The more unresolved trauma we carry (as background alarm), the more our perceptions will reflect that dangerous worldview—and the more we will perceive our environment as a place we need to be protected from. You will see more of what you already believe, and if you learned to take JABS at yourself as a child, you ingrain that mindset and "believe" or confirm negative things about yourself, and what's worse, you'll discount or simply ignore positive ones. Of course you're going to stockpile alarm energy!

I'll always remember the poignant way one of my patients, Carl, gave voice to some of the false beliefs he'd developed as a child to make sense of his pain. When Carl was young, his mother would fly into a rage every couple of weeks, then would lock herself in her room and typically not come out for two or three days, leaving Carl and his father at a complete loss. Carl told me each time she would withdraw, he would think, "I wonder if I've done something to upset her," or "She's hiding because of me." When he came to see me at the time he entered university, together we worked on shining the light of awareness on his belief that he was the cause of his mother's pain, and that belief was keeping him in alarm and anxiety. Because his mother's raging behavior started when Carl was a toddler, the belief that he was the cause was deep in him.

Now, here's the complicated part.

Body beliefs are not going to be changed by simply correcting them cognitively. If simply telling yourself not to believe something would actually heal it, a full course of psychotherapy would last about twenty-two minutes and cost about fifty bucks. We need to see those implicit, body beliefs in awareness first and then use a process to rewire them. That process is the ABCs. As you get more adept at the ABCs, you'll be able to use compassion to rewire your negative beliefs about yourself and the world.

We give our beliefs so much power, and in that power they are hard to change. On top of that, they hide in the shadows of our psyche so we don't consciously see them, so we unconsciously start to be them. *Without conscious awareness, we see our beliefs as who we are, and we are what we believe.* These beliefs form deep grooves because they have been ingrained by the ego dragon, scored in us since we were young children. Many of my protective beliefs were in me for more than fifty years!

When I left the practice of medicine, my ego dragon got all fired up because it had built up a belief that as long as I was a doctor I was protected (although in reality the opposite was more true). It wasn't until I was able to consciously see I held the belief "I am safe if I stay in medical practice" that I truly saw practicing medicine was killing me—and that's when I was able to make the compassionate choice to leave. Leaving medicine to pursue a career in helping others with anxiety has been the best life choice I have ever made.

THE POWER OF BELIEF

As you learned way back at the beginning of this book, your thoughts need to be believed to have any power over you. But if you struggle with anxiety, your alarm-based beliefs have been slow baked into your body since childhood and kept warm by your dragon. They lie beneath your awareness, yet it takes very little to fire them up.

A belief held outside of your awareness is a monstrous force. But once you make the unconscious conscious, you can choose not to be automatically led by your anxious thoughts. And simply bringing awareness defuses much of the pain behind the beliefs and anxious thoughts because it brings you into present-moment sensation and out of the pain body of your past and the worries of your projected future. You have a friend in your adult self to help you share the burden of that pain.

You know how you watch a movie like *Star Wars* with fantastical elements like laser swords or talking aliens in a bar and you're just supposed to suspend disbelief? Well, here, with your worries and ingrained false perceptions of yourself and your environment, I am asking you to *suspend belief.* You can think the thought, but allow it to sit in awareness before you compulsively believe everything you think.

This suspension of thinking is in contradiction to much of what I've read about healing or diffusing anxiety. I do not agree with authors who suggest critically appraising your thoughts for truth with the assumption that if you see your thoughts as false, those thoughts will disappear. It's like seeing that your odds of dying in a plane crash are one in eleven million will magically extinguish your anxiety about flying, or seeing your worries are irrational will somehow dissolve them. Spoiler alert: it won't. You just can't think your way out of a feeling problem—the more you think, the more you dig.

If you ask me, there's no point in trying to change your mind when you are in alarm—but I do see a lot of point in changing your body, because that is where your alarm and your implicit beliefs are stored. Your body must be calmed before your mind will change. A premise of somatic experiencing therapy is you cannot heal without a sense of safety. Your rational brain is paralyzed by the alarm in your body, so why are you trying to think when your mind is impaired? It's like trying to solve an algebra problem while you are being held at gunpoint.

Instead of trying to think while you are alarmed, wait to look at the objective facts of the situation *after you've gone through your ABCs.* Once you've moved out of your survival brain that is feeding your compulsive, future-based thinking and worry and change course into the awareness of present-moment sensation in your body, those things that appeared overwhelming will look much more manageable.

You can't think your way out of a feeling issue, but you can feel your way out. Let's stop reflexively bailing water trying to change the way we *think* and start reflectively patching the hole in the hull by changing the way we *feel.*

107

Faith Has No Victims and Victims Have No Faith

I had a profound awakening after I formed and committed to my intention to bring awareness to my anxious thoughts and my alarm. It was a deep realization that when my dad's trauma took my innocence as a child, it took my faith with it. When that happened, I lost the innocent, childlike view that I was whole and complete. I know now that in order to regain access to our innocent self, we must have faith in the inherent order and safety of the world. Without faith, we will be forever trapped in the ego-based protection of victimhood.

Simply and truthfully put, faith is often difficult for those of us who did not have secure attachment as children. It is hard for us to have faith in other people and the world when our trust was broken in our formative years by people who were supposed to have our best interests at heart. Without inherent faith that we are welcomed, supported, and loved, the fear bias of our human brains has nothing to balance out its bias to look for threats to our survival. Like fear and love being mutually exclusive in the box of your psyche, faith and danger have a similar mutually exclusive relationship. The more danger you put in (your worries), the more faith you push out; and the more faith you put in, the more worries you push out.

To put it in very simple terms, faith fosters trust and growth. Victimhood sparks alarm and protection. As long as you are a victim, you have no access to the soothing and healing power of faith because your dragon, in a misguided effort to protect you, will keep you locked in judgment, abandonment, blame, shame, resistance, defensive detachment, inability to receive, and compulsive thinking.

Until you choose to see it so you don't have to be it.

As a child, I developed a perceptual framework that the world was a dangerous place, and this framework was reinforced by my father's psychosis and the lack of trust in my caregivers to look after my emotional needs. As a result of this loss of faith in my caregivers or the world to provide a safe place for me (and throw in some bullying from my peers), I unconsciously transferred my safety to my ego dragon.

Children growing up in traumatic environments lose faith that the world has their backs and often resolve not to need anything and become highly self-sufficient—because this seems like a better option than dealing with the hurt of expecting support and being disappointed time and time again. As they get older, this self-denial is often accompanied by a coping strategy to be there for others, and they learn to become much more adept at meeting other people's needs over their own. This may give the illusion of being in control, but this lack of self-reference and self-care deepens background alarm because the child sees themselves as a victim starved for love and attention, especially from their very own selves. As we give to others while blocking our own ability to receive, we lose even more faith in the world and become more convinced we are victims. The worst part may be that we are victimizing ourselves.

One of the most damaging effects of childhood trauma is as we lose faith in others, we adopt the unconscious and damaging idea that everything is now up to us. Can you see how alarming it would be for a child to believe everything was up to them and know that they were still a powerless child?

Since people are wired to lovingly connect to other people, continually giving yourself the message that everything is up to you and you can't depend on anyone for anything, coupled with believing you are responsible for other people's needs over your own, makes the world feel like a very alarming place. When you are unable to access your SES, not only do you make it impossible to release the alarm you already have, but you create even more. As stated earlier, as alarm (sense of danger) increases, faith in the world diminishes in a vicious cycle.

Faith is fostered by a benevolent relationship with the world and the people in it. Can you see how you would have issues maintaining relationships if your alarm shut off your SES? Can you see how you might be able to feel close one minute and completely dissociated the next? Your relationship with other people can be no better than your relationship with yourself. If your alarm disengages your SES, you can't connect with yourself or others, and as a result, 1) you can't meet your own needs; 2) your relationships with others often become focused on meeting their needs; 3) the child in you feels abandoned from the inside; 4) the child in you feels abandoned and victimized by others (when it is you who defensively detaches from them); 5) it is child you who adopted the belief you must do it all yourself and won't trust your caregivers to look after you for fear that they will let you down once again. All five of these decrease your faith and increase your alarm.

Paradoxically, when you fully recognize that you can meet your own needs as an adult now, it also becomes okay to depend on other people.

You also get better at detecting which people to have faith in. You can even ask people for things and know you'll be able to handle it if they say no. Acting from a place of awareness and compassionate connection with yourself, you can take it one step at a time without spiraling into the repetition compulsion of reenacting your childhood pain of being abandoned. Whatever you focus on you'll see more of and that definitely goes for faith. Faith in yourself, faith in others, and faith in the world.

You don't have to have perfect faith right away. You can start with just a little. When you meet someone new and start to assume they'll eventually hurt you or disappoint you so it's not worth getting to know them, you can bring awareness to that thought, notice how it feels in your body, and have compassion for the child inside who was hurt so many times. And from that place, you can choose to take a chance and believe that this person just might be worth letting in—not necessarily every person in the whole wide world. You can start with just one person.

And that person is you. Having faith in your own compassionate connection to yourself by doing the ABCs on a regular basis will help reestablish the faith you lost as a child. What you seek is seeking you; you just have to have the faith to open up and allow it. As you see that you are not going to withdraw from yourself and that you are a consistent, loving, and compassionate presence for yourself, you learn to be the parent now you so wish you had back then. As your faith in yourself increases, you develop a stronger relationship internally, and that leads to a stronger relationship with others externally (and a significant and progressive decrease in your alarm).

Whatever you focus on, you'll get more of. Faith creates more faith, and victimhood creates more victimhood. Faith, along with being the antidote for uncertainty, is also the path to escape from victimhood. Faith in yourself and the world doesn't mean you aren't going to face challenges. It does mean that you don't have to know the outcome before the start of the game, and you don't have to do it all yourself. As you connect with yourself you will connect with others, and this eases your alarm. Your nervous system can learn, via neuroplasticity, that life is indeed about connection and safety, even in the face of uncertainty. Faith embraces uncertainty for it knows uncertainty is the mother of opportunity and growth. Victims pull back in the face of uncertainty and withdraw into protection and worry, just like when they faced painful uncertainty in their childhoods. In victim mentality, we rely on hope that someone or something external to us will come to our rescue, but as I have said before: nobody is coming to save you. It is up to you to save you. And that begins with faith.

> "Take a chance on faith—not religion, but faith.
> Not hope, but faith. I don't believe in hope.
> Hope is a beggar. Hope walks through the fire.
> Faith leaps over it."
>
> —JIM CARREY, MAHARISHI UNIVERSITY OF MANAGEMENT
> COMMENCEMENT ADDRESS, MAY 24, 2014

Victims cower in the face of uncertainty, as opposed to people with faith in themselves who can embrace it, even embracing the pain. Choose faith and courage and your brain chemicals will support more of that. Choose victimhood and withdrawal and your brain will create more of that.

I don't want to sound like I am blaming victims. In many ways, adopting victimhood was a way the childhood ego could survive, and I know that I was a victim for a very long time. Even now, when I feel alarmed, I can still drive myself straight into the Victimtown tavern for a few shots of JABS and a worry chaser. But in growing faith in my compassionate connection to myself, I recognize the old familiar road and my dragon, and I confer and choose to turn around much earlier.

When you have faith in your world things don't happen *to* you; they happen *for* you. This is a saying that people with faith tend to, well, have faith in. I know I perceived my Achilles rupture as one of the worst things that ever happened to me and getting into medical school as one of the best. The truth may well be the opposite. The Achilles rupture led me to growth and to have faith in myself to leave medicine and create a career I love and produce this book. Getting into medical school drove me deep into protection and really took what was just a sensitivity and predisposition to anxiety and alarm into a full-blown disorder.

If events in your life seem to form a repeating pattern, can you get curious about the repetition compulsion they might be trying to show you? The next time you find yourself thinking "Why does this always happen to me?" can you flip it to "How can I see this as happening *for* me?" or "What opportunity to rely on myself am I missing here?" or "What is this a replication of from my childhood?" (After doing your ABCs, of course, because the first question is a telltale sign you're in alarm.) I know this sounds a little Pollyanna, and "Turn that frown upside down, mister!" But I assure you, faith is a mindset, just as victimhood is a mindset. Like anything else, the more you focus on it, the more you'll see its influence in your life.

In short, having faith is the ability to not only let the uncertain remain uncertain but to embrace uncertainty as fertile ground for growth. And as you build up your track record of tolerating uncertainty, you also build your confidence that you'll be able to do so in the future. And you begin to see yourself as victor instead of victim.

When I speak of faith, it is not so much faith in a higher power (although that can help) as it is a faith in your own innocent self. Much of why we develop a victim mentality is because we have given over our power to something (like a dragon) or someone else. I am in no way against a belief in God, but as the psychologist, speaker, and author of *12 Rules for Life,* Jordan B. Peterson, points out (and I am paraphrasing), you can believe in God, but take responsibility for your own damn life.

The more I adopted victimhood as a coping strategy, the less I was able to take responsibility for my own damn life, and the more alarm I dumped into my system.

At its core, victimhood is making someone or something responsible for our circumstances and for changing them. As children we were victims in many ways because we had no choice, but we are not children anymore (but our amygdala didn't get the memo).

When our caregivers were unable to meet our needs, we never stopped hoping they would come back and do their job. This is how a traumatic childhood so often leads to a state of victimhood later in life—many of us are still waiting for our parents to see us, hear us, understand us, and protect us. As I said earlier, consciously we know that our parent is not going to change and start caring for us in the way we wanted, but unconsciously the child in us never gives up the ideal of the benevolent, loving, and connected parent. And often we don't take responsibility for our own needs, connections, and self-care because we unconsciously assume that one magical day our parent (or parent figure) is coming back to save us.

Again, no one is coming to save you—and by practicing what's in this book, eventually you will see that's a good thing. You could say when you stop hoping someone will come along and save you, this is happening for you and not to you. Instead of getting into yet another codependent relationship where you hope someone else will look after you and make you happy (which so many of us do when we have unresolved childhood trauma and alarm), you can step up and develop the emotional capacity to see you don't need anyone else to save you because *you* will save you. Note that this is different from the "lone wolf" denying connection that many of us adopted in childhood protection. It is the conscious intention that you will make a loving connection to your younger self and give them now what that child in you SHOULD have received long ago. I can tell you I feel some unconscious part of me is still waiting for my dad to return and give me the guidance and love to help me feel cared for, whole, and worthy—to be the teacher and protector he was in the first ten years of my life. There is a part of me that wants my father back the way he was when he was healthy and strong. I am aware of that part, and through the practice of making a conscious, compassionate connection to myself, I have taught myself to have faith in my own ability to give that lonely child in me the love, compassion, care, and teaching he needs. To have faith in myself to become my own wise father.

Waiting for a figure to come back and save us or putting that responsibility on a partner, friend, child, or anyone else locks us in a victim mentality where we depend on others to love us when all the while we won't love ourselves. In addition, I can tell you from personal experience that believing you will be quickly healed from decades of alarm by some doctor, treatment, supplement, patch, drug, psychedelic, hypnosis, meditation, or therapy is a fool's errand. As Dr. Nicole LePera, known as the Holistic Psychologist, says, and I unequivocally agree, "There is no quick fix." There is no doubt those things can help, but to truly heal on a deeper level, we need to relentlessly regain faith in our authentic, innocent selves and stop being victims by hoping that something or some magical "other" outside of us will come to our rescue. We must place the faith we need in ourselves. We must be our own magical figure and fiercely look after ourselves.

> *"What progress, you ask, have I made?*
> *I have begun to be a friend to myself."*
>
> —HECATO

Hope is a victim (victims hope to be rescued by someone or something outside of themselves). Victors keep the faith (faith in the moment being perfect for our growth and faith in ourselves for us to heal). We need to create faith that we can handle life and that the universe is a safe place regardless of our ego's relentless predictions to the contrary.

Look back at all the traumas you've had. Did you handle them? Are you still here? Sure, you may be suffering emotionally, but you made it through. And now you are reading a book that will show you how to empower yourself to begin to release your alarm and the subsequent anxiety that alarm creates. We need to realize we are not the alarmed children we once were.

We need to regain faith in our innocent selves again. We need to develop the faith in ourselves and the world that we lost as children. Taking responsibility for things you have no control over (the future) and that someone else will save you is a victim's hope-filled stance.

Taking responsibility for embracing uncertainty is an act of faith. I know that making a committed, conscious intention to have faith in the future—and to let the uncertain be gloriously uncertain—has been one of the best things I have done for my mental health. Instead of worry and rumination, I choose to use the ABCs and go into my body to find sensation and present-moment awareness instead of future-based doom.

I have faith in that process because it works, and it builds on itself, and it also builds faith in our connection with ourselves.

The more we stop being tricked by our dragon and come alongside it as a comrade in arms and find faith in all parts of our innocent selves, the more we break the devastating pattern of victimhood. With faith in our own connection to ourselves we can find our true power and embrace uncertainty in our body as opposed to running away from it in our mind. All anxiety is separation anxiety, and it's mostly separation from yourself. As you resolve the ingrained pattern of (self) separation from your childhood you will resolve your alarm and anxiety. Faith and courage are brothers in arms. Courage is facing and embracing the unknown. It will take courage and faith in yourself to embrace the ABC process and do it consistently, especially early on when your ego dragon resists and blocks your own loving connection to yourself. But when you tell the dragon, "I'm not a child anymore and I've got this," you remove its responsibility to protect you, and it has no choice but to recede. The dragon won't acquiesce without resistance, but although you may not know it, you are the dragon master. It must obey you and stand down if you command it with faith and courage, but if you fall back into victim mentality, the dragon will rise back up and burn you. We need the guidance from our ego dragon, but we don't want it to overwhelm us, we just need it to perch on our shoulder.

The tangible evidence I've observed by using the ABCs to regain faith in myself is that I look after my own needs much more—genuinely, pro-actively caring for myself with the achievable goal of growth, as opposed to worrying with the unattainable goal of protection. The more adept you get at the ABC process, the more you'll see yourself looking after your own needs—not just because you know that you should but because you truly want to.

Being compassionate and connected with your innocent self when you are alarmed is probably the opposite of what you have been doing all your life. It is an unfortunate feature of the human species that we deal with emotional threats in the same way we deal with physical ones: by moving into dorsal vagal survival physiology that locks out the ventral vagal system we so badly need to connect to our SES and resolve the emotional pain that sparked this survival physiology in the first place. Our alarm makes us unable to accept the love we need to heal the alarm. The ABCs help circumvent this evolutionary bug in the system.

When we train ourselves to connect with ourselves instead of withdrawing during emotional stresses, we break that old habit and can move toward thriving instead of being fixated on surviving. But thriving takes time and practice when you've been surviving for so long. We have to be patient and fully committed to our own connection with a hypervigilant focus on truly seeing our own innocence. To heal from anxiety and alarm, we must have faith in our ability to connect and nurture our younger, innocent selves.

"Be here now."

—RAM DASS

Faith is being present. Faith is consciousness. Faith is in us; we are faith; faith *is* us. As children, when we lost our innocence, we lost our faith as well, and that is one reason childhood trauma is so devastating. When we lose faith in the world, we lose touch with our true selves and part of us stops moving toward growth, so the only remaining option is to retreat into protection and alarm. We invent an omnipotent protector dragon that blocks some of the pain, but at the cost of blocking love and connection to ourselves and others (the worst deal ever). Without that connection and ability to be open and vulnerable, our nervous system is forged in protection, and like the Roach Motel ads in the 1980s where "roaches check in but they don't check out," alarm gets in but it can't get out. Unless we can return to seeing ourselves as innocent souls and truly let love back in to push out the fear, we will be trapped in protection, anxiety, and alarm forever.

Love is a path to faith, and faith can be a path to love. Faith in ourselves, to quote the title of a wonderful book by spiritual teacher Marianne Williamson, is "a return to love"—to consciously choose love and compassion over fear and protection. Faith, love, and connection are all linked and self-perpetuating, as are fear, worry, and alarm. When you see you are in anxiety or alarm, you can use the ABCs as a path to connect with and comfort the true, authentic self you left behind, and join your adult self to that child self to become whole again.

Moving from victimhood to faith at the level of thinking is short-lived. The ego dragon (like the Sirens) will always be able to seduce you back into victim mode of chronic worry, as there is not enough grounding resonance in thought alone. You can't overcome thinking with more thinking! The ABCs change your perception at the level of feeling, and feeling does have the resonance to keep you grounded—and as you do this more, your faith grows and you get better at feeling *and* feel better.

Throughout this book, I have maintained that protection and growth are mutually exclusive, but faith may be the place they intersect. Having faith both protects you and allows you to grow at the same time. Ego-based protection is an illusion because it exhausts you by relentlessly trying to predict the future from a place of fear. Ego-based protection has no substance to it because it is a prediction of the future that is, by definition, unknown. Faith, on the other hand, acknowledges that your compulsive, childlike need for protection is neither helpful nor necessary, for faith comes from inside of you and can never be taken away. Faith does not require an elaborate series of unpredictable events to be analyzed and protected against. The ego has a multitude of complex options to consider for the future, whereas faith is a single, simple pathway that is clearly present in every moment we choose to trust in it. It is awareness that allows us to see and choose the path of the ego or the path of faith.

In our awareness, we always have a choice to choose faith in every moment. Faith is always one conscious decision away in every circumstance. Faith is a singular path on the solid ground of courage and trust, grounding us in the reality of the present moment. Worry, on the other hand, is an infinite ocean surrounding us in all directions, in which we are treading water that chronically threatens to drown us in our own imaginings.

When we are in alarm and separate from ourselves, our need for ego protection dominates and we inadvertently create pain by trying to avoid pain. When we are connected to ourselves, we can rest in faith that we will deal with whatever arises, just as we have dealt with painful losses in our past.

Despite being a complete anxious mess upon entering medical school, I had faith in myself. Deep down I knew I could do it. My ego challenged me greatly, but through the pain of chronic, intense daily alarm, I had faith in myself—and I graduated four years later with two academic awards and as president of my graduating class. Like most worriers, as a victim I underestimated my abilities and overestimated my challenges, which is the exact opposite of faith.

I truly believe that faith in myself (facilitated by my ABC practice) has changed my physiology and my psychology. I am moving from a fear-based belief system that I created as a child, in which I needed my dragon to protect me, to a love-based belief system where I can be fed by my connection with my own true, innocent self. Faith allowed me to take responsibility for my own life and to live much more in growth and much less in protection. The more my physiology reflected confidence and safety, the easier it was to stay in the sensation down in my body and not be seduced into the victim mentality of compulsive worry and rumination up in my mind. My positive physiology then reflected my positive psychology. Faith allowed a grounded presence in my body so I no longer had to retreat into the trap of my mind.

For the first time in my life, the ABCs have given me a safe place to ground in my body.

Faith is embracing uncertainty and not going past the moment you are in. Faith is avoiding the need to predict or control. Your whole journey with anxiety and alarm stems from your child self's desire to control and avoid uncertainty because that uncertainty was excruciating. What if you just stopped trying to control it? A mantra for this is: "This is uncertain . . . and I can love that!"

But you can only allow and embrace the unknown from a place of faith in yourself, a grounded physiology that ultimately comes from knowing and fully believing in your own innocence. The call to explain and predict and control and worry has led you to immeasurable pain. But it is a habit of a child based in the need for protection. You have a choice to make that need for (over)protection no longer true for the adult you are now. In compassion for yourself, you see there is no anxious thought worth having and the most loving action is to let go, take the energy once used to follow the Siren song of your worries, and use that energy to create faith in the moment and yourself through the ABCs.

I cannot tell you the number of times in my life that I have been sure I was dying of some disease or condition, beyond panic, collapsed on my bed in terror that I was doomed. That went on for forty years.

Forty years.

What a relief it is to trade that alarm for faith. Faith in myself, faith in love, and faith that when my time comes, it is what it is. I do not have some magical power to change the future by worry and rumination, so instead, I leave it to faith in myself and in the safety and order that is inherent in the universe. This is the safety that your child self could not see—because it was not available to child you back then, but it is available to adult you now if you cultivate the faith to choose it.

There is no treatment, vitamin regimen, workshop, book, medication, drug, or exercise addiction that is going to heal you. You have to heal you, and you do that by minimizing separation from yourself.

As hard as it may be for you to believe, you do love yourself. You have always had love for yourself, but your protective ego dragon has blocked it under the guise of protecting you. Alarm (and anxiety) was created and magnified as you blocked love for yourself as a child. It is time to remove those blocks to loving yourself and to find connection and faith in your true, innocent self.

Choosing the ABCs over your ego dragon requires a leap of faith. And you can find the courage to make that leap when you get grounded in your body—when you get out of your thoughts and into your feelings.

Awareness is where your healing starts. Awareness is your biggest ally in breaking the alarm-anxiety cycle for good. You can't heal what you can't (or refuse to) see.

Once again, nobody is coming to save you. It is only you who can save you. It is going back to the child in you who created the overprotective dragon in the first place. What you seek is truly seeking you. The child in you is looking for you, and the alarm you feel is its beacon.

A victim runs from uncertainty, faith gives you the power to break through it, and the chemicals in your brain and body will support whatever path you pick. Once you have learned to embrace faith in uncertainty as the spice of life, your confidence increases in your own ability to overcome—to be victor instead of victim. By releasing the need to predict the future, you'll stop supplying energy to your powerless victim and, instead, redirect that energy into growing your faith and self-confidence. As you create a caring connection with your innocent self, increasing faith is a natural by-product of that loving commitment within you.

Before I leave this critical chapter, I want to show how faith takes the fire out of the ego dragon. In us worriers, discipline is absolutely critical when it comes to faith. The seduction to fall into worry is intense to say the very least, and you can use faith as an entry point to the ABCs, as well as develop faith as a practice of its own. Again, this is not faith in a higher power (but that can certainly help) so much as it is faith in your own self, but you must discipline yourself to avoid the seduction and repetition compulsion of your worries and move to a place of sensation over explanation.

One of the most powerful benefits of faith is that it grounds me in a safe place where I can suspend my belief in my worries. Worries have an urgency to them and make us feel we have to do something immediately. Faith provides the conscious space to do my ABCs, and that conscious connection with myself breaks my old unconscious connection to worry.

Because discipline is so important in employing faith, I want to use the same type of repetition here that we did when discussing discipline. The groove in the snow runs deep when it comes to defaulting to anxious thoughts, so we have to create a new groove.

Faith in yourself disarms self-judgment by focusing on the best in you.

Faith in yourself disarms self-abandonment by joining your child self to your adult self.

Faith in yourself disarms self-blame because it fosters responsibility over guilt.

Faith in yourself disarms self-shame because it creates forgiveness and understanding.

Faith in yourself disarms inability to receive by constantly giving to you.

Faith in yourself disarms defensive detachment because it attaches you to yourself.

Faith in yourself disarms compulsive thinking by showing thoughts are simply not needed.

Faith in yourself disarms resistance by providing a place to flow into the peace of the moment.

Faith in yourself disarms victim mentality by building your courage to move toward uncertainty.

Faith in yourself is faith in your innocence.

As a final critical point, faith allows you to sit with the uncertainty now that was unbearable back then. Like the smoker who wants to quit smoking but finds a cigarette in their mouth with no idea how it got there, we worriers will often fall onto the worry train so quickly and so insidiously we don't see a moment when we could have gotten off it. In a commitment to a practice of awareness and faith in ourselves, we can create that space between stimulus and response that Viktor Frankl talked about. In that space of awareness, there is choice to move down into the present-moment grounding of your body where before there was only the path up into future-based worry. If you can consistently fill that space with a commitment to faith in your connection to yourself, putting your hand on your chest and breathing in a loving connection, you will create a new, self-deepening groove that tracks you consistently toward faith in yourself and the ABCs and away from automatic and compulsive worry.

There is a reason this is the longest chapter. Faith really is the crux of everything. You need a leap of faith to jump over the fire of the ego dragon and reconnect with the innocent self the dragon hid inside the treasure chest so many years ago. This faith arises from your awareness and intention to access the chest and connect with the innocent child in you that was hurt so much they lost their faith and adopted the belief that everything was up to them.

Revisiting that traumatized child is hard, but relentless faith in bond to yourself and belief in your innocence are exactly the keys to your healing. By bringing that child in you out of the past amygdala-driven fear back then and into the present-moment sensation of connection with the adult in you today, you learn to heal your anxiety instead of just coping with it. Your younger, traumatized self is still in you, and that part needs to know you are there to comfort them in love and growth, as opposed to leaving them in the chest alone under the dragon's "protection." While you are split from yourself and your innocent self is sequestered away, you are powerless to overcome your alarm and anxiety. We heal in relationship, and there is no relationship more important than the one we have with ourselves.

The leap of faith comes when your adult self opens the chest, pulls out your innocent child self, and fully accepts, embraces, and loves them no matter what that child thought, said, or did (or failed to do). This allows us to learn that we are indeed safe in our own love and do not need the dragon's protection to face the world anymore. We have something infinitely more powerful: our faith in our connection to ourselves.

The ABC process connects your thinking adult self to your feeling child self and dissolves the separation that caused the alarm and anxiety in the first place. Whenever you are worried or alarmed, it is because you have become split and fallen back into the proverbial hole of believing you can think your way out of a feeling when really you're just digging yourself in deeper. When you get caught in the trap of overthinking, you lose connection with the feeling child in you. The ABCs are there to show you how your child self can feel their way out with your present-day love and connection supporting their growth.

A part of us stopped growing at the time of our trauma. When we are alarmed, our amygdala sends us straight back to the helpless child we once were. We need to go back and retrieve that child and build their nervous system now in a way that wasn't possible back then. Creating faith in our connection to that child starts that neuroplastic process and the ABCs deepen it. The more faith and effort we put into that connection, the more our child self sees they can trust our adult self, and our adult self sees they can trust our child self.

Anytime you become aware of anxiety and alarm, relief always starts with a connection to yourself. Having faith in your innocence of your whole being—no matter what you have ever thought, said, or done—will dissolve the separation that is at the root of your alarm and anxiety. A leap of faith to love and embrace your inner, younger self will accomplish what no medication, doctor, supplement, or spell will be able to do.

We heal by creating wholeness from the inside. Our commitment to faith in ourselves is what will heal the separation that is at the root of our alarm and anxiety. The ABCs at their core are a vehicle to develop an unwavering faith in our connection to ourselves.

If we worriers fear uncertainty most of all, faith—specifically, faith in ourselves—is our most powerful antidote. A simple touch of your hand to your chest and a deep breath in, reassuring yourself of your own presence, and assuring yourself "I am safe in this moment," can make the difference between a life spent in self-abandonment, alarm, and anxiety on the one hand, and a life spent in flow and connection with your authentic, innocent self on the other.

Using the ABCs trains you to consciously go to faith in your connection to yourself, creating a new groove that consistently and relentlessly tracks you away from worry. Ultimately, the worry was a distraction from the pain of alarm, and as you connect with yourself, that alarm dissolves, since the alarm was simply your younger self asking for your connection and love. If you give yourself that connection, the alarm is no longer needed.

I have no doubt this book will have helped you understand and heal from chronic anxiety and alarm. But the information is of limited benefit unless you make it a part of your daily life. Be warned, your ego dragon will try to trick you to abandon faith in your authentic self and slide back to the familiar groove of the alarm-anxiety cycle. That may simply look as insidious as abandoning the ABCs and just settling back into your old habit of worry. Worry will be your alarm signal that you have fallen back into the old childhood groove of fearing uncertainty.

Uncertainty will be your greatest teacher and your greatest opportunity to call on its antidote: faith. Know you will be faced with uncertainty and your ego's automatic reaction will be to transport you into alarm from your past or to start to worry about your future. In both cases, you abandon yourself because you leave the present moment. Staying with yourself, putting a hand on your chest, and taking a breath and staying in sensation (even if it hurts!) teaches you that uncertainty is bearable and you do not have to retreat into past alarm or leapfrog into future worries. Further, faith in the moment flows with, and completely embraces, the gift of uncertainty and shows you that uncertainty can be pleasurable because, perhaps for the first time in your life, there is truly nothing to do and nowhere to go!

At their core, anxiety and alarm thrive on intolerance of the uncertainty of our future. Over time, you teach yourself that uncertainty does not have to be a one-way superhighway to anxiety and alarm that it has been in your past.

Turning to faith in your present-moment connection to yourself when you are faced with uncertainty will always soothe you, no matter how much the worrying Sirens of your ego tell you otherwise. Faith shows you that the answer to "Am I safe in this moment?" is always "Yes, I am here *with* you and I am here *for* you."

Here is an exercise I draw on every . . . single . . . day. I know that worry and faith cannot coexist, so try this.

> When you become aware you are in worry, close your eyes, put your hand on your chest, do a few rounds of the physiological sigh, relax your shoulders and your jaw, and say to yourself, "I am just going to leave this to faith," and suspend thought by consciously directing your attention to a fierce intentional awareness of sensation. Keep breathing and stay with sensation.

Your focus on sensation will slow you down and that slowness is out of sync with the frenetic pace of your thoughts and worries, which starves those worries of energy.

After you do this a number of times it will become a safe go-to that gives you a sense of peace within your worries. Over time, you teach yourself to go to faith and stillness, and that is a place that worries have no power, because their only strength comes from your belief that you can predict the future. This sounds simple, and it is. It is one of my most trusted and effective strategies when I find I have slipped into worry.

Whew! This chapter just went on and on. I guess you're just going to have faith that I know what I'm doing. If you find that your anxiety and alarm rise up on you, just come back and read this one chapter. I have the ultimate faith that it will ground you and help you through.

108

Gratitude Is the End and the Beginning

So, we have our ABCDEs, and with *F* we added faith. To close this book, I will add *G* for gratitude.

Many people keep gratitude journals, and I do think that is a good idea, as it does change your physiology and psychology. Often this gratitude journal is for external things in your life that you're grateful for, like people or events. But I want you to develop a gratitude journal or practice specifically to capture and reflect on traits and characteristics you appreciate in yourself.

Make an intention to focus on, and really feel, compassion and love for yourself—and not just for you now, but gratitude for yourself at every age and stage of your life. Gratitude for the scared child who needed protection, and gratitude for the person you were who got through times you were lost in your anxiety and just doing the best you could. This process will supercharge your faith and connection with yourself.

Just as discipline and faith work together, the *C* and *G* in this alphabet can work together. If during your compassion practice you call to mind reasons you are proud of yourself, then when it's time for gratitude, you can bring those traits or accomplishments to mind and really feel into gratitude for the gifts you have. The key is to connect with the feeling and not just think (or say or write) the words. I can say to myself, "I am proud of you for writing this book," but if I take a breath, say it out loud, and commit to feeling that sense of pride, it will change my physiology—and I can feel it right away as my heart expands and my face starts to move into a smile.

If you are having a hard time finding things you love about yourself, please know that's not at all uncommon among worriers! Try searching online "list of positive traits" and choose the ones that resonate with you. And don't tell me you don't have positive traits, that's just your victim mentality talking.

In addition to reflecting on what you're grateful for in yourself right now, I would encourage you to set an intention to find qualities to be grateful for in your child self as well. You can tell yourself things like "I loved how sensitive and caring you were" or "I loved what a great swimmer you were" or "I loved how you took care of your dog"—and really feel each one. If you can say this to your picture on the bathroom mirror, all the better. It is critical to remember that the child your overprotective ego takes JABS at is also the source of your very best traits!

Building a positive self-image and connection to yourself helps you build faith. As you build faith in yourself, whatever you focus on you get more of, and your confidence increases and you see more of the positives of your innocent self. If all anxiety is separation anxiety and all alarm is separation alarm, then as you cultivate compassion, love, and gratitude for yourself, you heal the separation—and when the separation heals, the alarm heals too. As the alarm disappears, it takes the anxious thoughts with it.

When we were younger, uncertainty made us feel powerless, but it turns out that this is actually where our power lies: in our ability to embrace and love uncertainty and the unknown, to do our ABCs full of faith and gratitude; in our choice to see the innocence of our inner child and the innocence of life in general.

Seen from a grounded commitment to present-moment awareness, the unknown can now be a place of possibility and faith instead of apprehension. We can have gratitude for our ability to embrace uncertainty as part of the fun and feeling of life. When we view uncertainty this way, it has a peaceful, open quality, and loses the sense of fear that creates such alarm in us. We don't have to fill the gap in our uncertain future with worry—we don't actually have to fill it with *anything*, and not having to fill every moment with thought was a huge revelation for me. As the pain of uncertainty was our biggest challenge in childhood, it requires a special awareness in adulthood; when we see it, we do not have to be it.

You may get some help along the way from therapists and counselors—and the old wounds heal faster with the connection of another person, especially one who knows how to work with trauma stored in the body—but true healing is an inside job. After trying just about every kind of therapy, medication, plant medicine, yoga, and meditation, I found that healing is based in my adult self connecting to my child self and my mind connecting to my body. To heal my mind, I had to feel my body. To feel better, I had to get better at feeling.

Even today, I feel that frightened young boy looking out his bedroom window fifty years ago, watching his father being taken away. But I commit to seeing, hearing, opening to, understanding, loving, and defending that boy (the SHOULD acronym) as I bring him out of his past loneliness and into today. Rusty lives with me now, safe in the knowledge that we are present together, right here and right now. He never has to go back there by himself ever again. I see my younger self and my father, and I love them both. I love my dad for the kind, sensitive, innocent soul he was, and I love my younger self for the kind, sensitive soul he was (and still is). I can feel that my dad lives in me, and I see his best traits in me when I am a dad to my daughter. Instead of pushing my father and his pain away, I welcome and cherish his presence and know that we are connected in a loving and compassionate way. I can feel that Rusty also lives in me and that we are also connected in a loving and compassionate way. I love the innocent soul I found dead on that January day, who chose to exit the world with his last written words: "It's not your fault. It's no one's fault. Love, Dad." I also love the innocent soul that found him.

It truly was no one's fault. The world is innocent and we are innocent. It is only our self-created blocks and subjective perceptions that make it appear any other way.

EPILOGUE

I wrote this book so that my father's pain meant something. It helps me considerably to know that the absolute torture he went through created some good in the world. My life's work has been to help as many people suffering from anxiety as possible, using what I have learned myself and from my teachers along the way. I have often said that my life's work is to ensure that no one has to suffer with anxiety as I did. I absolutely believe this book and my MBRX program will change the way anxiety is understood and treated worldwide, but I reiterate: Your ego dragon is fiercely powerful and will encourage you to abandon or "forget" what you have learned here and return to your childhood default state of hypervigilance and worry.

Please do not let that happen.

With love, Russell Kennedy, MD, April 19, 2024.

109

The Final Bead

ACKNOWLEDGING MY TEACHERS AND GUIDES

When I returned home from India, my now wife, Cynthia, made me a mala, a string of beads I use in meditation to keep track of a phrase or intention that I repeat 108 times. She made it from 108 beads of rose quartz, the stone of unconditional love, and a slightly larger 109th bead of malachite, the stone of transformation. When one uses a mala, every time a mantra or intention is repeated, a bead is moved. When you finish the 108 repetitions and reach the larger 109th bead, it is a time to be grateful for your teachers and guides who have helped you on your journey.

As this is the 109th chapter, or final "bead" on my journey of writing this book, I want to acknowledge those who have helped me along the way and made this book possible.

My acknowledgment of my dad is bittersweet. As he is the most important influence in this book being produced, I feel it's only right to give him the longest acknowledgment. From the time I watched out my bedroom window as the ambulance took him away, I told myself I would make sense of this mess. I know my dad wanted much more from his life than his illness would allow. From his early days in radio, he had something special, and his sense of humor and intelligence shone through. But he was also handicapped by severe emotional and physical childhood trauma.

On October 5, 1934, my father was born Beverly Lorne Germa in Sudbury, Ontario, Canada. Beverly was a common boy's name until 1955, but as he grew older, it was more known as a girl's name. Another strike against him. He was born premature, weighing just over twenty-five ounces. Yes, twenty-five ounces. That is just over a pound and a half. I remember my grandmother telling the story of how she could get her wedding ring up to his shoulder and that they brought him home in a shoe box with the expectation he would not survive.

But he did survive. Babies born today at that weight have a very poor prognosis even with all the advancements in pediatric ICUs. He is a miracle.

I acknowledge his pain in just surviving. I do regret withdrawing emotionally from him in my late teens, as his psychotic breaks were often as heartbreaking as they were embarrassing. In many ways, I am much closer to him now than I was when he was alive. I see him in a different way now. I can see that it was his illness that I was seeing and not the man himself. But I have some shame in telling you that back then, I was embarrassed by my dad. When I got into medical school (a success of mine he never saw as he died six months before I learned I had been accepted), I changed my surname from Germa (my birth name) to Kennedy, my mother's maiden name.

I like to joke that Dr. Kennedy sounds infinitely better than Dr. Germa.

Jokes aside though, I remember him the way he was in his more functional days, taking me fishing, teaching me to play sports and billiards. In a way, I feel that I am fulfilling part of his destiny to make a difference in the world, in a way he could have never done personally. So if this book has made a difference for you, if you would take a second and send him some gratitude for his sacrifice, I would deeply appreciate it—and I know he would too!

My mother kept our household together, and I am very grateful for her. She emigrated to Canada from Scotland in 1958 and worked as a registered nurse. In fact, my father was one of her patients and that is how they met. My mother had been listening to my father on his radio show and was a fan and, soon after his recovery, became his wife.

My mother is tough. At the time I write this in February 2024 she is ninety years old, physically good but terribly anxious (or should I say alarmed!). Through so many of my father's suicide attempts, depressions, manic phases, and just general craziness, I only saw her cry a handful of times. We always had a place to live and food to eat because of her Scottish work ethic. She would often take extra shifts to help us make ends meet, and I have an immense amount of gratitude for my mother and her many sacrifices. Her life has not been an easy one, and she has always supported my brother and me in a selfless and relentless code of honor. The Kennedy clan motto is *avise la fin* (consider the end), and she always made sure we were safe in the end.

My mom has always supported me, and she supported me in this book. She knows exactly what anxiety and alarm feel like for she has felt them for close to nine decades. Throughout it all, she has maintained a brilliant sense of humor that I inherited to become a stand-up comedian, and many of the funny parts of this book come from her love of laughter.

My wife, Cynthia, essentially saved my life, and therefore played a big role in getting this book to you. It would have been very difficult to write this book if I were dead. In 2013, with a ruptured Achilles and a ruptured mind, I could not have envisioned this day when I would be able to put my knowledge into the world. At the start of this journey of healing, Cynthia was there for me, nursing me back to health. It is a gift to be able to learn with her as we have taken many trainings and workshops together. Being able to draw on her expertise as a somatic trauma therapist has been invaluable in the creation of this book. "Cyn-Cyn" is a truly beautiful soul and a gift beyond measure.

There are some family members I need to acknowledge. My brother Scott, who experienced our dad's craziness firsthand and has raised a thriving family of his own. My daughter, Leandra, who has had her own struggles with the anxiety monster (and the sea monster!), has always lovingly supported me in my personal and professional endeavors. Leandra also showed me love is safe, and her ability to make me laugh is second to none. She is also the mother of my two grandchildren, Avielle and Angus, who both have the Kennedy sense of humor.

To my teacher Gila Golub I am eternally grateful. I still remember the day in October 2014 that she and her right-hand man, Dave Romer, and right-hand woman, Britta Frombach, picked me up from an emotionally devastating journey on ayahuasca. The teachings and support I received from Gila, Britta, and Dave would set the stage for this book, and I will be forever grateful to them for giving me some hope in some very dark nights of the soul.

Dr. Gordon Neufeld has been an invaluable mentor. As I grew in emotional strength, I resonated deeply with Dr. Neufeld's teachings. Much of the basis of my theory of alarm comes from Dr. Neufeld. This book would not have the same resonance and depth without what I received from him and the Neufeld Institute.

There are some doctors who have made a real impact on me in my life and career. Dr. John Noseworthy (who is now the CEO of the Mayo Clinic) was one of the kindest and most compassionate doctors I have come across in supporting me over the years of medical school. Also, Dr. Bruce Yoneda of Victoria, British Columbia, a fellow physician (and a former ice hockey teammate), is a man of great character and help to others and really went above and beyond the call of duty to surgically repair my ruptured left Achilles tendon. Bruce really looked after me and helped me get back on my feet emotionally and physically. Dr. Saul Isserow and Dr. Michael Mulvey have also been outstanding physicians who have propped me up in some very dark times. Mike is a psychiatrist and has always been very supportive of my nontraditional theories! Also, thanks to Nima Rahmany, DC, for his friendship and our endless conversations about human emotion and healing from trauma, and to my Aussie pal and colleague Dr. Jen Draper for her wisdom and support.

I do have my more ethereal and spiritual side, and I am grateful to medium Debra Doerksen for helping me access my intuitive nature, which played a big role in understanding the messages needed for the creation of this book. Also, thanks to Edward Dangerfield for helping me to use my breath to access a deeper place of peace and wisdom that also shows up in these pages.

A special thanks to my fellow physician Dr. Keith Holden, who inspired me and blazed an unconventional trail in following his own atypical path to healing himself and others.

To my teachers and therapists Sophia Buchholz, Linda Stelte, Berns Galloway, Tait MacFarlane, and Ginger Henderson for helping me heal and formulate the ideas in this book, thank you!

Many people have helped me with this manuscript by giving me invaluable feedback and supporting me over the years, especially my good friend Angela Rinaldis. Thank you, Ang, you have always been there for me!

I am thankful to my Facebook friend Galina Singer, who encouraged my writing ten years ago when I asked her for advice. Galina planted the seed that I could actually become a good enough writer to write a book. Galina didn't know me from anyone but helped me for no other reason than she is a good person. You never know what simply helping someone can lead to!

I am also grateful for the teachings of Nicole LePera, PhD, also known as the Holistic Psychologist. Nicole's work has had a distinct impact on my own, and the world is fortunate to have her.

Amanda Johnson of Awaken Village Press played an invaluable role in bringing the first edition of this book to fruition, and the first edition really started my career as a writer. My friend Robyn Ellingson told me I had been working on this book before she suggested I go to Shakti Mhi's yoga teacher training program in 2007. Sixteen years later Robyn is still helping with edits and advice!

I am very grateful to Mel Robbins, Dr. Rangan Chatterjee, and Chris Williamson for having me on their podcasts to promote the book.

Anya Hayes at Ebury Press UK contacted me after seeing Dr. Chatterjee's show and birthed the idea of a second edition. Anya has been so supportive and I so appreciate her taking the initiative to get this second edition started.

Joel Fotinos and Emily Anderson at St. Martin's Press in the US have been an absolute joy to work with. Emily has been so very patient with me with all my last-minute changes!

My literary agent, Jeff Silberman, has gone above the call of duty on more occasions than I can count, talking me off the ledge and moving things forward. He's a true mensch!

I must thank my team at The Anxiety MD: Dimitra Emanuela Asimakis, Emi Geylan, and Leandra Yellowlees, as they have been invaluable in helping me build my message and get my work into the world.

Finally, I have seen people acknowledge their anxiety as a gift. While I'd love to say that my anxiety was a gift and that I am grateful for it, I'm not quite there yet. What I can say is, "I have anxiety, and I can love that about myself!"

What I am deeply grateful for, and anxiety and alarm have certainly helped me with this, is the opportunity to see and embrace my innocent self and to take Rusty with me wherever I go. Oh yes, thank you, Rusty, for your love and support.

Glossary of Terms

ALARM An activated energy buried in the body from old, unresolved trauma stored in the body. The root cause of the anxiety in the mind.

ALARM-ANXIETY CYCLE The self-reinforcing feedback loop the theory of this book is based on. Alarm stored in the body activates worrisome thoughts of the mind and the worries of the mind activate the alarm stored in the body.

AMYGDALA The bilateral, almond-shaped structure in the temporal lobes of the brain that is involved in virtually every real or imagined danger we face.

ANXIETY The warnings, what-ifs, and worst-case scenarios the mind compulsively creates in an effort to keep you up in your mind and therefore away from the old pain of alarm stored down in your body.

AUTONOMIC NERVOUS SYSTEM (ANS) A part of our peripheral nervous system that relays signals to and from the viscera, controlling the automatic, involuntary functions of the body. The ANS is typically separated into sympathetic (fight or flight) and parasympathetic (rest and digest) wings.

AWARENESS For the purposes of this book, the act of consciously directing attention to a present-moment sensation, feeling, emotion, thought, or worry.

BACKGROUND ALARM An uncomfortable energy that sits unconsciously in the background of our (mostly unconscious) awareness that drives the worries of our mind.

CALIBRATION With regards to this book, the process by which the autonomic nervous system learns to tune in and adjust itself automatically. The ANS can calibrate or tune itself to preferentially respond to safety or danger as an adaptation to the relative safety or danger of our childhood environment.

COGNITIVE Referring to the process of conscious thinking, reasoning, or remembering.

CONSCIOUS A volitional, intentional awareness or deliberately directed function.

DEFAULT MODE NETWORK (DMN) A network in the brain that creates an organized repeated pattern of neurological activity when we are not focused on a specific task. For those prone to anxiety and alarm, we may insidiously and automatically default into a place of self-referential thought and worry that may be mediated by the DMN.

DISSOCIATION An insidious process of disconnection of conscious awareness. A daydreaming type of defensive separation from distressing thoughts, feelings, or memories. Leaving the conscious awareness of your body and disappearing into a faraway place in the unconscious mind.

DORSAL VAGAL SHUTDOWN (DVS) A process in humans akin to a prey animal freezing and/or feigning death when cornered by a predator. In humans in DVS there is minimal eye contact, the voice becomes monotone, body movements are minimal, and the face loses color and expression. Essentially DVS is a complete loss of the social engagement system and is a form of dissociation.

EGO The hyper-protective, unconscious part of us that compulsively tries to avoid or block out anything that has ever caused us discomfort or pain.

EGO DRAGON A powerful but dumb mythical figure I invented to explain the ego's obstinate and powerful influence in our lives.

EMOTIONAL FREEDOM TECHNIQUE (EFT) A process of tapping or touching the body to create conscious physical sensation in the body to bring present-moment awareness to enable positive change in the nervous system.

EXTEROCEPTION The process by which we neurologically sense our external environment.

FOREGROUND ALARM The activity of the sympathetic wing of the autonomic nervous system. The fight, flight, or freeze response in the body in reaction to real or perceived threat.

INHERITED FAMILY TRAUMA Traumatic experiences that are passed down to offspring by epigenetic changes, learned behaviors, and environmental stressors in the internal and external environment of the mother and the father.

INSULA, OR INSULAR CORTEX For the purposes of this book, a part of the brain that modulates and recreates sensation in the body directly related to background alarm.

INTEGRATION The process by which disparate parts come together into a functional whole. Practically: joining the dysfunctional coping strategies of the child (e.g. chronic worrying) into a functional, adaptive whole in the adult.

INTERNAL FAMILY SYSTEMS (IFS) A type of therapy pioneered by Richard Schwartz, PhD, that uses "self-energy" to bring emotionally exiled parts of ourselves into a functional whole under the power of our higher self.

INTEROCEPTION The process by which we neurologically sense our internal environment. Through interoception the background alarm in the body drives the anxious thoughts of the mind.

LIMBIC SYSTEM A general term and construct referring to the more "emotional" parts of our brain.

MDMA also called ecstasy. A drug/chemical that creates a profound sense of being profoundly connected to love by hyperstimulation of serotonin pathways.

NEUROCEPTION The process by which we neurologically sense our internal and external environment.

PARASYMPATHETIC NERVOUS SYSTEM (PNS) The rest-and-digest wing of the autonomic nervous system. The PNS is involved in energy conservation and emotional and physical regulation. The vagus nerve is the primary nerve of this system.

PENDULATION An aspect of somatic therapy that oscillates a painful sensation with a pleasant or neutral one. This process shows the unconscious mind that the alarm isn't our entire existence (although it likely felt that way when we were young).

POLYVAGAL THEORY A construct that uses the evolutionary development in the vagus nerve to explain the ability of the ANS to adapt to trauma. Being in a "ventral vagal state" is engaging your social engagement system, while being in a "dorsal vagal state" is akin to dissociation, shutdown, and a distinct blunting of social connection.

POTENTIATION The process by which a neurological signal or pathway becomes stronger and easier to elicit the more that signal or pathway is activated.

PREFRONTAL CORTEX (PFC) For the purposes of this book, the area of our brain that is involved in reasoning and regulation of behavior and physiology.

PSYCHEDELICS A group of chemical compounds that includes psilocybin, ayahuasca, and LSD that removes the separation of the conscious from the unconscious and dissolves the feeling of an ego-based "self." The result is perceiving unconscious processes as if they were actually happening in conscious awareness. Losing a sense of ego-based self also can make a person feel that they are fluid with everything and not a separate "self."

REPETITION COMPULSION The Freudian term representing the powerful and unconscious urge to reproduce your childhood environment in your adult life.

SOCIAL ENGAGEMENT SYSTEM (SES) The human neurobiological network that connects one human being to another using eye contact, tone and prosody of voice, body language, and facial expression.

SOMATIC OR SOMA A general term that refers to the physical body.

SOMATIC EXPERIENCING (SE) A therapy pioneered by Peter Levine, PhD, using the awareness of sensation in the body to create regulation in the mind and nervous system.

STRESS HORMONES A general term for epinephrine, norepinephrine, and cortisol, three molecules that prepare our entire system for real or imagined threat. In the short term these chemicals are tolerated well, but long-term exposure can weaken the body and mind.

SYMPATHETIC NERVOUS SYSTEM (SNS) The wing of the autonomic nervous system that activates and energizes a state of action, often referred to as a fight-or-flight state. However, if the SNS is too strongly activated or activated for too long it can precipitate a freeze state.

UNCONSCIOUS A reservoir of energy outside of our conscious awareness that includes feelings, thoughts, memories, and drives. Also includes automatic programs for movement and behavior that have been programmed into us since childhood.

VAGUS NERVE The tenth cranial nerve and the main nerve of the parasympathetic (rest-and-digest) nervous system. Also the main player in the polyvagal theory.

WINDOW OF TOLERANCE The zone of arousal that a person can still maintain optimal functioning. Background alarm narrows this range of optimal responsiveness, making us more reactive and less able to stay present, rational, and grounded.

References

Bird, Nicola. 2019. *A Little Peace of Mind: The Revolutionary Solution for Freedom from Anxiety, Panic Attacks and Stress.* London: Hay House UK.

Block, Peter. 2003. *The Answer to How Is Yes: Acting on What Matters.* San Francisco: Berrett-Koehler Publishers.

Block, Peter. 2008. *Community: The Structure of Belonging.* San Francisco: Berrett-Koehler Publishers.

Bradshaw, John. 2005. *Healing the Shame That Binds You: Recovery Classics Edition.* Deerfield Beach: Health Communications, Inc.

Bradshaw, John. 1999. *Homecoming: Reclaiming and Championing Your Inner Child.* New York: Bantam Doubleday Dell Audio.

Bridges, William. 2003. *Managing Transitions: Making the Most of Change.* Boston: Da Capo Lifelong Books.

Brown, Brené. 2019. *Braving the Wilderness: The Quest for True Belonging and the Courage to Stand Alone.* New York: Random House.

Brown, Brené. 2013. *The Power of Vulnerability: Teachings of Authenticity, Connection, and Courage.* Louisville: Sounds True, Inc.

Brown, Brené. 2010. *The Gifts of Imperfection: Let Go of Who You Think You're Supposed to Be and Embrace Who You Are.* Center City: Hazelden Publishing.

Cease, Kyle. 2017. *I Hope I Screw This Up: How Falling in Love with Your Fears Can Change the World.* Webster: Audible Studios.

Chödrön, Pema. 2018. *The Places That Scare You: A Guide to Fearlessness in Difficult Times.* Boulder: Shambhala Publications.

Dana, Deb. 2018. *Polyvagal Theory in Therapy: Engaging the Rhythm of Regulation.* New York: W. W. Norton & Company.

Frankl, Viktor E. 2006. *Man's Search for Meaning.* Boston: Beacon Press.

Grof, Stanislav and Christina Grof. 2010. *Holotropic Breathwork: A New Approach to Self-Exploration and Therapy (SUNY Series in Transpersonal and Humanistic Psychology).* Albany: Excelsior Editions; Illustrated Edition.

Hanson, Rick and Richard Mendius. 2009. *Buddha's Brain: The Practical Neuroscience of Happiness, Love, and Wisdom.* Oakland: New Harbinger Publications.

Hawkins, David R. 2014. *Power vs. Force: The Hidden Determinants of Human Behavior.* Carlsbad: Hay House Publishing.

Huber, Cheri. 2014. *Unconditional Self-Acceptance: The Do-It-Yourself Course.* Louisville: Sounds True, Inc.

Jeffers, Susan. 2012. *Feel the Fear and Do It Anyway.* London: Vermilion.

LeDoux, Joseph. 2016. *Anxious: Using the Brain to Understand and Treat Fear and Anxiety.* New York: Penguin Books.

Levine, Amir and Rachel Heller. 2012. *Attached: The New Science of Adult Attachment and How It Can Help You Find—and Keep—Love.* New York: TarcherPerigee.

Levine, Peter A. 2008. *Healing Trauma: A Pioneering Program for Restoring the Wisdom of Your Body.* Louisville: Sounds True, Inc.

Levine, Peter A. and Ann Frederick. 1997. *Waking the Tiger: Healing Trauma.* Berkeley: North Atlantic Books.

Lewis, Thomas, Fari Amini, and Richard Lannon. 2001. *A General Theory of Love.* New York: Vintage Books.

Lipton, Bruce H. 2016. *The Biology Of Belief: Unleashing the Power of Consciousness, Matter & Miracles.* Carlsbad: Hay House, Inc.

Maté, Gabor. 2022. *The Myth of Normal: Trauma, Illness, and Healing in a Toxic Culture.* New York: Avery Publishing.

Miller, Alice. 2008. *The Drama of the Gifted Child: The Search for the True Self.* New York: Basic Books.

Miller, Alice. 2005. *The Body Never Lies: The Lingering Effects of Hurtful Parenting.* New York: W. W. Norton & Company.

Myss, Caroline. 1998. *Why People Don't Heal and How They Can.* New York: Harmony Books.

Paul, Sheryl. 2019. *The Wisdom of Anxiety: How Worry and Intrusive Thoughts Are Gifts to Help You Heal.* Louisville: Sounds True, Inc.

Peterson, Jordan B. 2018. *12 Rules for Life: An Antidote to Chaos.* Toronto: Random House Canada.

Porges, Stephen W. 2011. *The Polyvagal Theory: Neurophysiological Foundations of Emotions, Attachment, Communication, and Self-Regulation.* New York: W.W. Norton & Company.

Rankin, Lissa. 2016. *The Fear Cure: Cultivating Courage as Medicine for the Body, Mind, and Soul.* Carlsbad: Hay House, Inc.

Robbins, Mel. 2017. *The 5 Second Rule: Transform Your Life, Work, and Confidence with Everyday Courage.* Brentwood: Savio Republic.

Schaub, Friedemann. 2012. *The Fear and Anxiety Solution: A Breakthrough Process for Healing and Empowerment with Your Subconscious Mind.* Louisville: Sounds True, Inc.

Sharma, Robin. 2007. *The Monk Who Sold His Ferrari.* New York: HarperCollins Publishers.

Siegel, Daniel J. 2010. *Mindsight: The New Science of Personal Transformation.* New York: Bantam Books.

Siegel, Daniel J. 2011. *The Neurobiology of "We": How Relationships, the Mind, and the Brain Interact to Shape Who We Are.* Louisville: Sounds True, Inc.

Singer, Michael A. 2007. *The Untethered Soul: The Journey Beyond Yourself.* Oakland: New Harbinger Publications.

Tatkin, Stan. 2018. *Relationship Rx: Insights and Practices to Overcome Chronic Fighting and Return to Love.* Louisville: Sounds True, Inc.

Tolle, Eckhart. 2005. *A New Earth: Awakening to Your Life's Purpose.* New York: Penguin Books.

Tolle, Eckhart. 2004. *The Power of Now: A Guide to Spiritual Enlightenment.* Vancouver: Namaste Publishing.

Van der Kolk, Bessel A. 2015. *The Body Keeps the Score: Brain, Mind, and Body in the Healing of Trauma.* New York: Penguin Books.

Watt, Mélanie. 2006. *Scaredy Squirrel.* Toronto: Kids Can Press Ltd.

Wolynn, Mark. 2017. *It Didn't Start With You: How Inherited Family Trauma Shapes Who We Are and How to End the Cycle.* London: Vermilion.

About the Author

Dr. Russell Kennedy, also known as the Anxiety MD, is a medical doctor, anxiety expert, bestselling author, corporate speaker, yoga and meditation teacher, father, grandfather, and recovering hypochondriac.

Dr. Russ has earned university degrees in medicine and neuroscience, and he has had over one hundred thousand patient encounters in his medical career. In addition, he believes the vast majority of mental disease starts in childhood, and to that end, he has undergone master's-level training in developmental psychology at the Neufeld Institute in Vancouver.

Russ's own anxiety started as he was growing up in a chaotic and confusing household with a father who suffered from schizophrenia and bipolar illness. Once he became an adult, healing from his own anxiety took him on a long and frustrating road with plenty of dead ends. As a doctor, Russ had full access to the best methods and medications "modern" traditional psychology and psychiatry had to offer for many years, but traditional methods only provided limited relief. Desperate to find a solution, he forged an unconventional path, and many of his breakthroughs came from pursuing distinctly nontraditional, atypical, and counterintuitive sources.

He has often said he is driven by a need to help others in a way he could not help his father. He has also often said he does not want people to have to suffer as he did, and strives to make his father's painful life and death to mean something by helping other families heal from emotional illness. It's not all serious though, as for many years he was a doctor by day, comedian by night, performing in comedy clubs across the country.

A physician who is a stand-up comedian is unusual, but Russ freely admits to being atypical for a doctor. He studied meditation and intention while living at a temple in India, became a certified yoga and meditation teacher, practiced Holotropic Breathwork®, and has taken psychedelic (plant) medicines to see and experience as much of his mind as he possibly could. While under a therapeutic dose of LSD he discovered what his anxiety truly was and used that knowledge to develop a theory that would allow him to ultimately heal himself. That theory is found in his book, *Anxiety Rx*. There are no better guides than the ones who have been in the maze themselves and can show others the way out.

Continue the journey with Russ at www.theanxietymd.com.